Alternatives to Ankle Joint Replacement

Editor

WOO-CHUN LEE

FOOT AND ANKLE CLINICS

www.foot.theclinics.com

Consulting Editor
Cesar de Cesar Netto

March 2022 • Volume 27 • Number 1

ELSEVIER

1600 John F. Kennedy Boulevard • Suite 1800 • Philadelphia, Pennsylvania, 19103-2899

http://www.theclinics.com

FOOT AND ANKLE CLINICS Volume 27, Number 1
March 2022 ISSN 1083-7515, ISBN-978-0-323-81371-6

Editor: Megan Ashdown
Developmental Editor: Arlene B. Campos

Foot and Ankle Clinics (ISSN 1083-7515) is published quarterly by Elsevier, Inc., 360 Park Avenue South, New York, NY 10010-1710. Months of issue are March, June, September, and December. Periodicals postage paid at New York, NY, and additional mailing offices. Subscription price per year is $351.00 (US individuals), $763.00 (US institutions), $100.00 (US students), $378.00 (Canadian individuals), $786.00 (Canadian institutions), $100.00 (Canadian students), $489.00 (international individuals), $786.00 (international institutions), and $215.00 (international students). To receive student/resident rate, orders must be accompanied by name of affiliated institution, date of term, and the *signature* of program/residency coordinator on institution letterhead. Orders will be billed at individual rate until proof of status is received. Foreign air speed delivery is included in all *Clinics* subscription prices. All prices are subject to change without notice. **POSTMASTER:** Send address changes to *Foot and Ankle Clinics*, Elsevier Health Sciences Division, Subscription Customer Service, 3251 Riverport Lane, Maryland Heights, MO 63043. **Customer Service: 1-800-654-2452 (US and Canada). From outside of the United States and Canada, call 314-447-8871. Fax: 314-447-8029. E-mail: JournalsCustomerService-usa@ elsevier.com (for print support); JournalsOnlineSupport-usa@elsevier.com (for online support).**

Reprints. For copies of 100 or more, of articles in this publication, please contact the Commercial Reprints Department, Elsevier Inc., 360 Park Avenue South, New York, NY 10010-1710. Tel.: 212-633-3874; Fax: 212-633-3820; E-mail: reprints@elsevier.com.

Contributors

CONSULTING EDITOR

CESAR DE CESAR NETTO, MD, PhD
International Weight-Bearing CT Society, Assistant Professor, Department of Orthopedics and Rehabilitation, Carver College of Medicine, University of Iowa, Iowa City, Iowa, USA

EDITOR

WOO-CHUN LEE, MD, PhD
Seoul Foot and Ankle Center, Dubalo Orthopaedic Clinic, Dubalo Hospital, Gangnam-gu, Seoul, Repubic of Korea

AUTHORS

AHMAD ALAJLAN, MD
Swiss Ortho Center, Schmerzklinik Basel, Swiss Medical Network, Basel, Switzerland; Orthopaedic Department, Security Forces Hospital, Riyadh, Saudi Arabia

ALEXEJ BARG, MD
International Weight-Bearing CT Society, Department of Trauma, Hand and Reconstructive Surgery, University Medical Center Hamburg-Eppendorf, Hamburg, Germany

ARNE BURSSENS, MD
International Weight-Bearing CT Society, Department of Orthopaedics and Traumatology, University Hospital of Ghent, Gent, Belgium

CESAR DE CESAR NETTO, MD, PhD
International Weight-Bearing CT Society, Assistant Professor, Department of Orthopedics and Rehabilitation, Carver College of Medicine, University of Iowa, Iowa City, Iowa, USA

ALIRIO J. deMEIRELES, MD, MBA
Department of Orthopedic Surgery, Columbia University Irving Medical Center/NewYork-Presbyterian Hospital, New York, New York, USA

JACQUES du TOIT, MBChB, MSc Clin Epi, FCS (Orth)SA, PhD
Professor, Division of Orthopaedic Surgery, Faculty of Medicine and Health Sciences, Stellenbosch University, Tygerberg, South Africa

SCOTT ELLIS, MD
International Weight-Bearing CT Society, Orthopaedic Surgery, The Hospital for Special Surgery, New York, New York, USA

JOHN E. FEMINO, MD
Clinical Professor, Department of Orthopedics and Rehabilitation, University of Iowa, Iowa City, Iowa, USA

NAOKI HARAGUCHI, MD
Professor, Department of Orthopaedic Surgery, St. Marianna University Yokohama Seibu Hospital, Yokohama, Kanagawa, Japan

BEAT HINTERMANN, MD
Associate Professor and Chairman, Center of Excellence for Foot and Ankle Surgery, Kantonsspital Baselland, Liestal, Switzerland

TODD A. IRWIN, MD
OrthoCarolina Foot and Ankle Institute, Associate Professor, Atrium Health Musculoskeletal Institute, Charlotte, North Carolina, USA

JAEYOUNG KIM, MD
Department of Orthopaedic Surgery, Hospital for Special Surgery, New York, New York, USA

WOO-CHUN LEE, MD, PhD
Seoul Foot and Ankle Center, Dubalo Orthopaedic Clinic, Dubalo Hospital, Gangnam-gu, Seoul, Repubic of Korea

ANNA-KATHRIN LEUCHT, MD
Consultant, Department of Orthopaedics and Traumatology, Cantonal Hospital of Winterthur, Winterthur, Switzerland

XINGCHEN LI, MD
Department of Orthopaedics, Ruijin Hospital, Shanghai Jiaotong University School of Medicine, Shanghai, China

FRANCOIS LINTZ, MD
International Weight-Bearing CT Society, Clinique de l'Union, Foot and Ankle Surgery Centre, Toulouse, France

PILAR MARTÍNEZ-DE-ALBORNOZ, MD
Orthopaedic Foot and Ankle Unit, Orthopaedic and Trauma Department, Hospital Universitario Quirónsalud Madrid, Faculty Medicine UEM, Madrid, Spain

MANUEL MONTEAGUDO, MD
Orthopaedic Foot and Ankle Unit, Orthopaedic and Trauma Department, Hospital Universitario Quirónsalud Madrid, Faculty Medicine UEM, Madrid, Spain

MARTINUS RICHTER, MD, PhD
International Weight-Bearing CT Society, Department for Foot and Ankle Surgery, Rummelsberg and Nuremberg, Germany

ROXA RUIZ, MD
Senior Attending Surgeon, Center of Excellence for Foot and Ankle Surgery, Kantonsspital Baselland, Liestal, Switzerland

ALAN SHAMROCK, MD
Department of Orthopedics and Rehabilitation, University of Iowa, Iowa City, Iowa, USA

IGNATIUS P.S. TERBLANCHE, MBChB, FCS(Orth)SA
Division of Orthopaedic Surgery, Faculty of Medicine and Health Sciences, Stellenbosch University, Tygerberg, South Africa; CapeFootSurgery, Louis Leipoldt Mediclinic, Cape Town, South Africa

VICTOR VALDERRABANO, MD, PhD
Professor, Chairman, Swiss Ortho Center, Schmerzklinik Basel, Swiss Medical Network, Basel, Switzerland

ANDREA VELJKOVIC, MD, MPH(Harvard), BComm, FAOA, FRCSC
Associate Clinical Professor, Department of Orthopaedics, University of British, Partner, Footbridge Center for Integrated Foot and Ankle Care, Footbridge Clinic, Vancouver, British Columbia, Canada

DAVID VIER, MD
Baylor University Medical Center, Dallas, Texas, USA

ETTORE VULCANO, MD
Department of Orthopedic Surgery, Chief, Columbia University Orthopedics at Mount Sinai Medical Center, Miami Beach, Florida, USA

EMILIO WAGNER, MD
Staff Foot and Ankle Surgeon, Associate Professor, Universidad del Desarrollo, Clinica Alemana de Santiago, Santiago, Chile

PABLO WAGNER, MD
Staff Foot and Ankle Surgeon, Associate Professor, Universidad del Desarrollo, Clinica Alemana de Santiago, Santiago, Chile

XIANGYANG XU, MD, PhD
Department of Orthopaedics, Ruijin Hospital, Shanghai Jiaotong University School of Medicine, Shanghai, China

Editorial Advisory Board

Contents

Foreword: Let's Get to Work!   xv

Cesar de Cesar Netto

Preface: Alternatives to Ankle Joint Replacement   xvii

Woo-Chun Lee

Analysis of Whole Limb Alignment in Ankle Arthritis   1

Naoki Haraguchi

> A full-length standing posteroanterior radiograph that includes the calcaneus (hip-to-calcaneus radiograph) is obtained for evaluation of the mechanical axis of the entire lower limb in patients with a lower limb condition involving malalignment. Such evaluation clarifies several pathomechanical aspects of hindfoot disorders, facilitates surgical planning, and elucidates factors contributing to unsatisfactory results of a particular operation. Whole limb alignment is influenced not only by the knee joint but also by the ankle joint; thus, knee realignment influences hindfoot alignment and vice versa. It is essential to analyze alignment of the whole limb in planning corrective lower limb surgery.

The Assessment of Ankle Osteoarthritis with Weight-Bearing Computed Tomography   13

Martinus Richter, Cesar de Cesar Netto, Francois Lintz, Alexej Barg, Arne Burssens, and Scott Ellis

> The standard for diagnostic radiographic imaging in foot and ankle surgery was until 2012 radiographs with full weight-bearing without any useful alternative. Weight-bearing cone-beam computed tomography (WBCT) was introduced 2012 for foot and ankle use as a new technology that allows 3D imaging with full weight-bearing which should be not influenced by projection and/or foot orientation. The assessment of ankle osteoarthritis with WBCT including the description of healthy status, effect of alignment and7or (in)stability is extensively illustrated in this review article.

Joint Preservation Strategies for Managing Varus Ankle Deformities   37

Beat Hintermann and Roxa Ruiz

> Joint preserving strategies have evolved to a successful treatment option in early and midstage medial ankle OA caused by varus deformity. Though talar tilt can often not be fully corrected, it provides substantial postoperative pain relief, functional improvement, and slowing of the degenerative process. Osseous balancing with osteotomies is the main step for restoration of ankle mechanics and normalization of joint load. Overall, the key for success is to understand the underlying causes that have contributed to the varus OA in each case, and to use all treatment modalities necessary to restore appropriate alignment of the hindfoot complex.

Joint Preserving Surgery for Valgus Ankle Osteoarthritis   57

Ahmad Alajlan and Victor Valderrabano

Valgus ankle OA is a complex problem with multiple etiologies that can either be isolated or superimposed on top of other medical or musculo-skeletal disorders. Proper medical history, physical, and preoperative radiological examinations are crucial in deciding on surgery and planning the surgical approach. JPS, especially the varisating medial closing-wedge SMOT with solid plate fixation, has been consistently associated with good outcomes for patients with valgus ankle OA. To further improve JPS for valgus ankle OA, further clinical and biomechanical studies are required to address the long-term clinical and functional outcomes and complications.

Joint Preservation for Posttraumatic Ankle Arthritis After Tibial Plafond Fracture   73

Xingchen Li and Xiangyang Xu

Management of posttraumatic ankle arthritis due to tibial plafond fracture is technically demanding. The distal tibial plafond-plasty could be an alter-native to preserve the ankle joint for young patients with limited ankle arthritis. The surgical principles are to realign the mechanical axis, recon-struct the articular surface of the distal tibial plafond, and achieve a congruent and stable ankle joint. In addition to the anteroposterior view of the ankle joint, the lateral view was also paramount for surgeons to fully evaluate the reduction quality. The revision procedures are as follows: os-teotomy for exposure, articular surface reconstruction, bone grafting, and osteotomy fixation.

Correction of the Valgus Ankle with a Joint Sparing Supra-Malleolar Osteotomy: The Modified Wiltse Technique   91

Ignatius P.S. Terblanche and Jacques du Toit

The valgus ankle is a common cause of pain, deformity, and disability in patients. Addressing these deformities with extraarticular osteotomies is a valuable, joint-sparing treatment option. The modified Wiltse osteotomy provides correction of the mechanical alignment as well as allowing inherent stability. Accurate templating of the Wiltse triangle enables repro-ducible, accurate intraoperative results.

Joint Preservation Surgery for Varus and Posterior Ankle Arthritis Associated with Flatfoot Deformity   115

Jaeyoung Kim and Woo-Chun Lee

This article introduces novel types of ankle arthritis related to a flatfoot deformity. There has been a long-held belief that severe unmanaged flat-foot deformity leads to valgus ankle arthritis, due to deltoid ligament insuf-ficiency. However, flatfoot deformity can also give rise to varus ankle arthritis as the talus and calcaneus subluxate into opposite directions. Plantarflexion and posterior translation of the talus in the sagittal plane contributes to the eccentric narrowing of the posterior aspect of the tibio-talar joint, which the authors termed posterior ankle arthritis. Subtalar arthrodesis was performed to address the opposing dynamics of the talus and calcaneus, and was combined with a medial longitudinal arch reconstruction in most cases of posterior ankle arthritis and in selected cases of varus ankle arthritis, and satisfactory clinical and radiological results were achieved.

Correction of Sagittal Plane Deformity of the Distal Tibia   129

Emilio Wagner and Pablo Wagner

Distal tibia sagittal plane deformities are a frequent finding in tibial malunions (antecurvatum or recurvatum) or ankle posttraumatic arthritis (anterior or posterior ankle arthritis). They should be evaluated in all deformities using long leg and tibia radiographs. Measuring the anterior distal tibia angle is necessary to evaluate the deformity severity. To evaluate the magnitude of secondary talar anterior or posterior displacement, the tibial axis to talus ratio and/or the talar lateral process position relative to the tibia axis should be measured. Anterior closing or opening wedge osteotomies are the recommended treatment options for posterior ankle arthritis or anterior ankle arthritis, respectively.

The Role of Distraction Arthroplasty in Managing Ankle Osteoarthritis   145

Alirio J. deMeireles and Ettore Vulcano

Ankle distraction arthroplasty (DA) is a joint-preserving option for the treatment of ankle osteoarthritis. The ideal patient is a young, active person who is compliant with follow-up and understands that clinical improvements may not be fully evident until 1 year after surgery. The procedure promotes cartilage healing and regeneration by removing mechanical stress at the joint surface through the application of a joint-spanning external fixator. There is an array of adjuvant procedures commonly performed to optimize healing potential—including microfracture, osteophyte removal, osteotomies, and soft tissue balancing procedures. Short- and intermediate-term studies have been promising, though there is a wide variance in reported failure and complication rates.

The Role of Anterior Ankle Arthroscopy in the Management of Ankle Arthritis: Literature Review, Patient Evaluation, Goals of Treatment and Technique   159

John E. Femino and Alan Shamrock

The current body of literature regarding anterior ankle arthroscopic debridement for anterior ankle impingement (AAI) cases with ankle osteoarthritis (OA) has significant limitations. The reported poor outcomes lack the necessary rigor in patient selection, preoperative evaluations and in most reports, the use of a systematic operative approach. Furthermore, the lack of postoperative evaluation by authors using physical examination and radiologic studies to determine the etiology of ongoing pain leaves open the possibility that treatment of impingement was incomplete. For these reasons, it would be inappropriate to conclude that anterior arthroscopic debridement has no role in the treatment of ankle OA. Critical analysis of some studies provides encouragement that this can be a useful intermediate treatment of appropriately selected patients with AAI and ankle OA. The level of required detail in the physical examination and radiologic evaluation is much greater than for more straight-forward cases of soft tissue impingement or simple osteophyte impingement in otherwise healthy joints. The success of the treatment requires a systematic approach to the evaluation and performance of the procedure, which is perhaps why results in the literature have been suboptimal in most series. Future studies should apply this rigorous approach to patient selection, procedure performance, and postoperative analysis to best clarify which patients can be best served with this procedure as part of the various intermediate treatment options for ankle OA.

Arthroscopic Ankle Arthrodesis   175

Anna-Kathrin Leucht and Andrea Veljkovic

End-stage ankle arthritis typically affects an active younger patient population as compared with hip and knee arthritis. The optimal surgical treatment depends on several patient-specific factors. Open ankle arthrodesis has achieved reliable outcomes for this condition over years; however, arthroscopic techniques seem to be advantageous and feasible even in cases with significant intraarticular deformity. This article describes the surgical technique of arthroscopic ankle arthrodesis and discusses the outcome compared with that of open ankle fusion and total ankle replacement.

Open Ankle Arthrodesis for Deformity Correction   199

David Vier and Todd A. Irwin

Open ankle arthrodesis remains a reliable solution for ankle arthritis, especially in the setting of deformity. Careful preoperative evaluation needs to be performed, both clinically and radiographically. The specific deformity present helps determine the approach used and the fixation choices. Deformity is most commonly seen intraarticularly, though deformity can also be present anywhere along the lower extremity, including compensatory deformity in the foot. Multiple different techniques can be used to address both the deformity and achieve a successful ankle arthrodesis. Patient outcomes reported in the literature are generally good, with high union rates and improved functional outcomes.

Deciding Between Ankle and Tibiotalocalcaneal Arthrodesis for Isolated Ankle Arthritis   217

Manuel Monteagudo and Pilar Martínez-de-Albornoz

 Video content accompanies this article at http://foot.theclinics.com.

After isolated ankle (tibiotalar) arthrodesis, the triceps progressively shifts the subtalar joint into varus thus blocking compensatory motion from the midtarsal joints. In a tibiotalocalcaneal arthrodesis, the subtalar may be fixed with the correct valgus. Comparison between ankle and tibiotalocalcaneal arthrodesis does not clearly favor one over another for pain relief, satisfaction, and gait analysis. Compensatory sagittal plane motion through the midtarsal joints when the subtalar is fixed in valgus may be responsible for these results. Tibiotalocalcaneal arthrodesis has become our procedure of choice over isolated tibiotalar for end-stage ankle arthritis regardless of the radiographic state of the subtalar.

FOOT AND ANKLE CLINICS

FORTHCOMING ISSUES

June 2022
Managing Complications of Foot and Ankle Surgery
Scott Ellis, *Editor*

September 2022
Managing Challenging Deformities with Arthrodesis of the Foot and Ankle
Manuel Monteagudo, *Editor*

December 2022
The Diabetic Foot
Fabian Krause, *Editor*

RECENT ISSUES

December 2021
Foot Ankle Deformity in the Child
Maurizio De Pellegrin, *Editor*

September 2021
Controversies in Managing the Progressive Collapsing Foot Deformity (PCFD)
Cesar de Cesar Netto, *Editor*

June 2021
Advances in the Treatment of Athletic Injury
Mark S. Myerson, *Editor*

RELATED SERIES

Orthopedic Clinics
Clinics in Sports Medicine
Physical Medicine and Rehabilitation Clinics

THE CLINICS ARE NOW AVAILABLE ONLINE!
Access your subscription at:
www.theclinics.com

Foreword
Let's Get to Work!

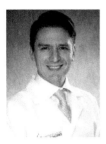

Cesar de Cesar Netto, MD, PhD
Consulting Editor

Dear Foot and Ankle Clinics of North America Colleagues and Friends,

During these unparalleled times of uncertainty and suffering to the whole world, I make wishes and prayers that we can all have a better and healthier year in 2022. Happy New Year!

We have been working behind the scenes with our editorial team to come up with exciting innovations, foot and ankle topics, and stellar foot and ankle surgeons and researchers to serve as guest editors and authors of our journal's articles. To convey new perspectives, I decided to change the format and the members of our Editorial Board, bringing on board some fresh eyes to our team. The new members are close life references to me and are well-recognized leaders in the Foot and Ankle Surgery Community.

Before announcing the new members of the Editorial Board, I'd like to recognize the outstanding work performed by the members that are temporarily pausing their editorial services: Dr Kent Ellington, Dr Stefan Rammelt, Dr Jeffrey Seybold, and Dr Federico Usuelli. Thank you so much for all the hard and excellent work you provided for several years. We definitely count on your constant future support to the journal, and I'm sure we will cross paths again shortly.

We also take this opportunity to welcome the new Associate Editor Members: Dr Alexej Barg, representing Europe; Dr Caio Augusto de Souza Nery, representing Latin America; and Dr Shuyuan Li (continuing as Editorial Member), representing Asia. Thank you for agreeing to be part of this great team and for the extensive experience and networking you bring to the journal. Let's get to work!

I hope you all enjoy the articles of this current *Foot and Ankle Clinics of North America* issue! I'm also thrilled to introduce Dr Woo-Chun Lee as the Guest Editor for this current issue on joint-preserving treatment for end-stage ankle arthritis. Dr Lee is a world-recognized orthopedic foot and ankle surgeon, researcher, and innovator and has served as a mentor to hundreds of South-Korean and international

Foot Ankle Clin N Am 27 (2022) xv–xvi
https://doi.org/10.1016/j.fcl.2022.01.001
1083-7515/22/© 2022 Published by Elsevier Inc.

trainees and is a role model to all of us. He has put together a world-class team of authors with extensive experience in the treatment of ankle arthritis.

Stay safe!

Regards,

Cesar de Cesar Netto, MD, PhD
Department of Orthopaedics and Rehabilitation
University of Iowa
Iowa City, IA 52242, USA

E-mail address:
cesar-netto@uiowa.edu

Preface

Alternatives to Ankle Joint Replacement

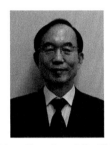

Woo-Chun Lee, MD, PhD
Editor

The gradual and continuous increase in frequency of total ankle replacement (TAR) implies its favorable results compared with other options for management of end-stage ankle arthritis. However, long-term results following TAR are not known, and comparisons with conventional treatments, such as ankle arthrodesis, do not show a definitive advantage of TAR over ankle arthrodesis. Considering the relatively young age of patients with ankle arthritis coupled with the uncertainty of TAR longevity, it would seem that preventing or halting the progression of ankle arthritis in its earlier stages is of utmost importance. Therefore, several different approaches for joint preservation have been developed for each specific type and stage of ankle arthritis.

In this issue, various joint-preservation methods, including arthroscopic measures for early ankle arthritis, are presented following previous articles detailing the assessment of whole-limb alignment and the usefulness of weight-bearing computed tomographic (CT) scans. Then, joint-preservation methods for different types of eccentric ankle arthritis are elaborated, including eccentric arthritis in the sagittal plane. Pathomechanisms and detailed surgical decision-making processes for each specific ankle arthritis will help readers of this journal for the benefit of their patients with ankle arthritis.

Regarding end-stage arthritis, ankle arthrodesis is still more commonly performed than TAR in many hospitals around the world, and distraction arthroplasty is another treatment option in younger patients for delaying joint-sacrificing procedures or as a definitive measure. Pros and cons of arthroscopic and open ankle arthrodesis will be more easily understood after reading these relevant articles. Finally, indications for tibiotalocalcaneal arthrodesis are described.

I really appreciate all the authors of every article in this issue for their effort to complete their article based on their extensive experience and comprehensive review of the literature. Appropriate radiographs, photographs, and drawings by the authors have

Foot Ankle Clin N Am 27 (2022) xvii–xviii
https://doi.org/10.1016/j.fcl.2021.11.013
1083-7515/22/© 2021 Published by Elsevier Inc.

foot.theclinics.com

made the articles more easily understood, and I also personally learned a lot through their contributions.

Note that that this issue of *Foot and Ankle Clinics of North America* includes various review articles from assessments based on whole-limb alignment and the usefulness of weight-bearing CT on degenerative ankle arthritis. I believe this issue will provide the readers of *Foot and Ankle Clinics of North America* with comprehensive and detailed knowledge of the complexity and treatment options for ankle arthritis.

Diverse joint-preservation methods for different types and stages of ankle arthritis are described in seven articles. Coronal plane eccentric ankle arthritis has been relatively widely investigated regarding its etiology and treatment, which includes various methods to unload the degenerated area and shift the load-bearing to the uninvolved area.

Correction of talar tilt in the coronal plane is reviewed based on the authors' experience and published articles. Details of Wiltse osteotomy are elaborated in one article, which may be helpful for specific types of ankle arthritis.

In contrast to eccentric arthritis in the coronal plane, eccentric arthritis in the sagittal plane has not been extensively detailed in the existing literature. In this issue, three articles elaborate sagittal plane deformity correction, posttraumatic arthritis, and arthritis associated with flatfoot and sagittal plane correction.

Furthermore, the role of arthroscopic approaches for early ankle arthritis is described in this issue.

Distraction arthroplasty has a distinctive role in the armamentarium to treat end-stage ankle arthritis. Arthrodesis of the ankle is still the standard treatment for end-stage ankle arthritis. Both arthroscopic and the open method of ankle arthrodesis are described in detail. Extended arthrodesis to the subtalar joint is also included.

I genuinely appreciate the authors of each article for their comprehensive review of and collective experience. In addition, the effort to include as many figures as appropriate to increase the readability of these articles is much appreciated.

Woo-Chun Lee, MD, PhD
Seoul Foot and Ankle Center
Dubalo Hospital
45, Apgujeong-ro 30 gil, FL 2-4
Gangnam-gu, Seoul
Republic of Korea

E-mail address:
leewoochun@gmail.com

Analysis of Whole Limb Alignment in Ankle Arthritis

Naoki Haraguchi, MD

KEYWORDS

- Whole limb alignment • Ankle arthritis • Hip-to-calcaneus radiograph
- Flatfoot deformity • Total ankle arthroplasty

KEY POINTS

- A full-length standing posteroanterior radiograph that includes the calcaneus (hip-to-calcaneus radiograph), obtained with the patient in a bipedal stance on a radiolucent platform and facing the long film cassette, can be used to evaluate the mechanical axis of the lower limb and hindfoot alignment.
- This simple radiograph clarifies various pathomechanical aspects of hindfoot disorders, facilitates preoperative surgical planning, and sheds light on factors contributing to unsatisfactory results of a particular operation.
- Knee realignment surgery influences hindfoot alignment and vice versa.
- It is essential to evaluate whole limb alignment in planning corrective lower limb surgery.

INTRODUCTION

Various hindfoot disorders, such as ankle osteoarthritis, flatfoot deformity, rheumatoid hindfoot, hindfoot deformity associated with cavus foot, posttraumatic deformity, congenital deformity, and paralytic foot, lead to hindfoot malalignment. With weight-bearing being the main function of the lower limbs, analyzing changes in the mechanical axis resulting from malalignment in the diagnosis and treatment of lower limb disorders is imperative.

The mechanical axis of the lower limb has, traditionally, been taken as a line on a full-length standing anteroposterior radiograph extending from the center of the femoral head to the center of the tibial plafond (Mikulicz line), and it has been considered key to understanding malalignment and deformity from the hip to the lowest part of the tibia. Assessing the mechanical axis of the lower limb based on this line is mandatory for reconstructive surgery on the lower limb, such as total knee replacement, high tibial osteotomy, or corrective osteotomy for a malunited fracture of the femur or tibia. However, use of the Mikuliczline does not allow for identification of the point at which the mechanical axis of the lower limb passes through the tibial plafond.

Department of Orthopaedic Surgery, St. Marianna University Yokohama Seibu Hospital, 1197-1 Yasashicho, Asahi-ku, Yokohama, Kanagawa 241-0811, Japan
E-mail address: naoki.haraguchi@marianna-u.ac.jp

Foot Ankle Clin N Am 27 (2022) 1–12
https://doi.org/10.1016/j.fcl.2021.11.014
1083-7515/22/© 2021 Elsevier Inc. All rights reserved.

A line from the center of the femoral head to the lowest point of the calcaneus, not to the center of the tibial plafond, should be taken as the true mechanical axis of the lower limb. Only by drawing such a line can the point at which the mechanical axis of the lower limb passes through the tibial plafond be determined. For this, a radiograph that extends from the center of the femoral head to the lowest point of the calcaneus, which itself must be clearly visualized, is needed (**Fig. 1**).

I have described use of a full-length standing posteroanterior radiograph that includes the calcaneus for assessment of both the mechanical axis of the lower limb and hindfoot alignment.[1] Use of this "hip-to-calcaneus radiograph" has clarified various pathomechanical aspects of hindfoot disorders. Herein I describe how such a radiograph is obtained, how the mechanical axis of the lower limb is identified, especially the point at which the mechanical axis passes through the ankle joint, and various conditions and procedures for which analyzing the mechanical axis of the lower limb is applicable.

The author declare they have no commercial or financial relationship that can be considered a conflict of interest and that the study was funded solely by departmental resources.

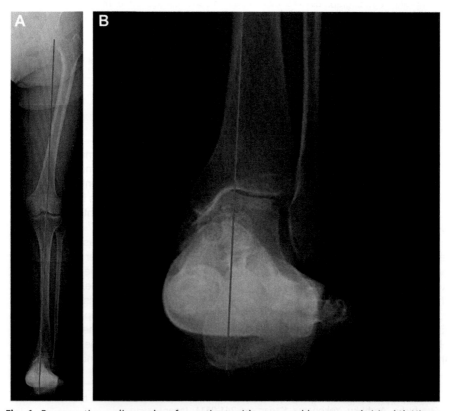

Fig. 1. Preoperative radiographs of a patient with varus ankle osteoarthritis. (*A*) Hip-to-calcaneus radiograph. (*B*) The lower part of the preoperative hip-to-calcaneus radiograph shows obliteration of the joint space between the medial malleolus and the medial facet of the talus with subchondral bone contact and that the mechanical axis (*red line*) passes through the medial part of the ankle joint.

OBTAINING THE HIP-TO-CALCANEUS RADIOGRAPH AND IDENTIFYING THE MECHANICAL AXIS OF THE LOWER LIMB, INCLUDING THE POINT AT WHICH IT PASSES THROUGH THE ANKLE JOINT

The hip-to-calcaneus radiograph is obtained with the patient maintaining a bipedal stance on a radiolucent platform and facing a so-called long-length film cassette,[1] as shown in **Fig. 2**. For the lowest point of the calcaneus to be captured on the radiograph, the cassette is slid into position, with its lower edge advanced beyond the edge of the platform. The patient's patella is oriented forward, and the x-ray beam is centered on the knee of the imaged leg from a distance of 2 m. Voltage is typically 200 mA, and current is typically 85 kV.

Once the radiograph is obtained, a line is drawn from the center of the femoral head to the lowest point of the calcaneus, and the point at which the mechanical axis crosses the tibial plafond is easily identified. This point, referred to as the mechanical

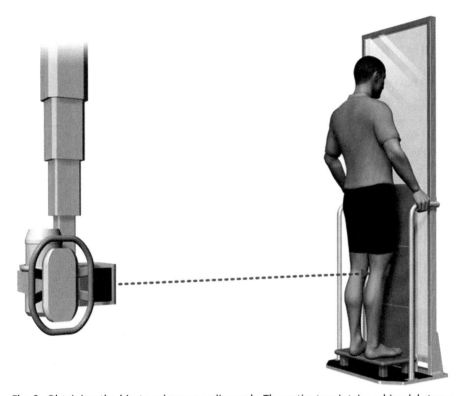

Fig. 2. Obtaining the hip-to-calcaneus radiograph. The patient maintains a bipedal stance on a radiolucent platform and faces the long film cassette. For the lowest point of the calcaneus to be visualized on the radiograph, the cassette is slid into position with its lower edge passing the edge of the platform. The patient's patella is oriented forward. The x-ray beam is centered on the knee of the imaged leg from a distance of 2 m. Voltage and current are 200 mA and 85 kV, respectively. It is important to confirm on the radiograph that the patella is centered between the femoral condyles. (Reprinted with permission from Haraguchi N, Ota K, Tsunoda N, Seike K, Kanetake Y, Tsutaya A. Weight-bearing-line analysis in supramalleolar osteotomy for varus-type osteoarthritis of the ankle. J Bone Joint Surg Am. 2015;97:333-339).

ankle joint axis point, is expressed as a percentage of the measured length of the pla-fond in the coronal plane (**Fig. 3**A), with the medial and lateral edges of the tibial pla-fond taken as 0% and 100%, respectively. Thus, a negative value indicates that the mechanical ankle joint axis point lies medially beyond the medial corner of the plafond, and a value of greater than 100% indicates that the point lies laterally beyond the lateral edge of the plafond (**Fig. 3**B).

The mechanical ankle joint axis point is affected by the position of the heel contact point, which is directly influenced by rotation of the lower limb. External rotation of the lower limb moves the heel contact point medially, and internal rotation of the lower limb moves the heel contact point laterally. Traditionally, the axis of the foot is used to control rotation of the lower limb in obtaining radiographs for hindfoot evaluation, for example, with the foot placed with its axis parallel to the x-ray beam. However, the long axis of the foot is often deviated in patients with foot and ankle malalignment. Likewise, if the transmalleolar axis is used to control limb rotation, by positioning the ankle so that the transmalleolar axis is perpendicular to the x-ray beam, the lower limb is rotated internally because the transmalleolar axis is rotated externally in relation to the transepicondylar axis of the femur. I have found it best to use the patella rather than the foot or ankle to control rotation of the lower limb. It is important to confirm on the radiograph that the patella is centered between the femoral condyles.

OSTEOTOMY FOR VARUS ANKLE OSTEOARTHRITIS

Varus ankle osteoarthritis is often treated by supramalleolar tibial osteotomy, a reliable joint-preserving procedure.[2–11] For some patients, however, clinical and radiological outcomes are not satisfactory. In performing this procedure, the tibial correction angle has been traditionally determined based on the tibial ankle surface (TAS) angle, defined as the angle between the tibial shaft and its distal joint surface on the antero-posterior radiograph.[8] Slight overcorrection is recommended for such osteotomy, but the target TAS angle is based primarily on the surgeon's experience, and it varies from one group to another.[3,6,8–10] The purpose of supramalleolar osteotomy for varus ankle osteoarthritis is transfer of the weight-bearing line from the medial to the lateral side of the ankle, which is expected to open the medial side of the ankle joint. However, there has been little preoperative and postoperative analysis of the weight-bearing line in the ankle. Thus, the target mechanical axis point at the ankle remains unknown.

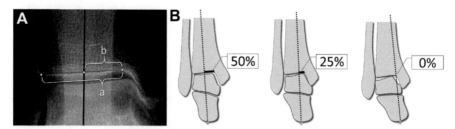

Fig. 3. Mechanical ankle joint axis point. (A) The mechanical ankle joint axis point is ex-pressed as the ratio representing the division of the coronal length of the plafond by the axis and is a radiographic measure of the distance of this point from the medial corner of the plafond (ie, b/a × 100). (B) The medial and lateral edges of the tibial plafond are taken as 0% and 100%, respectively. Thus, a negative value indicates that the mechanical ankle joint axis point lies medially beyond the medial corner of the plafond, and a value of greater than 100% indicates that the point lies laterally beyond the lateral edge of the plafond.

For patients with varus ankle osteoarthritis, I have used our radiographic method to determine, both before and after traditional supramalleolar osteotomy, the mechanical ankle joint axis point.[1] I have assessed correlation between the mechanical ankle joint axis point and clinical outcomes of the surgery. I found marked postoperative variation in the location of the mechanical ankle joint axis point and that when this axis point was found, preoperatively, to be medial to the edge of the tibial plafond, the surgery resulted in insufficient lateral movement of the axis point and a less than satisfactory clinical outcome.

Factors that can contribute to the excessively medial position of the mechanical ankle joint axis point in cases of varus ankle osteoarthritis include varus tilt of the tibial plafond, varus tilt of the talus within the ankle mortise, wearing of the articular cartilage and subchondral bone of the medial part of the of the plafond and the medial gutter, and inward deviation of the medial malleolus resulting in an abnormally wide angle between the articular surfaces of the medial malleolus and tibial plafond. Thus, I continue to use a TAS angle of 98° as our supramalleolar osteotomy target, but in some patients I use a target TAS angle of a little more than 98° and add lateral sliding calcaneal osteotomy and/or opening-wedge medial malleolar osteotomy[12] (**Fig. 4**) to further move the mechanical axis laterally. The medial malleolar osteotomy is performed to prevent postoperative medial translation of the talus, which can lead to medial positioning of the mechanical axis point. Adding lateral sliding calcaneal osteotomy further moves the lowest point of the calcaneus laterally and contributes to proper lateral positioning of the mechanical axis point. These additional procedures also add a hindfoot valgus moment arm.

Thus far, I have found that adding these procedures for ankles for which the mechanical axis point is in an excessively medial position (mainly in cases of Takakura stage 3b ankle osteoarthritis) moves the mechanical axis point laterally, more so

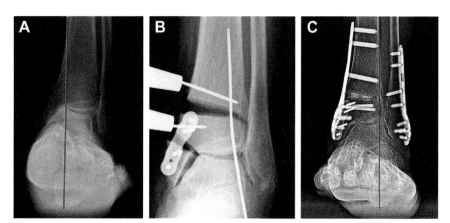

Fig. 4. Images of a patient who underwent supramalleolar osteotomy combined with ankle mortise reconstruction for varus ankle osteoarthritis. (*A*) The lower part of the preoperative hip-to-calcaneus radiograph shows subchondral bone contact that extends to the roof of the talar dome (Takakura stage 3b osteoarthritis). The mechanical ankle joint axis point is 0%. (*B*) Intraoperative image obtained during opening-wedge osteotomy of the medial malleolus performed to reconstruct the ankle mortise. (C) The lower part of the postoperative hip-to-calcaneus radiograph shows that the mechanical axis (*red line*) has been transferred to the lateral part of the ankle, with the mechanical ankle joint axis point being 100%, and the joint space has opened up.

than can be accomplished by traditional supramalleolar osteotomy alone, and thus better clinical outcomes are achieved. Correcting the talar tilt in ankles with stage 3b osteoarthritis is challenging. According to our experience, however, sufficient translation of the mechanical axis point is, with respect to long-term outcomes, much more influential than residual talar tilt.

Notably, evaluating the mechanical ankle joint axis point is also useful in cases of valgus ankle osteoarthritis (**Fig. 5**). An investigation aimed at determining the target mechanical ankle joint axis point when supramalleolar osteotomy is performed for valgus ankle osteoarthritis is under way.

RECONSTRUCTION OF STAGE IV-A ADULT-ACQUIRED FLATFOOT DEFORMITY

Hindfoot malalignment is seen in many individuals with adult-acquired flatfoot deformity. The valgus malalignment is especially severe in cases that have reached stage IV. In the original Myerson classification system, stage IV was defined as valgus angulation of the talus and early degeneration of the ankle joint.[13] Reconstruction in cases of stage IV deformity remains a substantial surgical challenge. Tibiotalocalcaneal arthrodesis has been recommended for stage IV deformity[13]; however, patient satisfaction tends to be quite low.

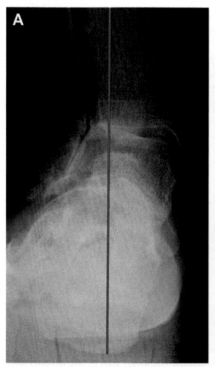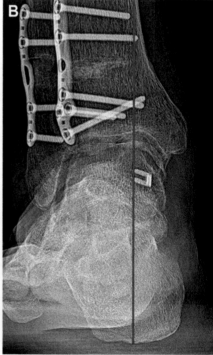

Fig. 5. Radiographs obtained in a case of valgus ankle osteoarthritis. (*A*) The lower part of the preoperative hip-to-calcaneus radiograph shows obliteration of the joint space in the lateral part of the ankle with subchondral bone contact and the mechanical axis (*red line*) passing through the lateral part of the ankle joint. (*B*) The lower part of the postoperative hip-to-calcaneus radiograph obtained 3 years after opening-wedge supramalleolar osteotomy for valgus ankle osteoarthritis shows that the mechanical axis (*red line*) has been transferred to the medal part of the ankle, and the joint space has opened up.

Stage IV adult-acquired flatfoot deformity[13] was eventually subdivided into stage IV-A, in which the ankle valgus is flexible, and stage IV-B, in which the valgus is rigid.[14,15] Stage IV-A deformity can sometimes be treated by means of a joint-sparing procedure such as deltoid ligament reconstruction in conjunction with triple arthrodesis[16] or deltoid ligament reconstruction in conjunction with calcaneal osteotomy, flexor digitorum longus tendon transfer, and lateral column lengthening[17]; however, clinical results of these procedures have been suboptimal. In some cases in which deltoid ligament reconstruction was performed in conjunction with triple arthrodesis, correction was lost over time, indicating that reconstruction of the deltoid ligament is not adequate for sustained correction of marked tibiotalar valgus deformity.[16]

In stage IV-A adult-acquired flatfoot deformity, the mechanical ankle joint axis point is in an excessively lateral position due to heel valgus and talar tilting. Furthermore, stage IV-A covers ankle osteoarthritis of various degrees. Because of these factors, I now perform supramalleolar osteotomy in addition to flatfoot reconstruction procedures, such as flexor digitorum longus tendon transfer, medializing calcaneal osteotomy, and/or Cotton osteotomy, for stage IV-A adult-acquired flatfoot deformity. In this operation, the distal aspect of the fibula and distal aspect of the tibia are exposed through a single incision on the anterolateral side of the ankle. Lateral opening-wedge tibial osteotomy is performed, along with oblique fibular osteotomy at the same level. A locking plate is used for tibial and fibular fixation. The gap created by the opening-wedge tibial osteotomy is filled with beta-tricalcium phosphate.

TOTAL ANKLE ARTHROPLASTY

One of the important technical principles of total knee arthroplasty (TKA) is restoration of neutral mechanical alignment, which is achieved when the mechanical axis of the lower extremity passes through the center of the knee joint.[18,19] In total ankle arthroplasty, as well, restoration of neutral mechanical alignment is important because increased edge loading due to hindfoot malalignment can lead to prosthesis loosening or breakage.[20,21] Yi and colleagues[22] reported association of medial malleolar impingement, delayed malleolar fracture, implant overhang, insert dislocation, and edge loading with talar translation, and that these factors are known causes of prosthetic failure after total ankle replacement. Deviation of the mechanical axis (angle between the mechanical axis of the lower limb and the tibial axis), lateral distal tibial angle, and hindfoot alignment are factors strongly associated with talar translation. Hence, the authors concluded that, in patients with a preoperative medial or lateral translation of the talus along with a great degree of hindfoot malalignment, simultaneous correction of the hindfoot malalignment should be considered.[22]

Studies of the mechanical axis at the ankle joint before and after total ankle arthroplasty are scarce. The mechanical ankle joint axis point reflects both mechanical axis deviation and hindfoot alignment. Hirao and colleagues,[23] in describing total ankle arthroplasty performed for patients with rheumatoid arthritis, reported that the angle that must be corrected for proper adjustment of the weight-bearing line in the ankle joint, is seen on the hip-to-calcaneus radiograph as the angle created by the lines connecting the center of the plafond and the calcaneal tip and the ideal loading axis (**Fig. 6**).

On rare occasion, I perform supramalleolar osteotomy after total ankle arthroplasty. This is needed in cases in which the postoperative hip-to-calcaneus radiograph shows malalignment of the ankle prosthesis, that is, deviation of the mechanical ankle joint axis point from the center of the ankle joint (**Fig. 7**).

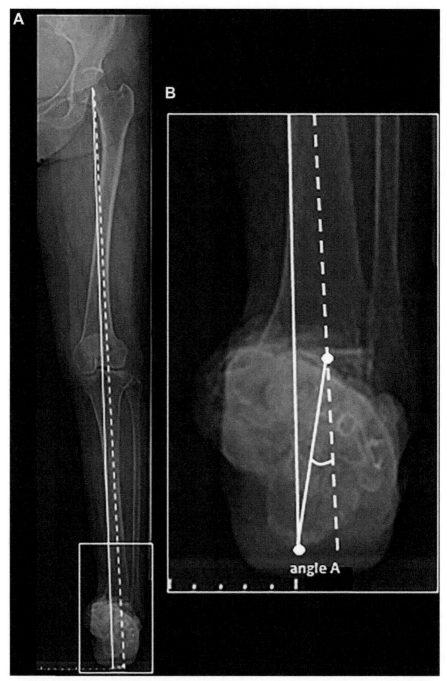

Fig. 6. Preoperative radiographs used in planning total ankle arthroplasty. (*A*) Hip-to-calcaneus radiograph. The solid line shows the preoperative calcaneal tip and loading axis. The dashed line shows the ideal loading axis, which passes through the center of the distal tibial plafond. (*B*) Angle A (created by the *lines* connecting the center of the plafond and the calcaneal tip and the ideal loading axis) is defined as the angle that must be

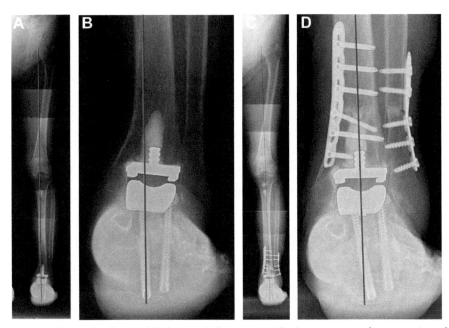

Fig. 7. Radiographs obtained before and after supramalleolar osteotomy for correction of malalignment after total ankle replacement in a patient with rheumatoid arthritis. (*A*) Preoperative hip-to-calcaneus radiograph. (*B*) The lower part of the preoperative hip-to-calcaneus radiograph shows that the mechanical axis (*red line*) passing through the lateral part of the ankle joint. (*C*) Postoperative hip-to-calcaneus radiograph. (*D*) The lower part of the postoperative hip-to-calcaneus radiograph shows the mechanical axis (red *line*) passing through the center of the ankle joint. (Reprinted with permission from Haraguchi N, Hip to calcaneus view for treatment planning and evaluation of hindfoot disorders. Bone Joint Nerve. 2012;2:569–575.)

REALIGNMENT OF THE OSTEOARTHRITIC KNEE AND ITS RELATION TO ANKLE JOINT ALIGNMENT

Ankle osteoarthritis is sometimes found in patients with knee osteoarthritis, and the ankle symptoms can either improve or worsen after knee surgery, such as total knee replacement or high tibial osteotomy. Norton and colleagues[24] showed compensatory hindfoot alignment for a given varus deformity of the knee; that is, as the mechanical axis angle becomes more varus, the hindfoot will subsequently become more valgus. They stated that patients undergoing TKA should be advised that their hindfoot symptoms might worsen afterward. Choi and colleagues[25] found that, after high tibial osteotomy performed in patients with medial compartment osteoarthritis with a varus deformity at the knee, the hindfoot valgus deviation observed preoperatively decreased significantly by 12 months, approaching normal values. Chang and

corrected for proper alignment of the weight-bearing line in the ankle joint. (Reprinted with permission from Hirao M, Hashimoto J, Tsuboi H, Ebina K, Nampei A, Noguchi T, Tsuji S, Nishimoto N, Yoshikawa H. Total ankle arthroplasty for rheumatoid arthritis in Japanese patients: a retrospective study of intermediate to long-term follow-up. JB JS Open Access. 2017;2:e0033).

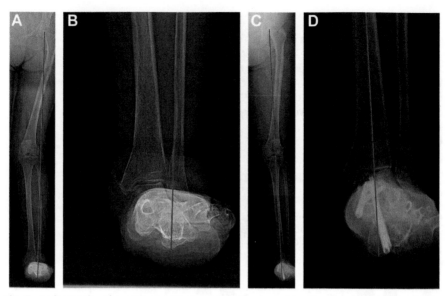

Fig. 8. Radiographs of a patient with stage-3 flatfoot combined with vulgus knee osteoarthritis. (*A*) Preoperative hip-to-calcaneus radiograph of a patient with stage 3 flatfoot and concomitant vulgus knee osteoarthritis. The hip-knee ankle angle is −10°. (*B*) The lower part of the preoperative hip-to-calcaneus radiograph shows hindfoot valgus and that the mechanical axis lies laterally beyond the lateral edge of the tibial plafond. (*C*) The knee vulgus resolved (hip-knee-ankle angle of −2°) as a result of triple arthrodesis performed for the flatfoot. (*D*) The lower part of the postoperative hip-to-calcaneus radiograph shows neutral hindfoot alignment and that the mechanical axis passes through the center of the tibial plafond.

colleagues[26] reviewed the cases of 24 patients who underwent TKA and had concomitant varus ankle osteoarthritis, and they found, as a result of the correction of the varus malalignment of the lower limb following TKA, that radiographic profiles of the ankle joint (eg, orientation of the joint line relative to the ground and medial joint space) had improved. However, although the radiographic features of the ankle joint had improved, many patients experienced increased ankle pain following TKA. The investigators speculated that drastic change in the alignment of the ankle joint could have an adverse effect on the tension of the ligaments that surround the ankle.[26] On the other hand, Takeuchi and colleagues[27] reported clinical outcomes of valgus high tibial osteotomy performed for patients with varus knee osteoarthritis accompanied by ipsilateral varus ankle osteoarthritis. The high tibial osteotomy led to improved American Orthopaedic Foot and Ankle Society Ankle-Hindfoot scores and ankle joint congruency in their patients.

I have found great variation in locations of the mechanical ankle joint axis point in patients with medial compartment osteoarthritis and almost no correlation between the hip-knee-ankle angle and the location of the mechanical ankle joint axis point (data unpublished). When undertaking knee surgery, surgeons should check the patient's mechanical ankle joint axis point preoperatively to evaluate whether the patient's ankle symptoms will worsen or improve.

Needless to say, lower limb alignment is influenced not only by the knee joint but also by the ankle joint. Knee realignment surgery influences hindfoot alignment and vice versa (**Fig. 8**).

SUMMARY

Analyzing the mechanical axis of the lower limb as a line from the center of the femoral head to the lowest point of the calcaneus clarifies the pathogenesis of various hindfoot disorders. Such analysis also facilitates surgical planning. Further, the analysis can clarify the cause of an unsatisfactory outcome of corrective surgery in particular cases. I believe it essential to analyze alignment of the whole limb when planning reconstructive surgery for lower limb conditions involving malalignment.

CLINICS CARE POINTS

- When planning reconstructive surgery of lower limbs with malalignment, it is essential to analyze the alignment of the whole limb prior to surgery.
- When obtaining hip-to-calcaneus radiographs, it is best to use the patella rather than the foot or ankle to control rotation of the lower limb. It is also important to confirm by radiograph that the patella is centered between the femoral condyles.
- When performing supramalleolar osteotomy for patients with a mechanical ankle joint axis point to be medial to the edge of the tibial plafond, use a target TAS angle slightly over 98° and add lateral sliding calcaneal osteotomy and/or opening-wedge medial malleolar osteotomy to further move the mechanical axis laterally.
- Before undertaking realignment surgery of the knee joint, surgeons should check the patient's mechanical ankle joint axis point to evaluate whether the patient's ankle condition will worsen or improve after surgery.

DISCLOSURE

The authors have nothing to disclose.

REFERENCES

1. Haraguchi N, OtaK TN, Seike K, et al. Weight-bearing-line analysis in supramalleolar osteotomy for varus-type osteoarthritis of the ankle. J Bone Joint Surg Am 2015;97:333–9.
2. Tanaka Y. The concept of ankle joint preserving surgery: why does supramalleolar osteotomy work and how to decide when to do an osteotomy or joint replacement. Foot Ankle Clin 2012;17:545–53.
3. Knupp M, Hintermann B. Treatment of asymmetric arthritis of the ankle joint with supramalleolar osteotomies. Foot Ankle Int 2012;33:250–2.
4. Knupp M, Stufkens SA, Bolliger L, et al. Classification and treatment of supramalleolar deformities. Foot Ankle Int 2011;32:1023–31.
5. Lee WC, Moon JS, Lee K, et al. Indications for supramalleolar osteotomy in patients with ankle osteoarthritis and varus deformity. J Bone Joint Surg Am 2011; 93:1243–8.
6. Harstall R, Lehmann O, Krause F, et al. Supramalleolar lateral closing wedge osteotomy for the treatment of varus ankle arthrosis. Foot Ankle Int 2007;28:542–8.
7. Stamatis ED, Cooper PS, Myerson MS. Supramalleolar osteotomy for the treatment of distal tibial angular deformities and arthritis of the ankle joint. Foot Ankle Int 2003;24:754–64.
8. Tanaka Y, Takakura Y, Hayashi K, et al. Low tibial osteotomy for varus-type osteoarthritis of the ankle. J Bone Joint Surg Br 2006;88:909–13.

9. Pagenstert GI, Hintermann B, Barg A, et al. Realignment surgery as alternative treatment of varus and valgus ankle osteoarthritis. Clin Orthop Relat Res 2007; 462:156–68.

10. Cheng YM, Huang PJ, Hong SH, et al. Low tibial osteotomy for moderate ankle arthritis. Arch Orthop Trauma Surg 2001;121:355–8.

11. Hintermann B, Knupp M, Barg A. Supramalleolar osteotomies for the treatment of ankle arthritis. J Am Acad Orthop Surg 2016;24:424–32.

12. Hasegawa A, Kaneko H, Yanagawa T, et al. Arthroplasty for the arthrosis deformans of the ankle. J Jpn Soc Surg Foot 1997;18:101–8.

13. Myerson MS. Adult acquired flatfoot deformity: treatment of dysfunction of the posterior tibial tendon. Instr Course Lect 1997;46:393–405.

14. Bluman EM, Title CI, Myerson MS. Posterior tibial tendon rupture: a refined classification system. Foot Ankle Clin 2007;12:233–49.

15. Haddad SL, Myerson MS, Younger A, et al. Symposium: adult acquired flatfoot deformity. Foot Ankle Int 2011;32:95–111.

16. Jeng CL, Bluman EM, Myerson MS. Minimally invasive deltoid ligament reconstruction for stage IV flatfoot deformity. Foot Ankle Int 2011;32:21–30.

17. Ellis SJ, Williams BR, Wagshul AD, et al. Deltoid ligament reconstruction with peroneus longus autograft in flatfoot deformity. Foot Ankle Int 2010;31:781–9.

18. Tanzer M, Makhdom AM. Preoperative planning in primary total knee arthroplasty. J Am Acad Orthop Surg 2016;24:220–30.

19. Jaffe WL, Dundon JM, Camus T. Alignment and balance methods in total knee arthroplasty. J Am Acad Orthop Surg 2018;26:709–16.

20. Haskell A, Mann RA. Ankle arthroplasty with preoperative coronal plane deformity: short- term results. Clin Orthop Relat Res 2004;424:98–103.

21. Wood PL, Deakin S. Total ankle replacement. The results in 200 ankles. J Bone Joint Surg Br 2003;85:334–41.

22. Yi Y, Cho JH, Kim JB, et al. Change in talar translation in the coronal plane after mobile-bearing total ankle replacement and its association with lower-limb and hindfoot alignment. J Bone Joint Surg Am 2017;99:e13.

23. Hirao M, Hashimoto J, Tsuboi H, et al. Total ankle arthroplasty for rheumatoid arthritis in Japanese patients: a retrospective study of intermediate to long-term follow-up. JB JS Open Access 2017;2:e0033.

24. Norton AA, Callaghan JJ, Amendola A, et al. Correlation of knee and hindfoot deformities in advanced knee OA: compensatory hindfoot alignment and where it occurs. Clin Orthop Relat Res 2015;473:166–74.

25. Choi JY, Song SJ, Kim SJ, et al. Changes in hindfoot alignment after high or low tibial osteotomy. Foot Ankle Int 2018;39:1097–105.

26. Chang CB, Jeong JH, Chang MJ, et al. Concomitant ankle osteoarthritis is related to increased ankle pain and a worse clinical outcome following total knee arthroplasty. J Bone Joint Surg Am 2018;100:735–41.

27. Takeuchi R, Saito T, Koshino T. Clinical results of a valgus high tibial osteotomy for the treatment of osteoarthritis of the knee and the ipsilateral ankle. Knee 2008;15: 196–200.

The Assessment of Ankle Osteoarthritis with Weight-Bearing Computed Tomography

Martinus Richter, MD, PhD[a,b,*], Cesar de Cesar Netto, MD[a,c], Francois Lintz, MD[a,d], Alexej Barg, MD[a,e], Arne Burssens, MD[a,f], Scott Ellis, MD[a,g]

KEYWORDS

• Ankle • Osteoarthritis • Weight-bearing CT • WBCT • Alignment

KEY POINTS

• The cone beam technology as such is similar to previous applications as for example intra-operative 3D-imaging.
• The accuracy of the bone position assessment, i.e. different measurement of angles between bones or position of bones have been investigated in many studies.
• The assessment of the hindfoot axis, position of the fibula in relation to the tibia and joint space analysis are important for the assessment of ankle osteoarthritis (AOA) and for treatment planning.

INTRODUCTION

Weight-Bearing CT (WBCT) was not especially invented for the assessment of ankle osteoarthritis (AOA). The principles of the technology and the evolvement of use are also the basis for the assessment of AOA as described in the following. The standard for diagnostic radiographic imaging in foot and ankle surgery was until 2012 radiographs with full weight-bearing without any useful alternative.[1–3] The three-dimensional position of bones and relationships between bones in the foot (for example angles) are difficult to assess with standard radiographs due to the

[a] International Weight-Bearing CT Society; [b] Department for Foot and Ankle Surgery Rummelsberg and Nuremberg, Rummelsberg 71, 90592 Schwarzenbruck, Germany; [c] Department of Orthopedics and Rehabilitation, Carver College of Medicine, University of Iowa, 200 Hawkins Dr, Iowa City, IA 52242, USA; [d] Clinique de l'Union, Foot and Ankle Surgery Centre, Boulevard de Ratalens, 31240, Saint-Jean, Toulouse, France; [e] Department of Trauma-, Hand- and Reconstructive Surgery, University Medical Center Hamburg-Eppendorf, Hamburg, Germany; [f] Department of Orthopaedics and Traumatology, University Hospital of Ghent, Corneel Heymanslaan 10, 9000 Gent, Oost-Vlaanderen, België; [g] The Hospital for Special Surgery, 535 East 70th Street, New York, NY 10021, USA
* Corresponding author. Department for Foot and Ankle Surgery Rummelsberg and Nuremberg, Location Hospital Rummelsberg, Rummelsberg 71, Schwarzenbruck 90592, Germany.
E-mail address: martinus.richter@sana.de

Foot Ankle Clin N Am 27 (2022) 13–36
https://doi.org/10.1016/j.fcl.2021.11.001
1083-7515/22/© 2021 Elsevier Inc. All rights reserved.

foot.theclinics.com

superimposition of the different bones.[1,4] The reason is the "reduction" of a three-dimensional body (foot) to a two-dimensional image (conventional radiograph). Angle measurements with conventional radiographs could be inaccurate due to inaccuracies of the projection (orientation of (central) beam) and/or foot orientation (**Fig. 1**).[1,3,5–7] 3D imaging with conventional computed tomography (CT) allows for exact analysis within the 3D data that is not influenced by projection and/or foot orientation but lacks weight-bearing (**Fig. 2**).[1,3,4,8] WBCT was introduced 2012 for foot and ankle use as a new technology that allows 3D imaging with full weight-bearing which should be not influenced by projection and/or foot orientation.[1] The cone-beam technology as such is similar to previous applications as for example, intraoperative 3D imaging (**Fig. 3**).[3,9] Different devices from different companies became available. Several measurement possibilities had been provided with different software solutions (**Tables 1** and **2**).[1–3] Many clinical application possibilities have been shown.[1–3] From the very beginning of the device availability, scientific studies have been used.[1–3] Most of the studies investigated the accuracy of the bone position assessment, that is, different measurement of angles between bones or position of bones.[1–3] Shortly after, additional measurements as for example, pedography were added.[10,11] From the previously described parameter, especially the assessment of the hindfoot axis, position of the fibula in relation to the tibia and joint space analysis is important for the assessment of AOA and for treatment planning.

STATUS IN HEALTHY SUBJECTS

The main purpose of WBCT is exact and detailed evaluation of foot and ankle pathologies including alignment and degenerative in natural standing position. However, WBCT can also be used in healthy persons for a better understanding of complex anatomy and biomechanics.[12,13]Lepojarvi and colleagues investigated the rotational

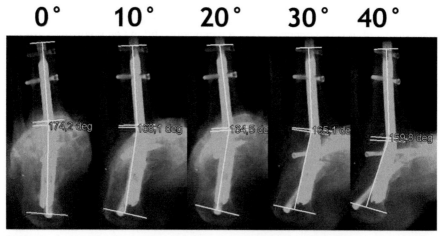

Fig. 1. Conventional radiographs for measurement of hindfoot alignment in a patient with healed tibio-talo-calcaneal arthrodesis with retrograde nail. The healed arthrodesis ensures uniform hindfoot position during repetitive radiographic assessment. Radiographs with different internal rotations (0°–40°) of the foot in relation to the central beam were obtained and the hindfoot angle was measured. The measured hindfoot angles ranged from 5.8° to 21.2°. The different angles are not influenced by the "real" hindfoot angle (healed arthrodesis plus nail) but only by different orientation (internal rotation) of the foot and ankle during radiographic assessment.

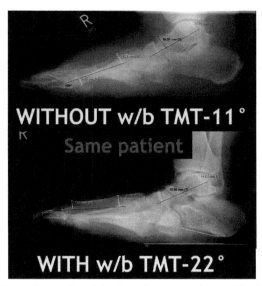

Fig. 2. Lateral radiographs of the right foot from a patient with Charcot arthropathy without weight-bearing (top) and with weight-bearing (bottom). The lateral talo-1st meta-tarsal-angle (TMT) was measured. This was −11° without and −22° with weight-bearing showing the influence of weight-bearing on the relationship of the bones (angles).

dynamics of the distal tibiofibular joint by analysis of fibula position in axial plane.[13] In neutrally aligned ankle under weight-bearing conditions, the fibula was found anteriorly in the tibial incisura in 88% of all subjects. Internal and external rotation with a mean moment of 30 Nm resulted in a mean sagittal translation of the fibula of 1.5 ± 1.2 mm and in mean fibula rotation of 3.2 ± 2.8°.[13] In their second study, rotational dynamics of the talus were analyzed in the same healthy subjects.[13] The rotation of the talus, as well as radiographic alignment of mortise, were measured while standing with versus without rotation. Internal and external rotation resulted in significant changes of talus rotation of 10.0 ± 5.8° with any substantial changes in the medial clear space.[13] The anatomy and kinematics of the distal tibiofibular syndesmosis have been the subject of several studies recently. Hagemeijer and colleagues analyzed 24 healthy ankles

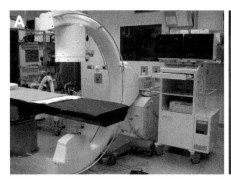
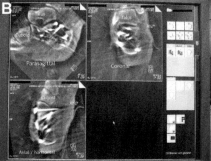

Fig. 3. (*A*, *B*) Cone-beam technology application for intraoperative 3D imaging (ISO-C-3D, Siemens, Erlangen, Germany). (*A*) shows the device in the operating theater and (*B*) a monitor view example. The monitor shows intraoperative imaging after open reduction and internal fixation of a calcaneal fracture. 3D reformations are shown (parasagittal, top left; coronal, top right; axial, bottom).

Table 1
Radiographic assessment of the forefoot using weight-bearing computed tomography [1,56–59]

Radiographic Measurement	Interobserver Reliability	Intraobserver Reliability	Correlation with Other Measurements	Clinical Findings
α angle (1st MT pronation angle)	n.a.	n.a.	■ vs. HVA[55]: .076[a], P value < .1 ■ vs. IMA.[55]: .144[a], P value < .1 ■ vs. sesamoid position.[55]: .019[a], P value < .1	■ HV group: 21.9°, control group: 13.8°[55] ■ HV group: 8° ± 2° (4°–12°), control group: 2° ± 3° (−4°–8°)[2] ■ HV group: 17.7° ± 6.9, control group: 14° ± 7.8°[57]
1st MT/ground angle	n.a.	n.a.	n.a.	• HV group: 18° ± 1°, control group: 21° ± 1°[56]
HVA (2D)	n.a.	n.a.	n.a.	• HV group: 35° ± 3°, control group: 13° ± 4°[56] ■ HV group: 39.8° ± 8.6°, control group: 14.7° ± 3.1°[58] ■ HV group: 30.7° ± 8°, control group: 11° ± 3.8°[57]
HVA (3D)	n.a.	n.a.	• vs. HVA on plain radiographs.[56]: .95[b], P value < .05 • vs. HVA (2D).[56]: .94[b], P value < .05	• HV group: 35° ± 3° (WB), 46° ± 5° (NWB), control group: 15° ± 4° (WB), 32° ± 8° (NWB)[56]
IMA (2D)	n.a.	n.a.	n.a.	• HV group: 19° ± 1°, control group: 11° ± 1°[56] ■ HV group: 22.2° ± 4.4°, control group: 8.7° ± 1.0°[4] ■ HV group: 14.6° ± 4.4°, control group: 10.5° ± 2.5°[57]
IMA (3D)	n.a.	n.a.	• vs. IMA on plain radiographs.[56]: .72[b], P value < .05 • vs. IMA (2D).[56]: .81[b], P value < .05	• HV group: 17° ± 1° (WB), 14° ± 1° (NWB), control group: 11° ± 1° (WB), 8° ± 2° (NWB)[56] • 9.3° ± 3.5° (WB), 7.8° ± 3.9° (NWB)[56]

Max. horizontal width (mm)	n.a.	n.a.	n.a.	HV group: 98 ± 1 (WB), 89 ± 2 (NWB), control group: 86 ± 2 (WB), 78 ± 3 (NWB)[56]
Sesamoid position in coronal plane	n.a.	n.a.	■ vs. α angle.[55]: 019[a], P value < .1 ■ vs. HVA.[1]: 477[a], P value < .01	■ HV group: true sesamoid subluxation 71.7%, no sesamoid subluxation 28.3%[55]
TMT angle dorsoplantar	n.a.	n.a.	n.a.	• -5.0° ± 12.0° (WB), 4.3° ± 10.0° (NWB)[1]
TMT angle lateral	n.a.	n.a.	n.a.	• -7.6° ± 8.2° (WB), 0.5° ± 8.4 (NWB)[1]

Abbreviations: HV, hallux valgus; HVA, hallux valgus angle; IMA, intermetatarsal angle; metatarsal, MT; metatarsal, n. a., not available; NWB, non-weight-bearing; TMT, talo-1st metatarsal; WB, weight-bearing.
[a] Spearman Rank Correlation Coefficient.
[b] Pearson Correlation Coefficient.

Table 2
Radiographic Assessment of the Midfoot and Hindfoot using Weight-Bearing Computed Tomography[14,22,27,32,45,55,60–62]

Radiographic Measurement	Interobserver Reliability	Intraobserver Reliability	Correlation with Other Measurements	Clinical Findings
Calcaneal pitch angle	n.a.	n.a.	n.a.	• 17.8° ± 5.4° (WB), 16.5° ± 5.0° (NWB)[59]
Calcaneofibular distance (mm)	0.61[a,2]	n.a.	n.a.	• 0.3 ± 6.0 (WB), 3.6 ± 5.2 (NWB)[2]
Fibular rotation	n.a.	n.a.	n.a.	▪ syndesmosis injury: 8.4° ± 7.0°[27,59] ▪ control group: 10.3° ± 5.5°[27,59]
Foot and ankle offset (%)	0.99 ± 0.00[c,4]	0.97 ± 0.02	n.a.	• 2.3 ± 2.9 (95%CI: 1.5–3.1) (patients with neutral alignment)[27] • −11.6 ± 6.9 (95%CI: −13.9 to −9.4) (patients with varus alignment)[27] • 11.4 ± 5.7 (95%CI: 9.6–13.3) (patients with valgus alignment)[27]
HAA	0.83[a,2]	n.a.	n.a.	• 21.0° ± 7.9 (WB), 19.0° ± 9.0° (NWB)[60] • 10.1° ± 7.1° (WB), 5.4° ± 5.6° (NWB)[59]
HAA$_{CL}$	0.72 (valgus), 0.69 (varus)[c,5]	0.73 (valgus), 0.67 (varus)[5]	n.a.	• 25.2° (valgus), 22° (varus)[5]
HAA$_{LA}$	0.7 (valgus), 0.71 (varus)[c,5]	0.71 (valgus), 0.72 (varus)[5]	n.a.	• 16.4° (valgus), 11.9° (varus)[5]
HAA$_{NOV}$	0.69 (valgus), 0.6 (varus)[c,5]	0.67 (valgus), 0.67 (varus)[5]	n.a.	• 17.7° (valgus), 13.5° (varus)[22]
Lateral talocalcaneal joint space width (mm)	0.82[a,2]	n.a.	n.a.	• 2.2 ± 1.1 (WB), 2.9 ± 1.7 (NWB)[60]
Middle facet percentage of uncoverage	0.75 (0.53–0.87)[6]	0.90 (0.81–0.95)[6]	n.a.	▪ 45.3% (AAFD), 4.8% (controls)[32]

Middle facet incongruence angle	0.93 (0.85–0.96)[6]	0.95 (0.91–0.98)[6]	n.a.	■ 17.3° (AAFD), 0.3° (controls)[32]
Naviculocalcaneal distance (mm)	0.85[a,2]	n.a.	n.a.	● 15.3 ± 4.7 (WB), 13.5 ± 4.0 (NWB)[60]
Subtalar inferior facet-horizontal angle	n.a.	n.a.	■ no correlation with any weight-bearing radiographic measures[7]	■ stage II AAFD group: 15.9° ± 5.7°, control group: 5.7° ± 6.7°[45]
Subtalar inferior-superior facets angle	n.a.	n.a.	■ vs AP coverage angle[7]: P value .003; ■ vs. AP talar-1st MT angle[7]: P value .003; ■ vs. calcaneal pitch[7]: P value .014; ■ vs. Meary's angle[7]: P value < .001; ■ vs medial column height[7]: P value .007	■ stage II AAFD group: 21.2° ± 6.7°, control group: 10.7° ± 6.4°[45]
Subtalar vertical angle	● 0.975[a,5]; ● 0.72 (valgus), 0.73 (varus)[c,5]	● 0.989[8]; ● 0.77 (valgus), 0.78 (varus)[5]	n.a.	● 91° (72°–109°) (varus OA group), 109° (97°–120°) (valgus OA group), 98° (85°–114°) (controls)[61]; ● 74.3° (valgus), 69.1° (varus)[5]
Syndesmosis area	n.a.	n.a.	n.a.	■ syndesmosis injury: 164.8 ± 46.8 cm[3,60]; ■ control group: 118.7 ± 37.7 cm[14,60]
Syndesmosis volume	n.a.	n.a.	n.a.	■ syndesmosis injury: 5.5 cm[60] (3 cm above TP), 14.1 cm[60] (5 cm above TP), 33.5 cm[60] (10 cm above TP)[54]

(continued on next page)

Table 2
(continued)

Radiographic Measurement	Interobserver Reliability	Intraobserver Reliability	Correlation with Other Measurements	Clinical Findings
				■ control group: 4.7 cm[60] (3 cm above TP), 7.9 cm[60] (5 cm above TP), 23.3 cm[60] (10 cm above TP)[54]
Talar tilt	0.92 (valgus), 0.89 (varus)[c,5]	0.89 (valgus), 0.89 (varus)[5]	n.a.	• 5.9° (valgus), 4.8° (varus)[5]
Talar translation (mm)	0.86 (valgus), 0.82 (varus)[c,5]	0.87 (valgus), 0.88 (varus)[5]	n.a.	• 21 (valgus), 19 (varus)[5]
Talocalcaneal overlap (mm)	0.81[b]	n.a.	n.a.	• 1.4 ± 3.9 (WB), 4.1 ± 3.9 (NWB)[60]
Tibiocalcaneal distance (mm)	0.72[b,2]	n.a.	n.a.	• 20.6 ± 4.2 (WB), 21.7 ± 6.2 (NWB)[60]

Abbreviations: AAFD, adult-acquired flatfoot deformity; AP, antero-posterior; HAA, hindfoot alignment angle; HAA$_{CL}$, hindfoot alignment angle measured by the bisector of the Achilles tendon and the calcaneus; HAA$_{LA}$, hindfoot alignment angle measured using an inclination set at 45° to simulate the long axial view; HAA$_{NOV}$, hindfoot alignment angle measured by combining the inclination of the tibia (anatomic axis) and inclination of the talus and calcaneus (talocal-caneal angle); MT, metatarsal; n.a., not available; NWB, non–weight-bearing; TP, tibial plafond; WB, weight-bearing.

[a] Intraclass correlation coefficient to assess the interobserver reliability (measurements of one orthopedic resident, one medical student, and one scientific associate).

[b] Intraclass correlation coefficient to assess the interobserver reliability (measurements of 2 musculoskeletal radiologists).

[c] Intraclass correlation coefficient to assess the interobserver reliability (measurement of 2 independent observers)

and found the mean fibular sagittal plane position of 1.8 ± 1.0 mm as well as mean fibular rotation of 11.5 ± 5.2°.[14] Malhotra and colleagues addressed the effect of weight-bearing on the measurements of the distal tibiofibular syndesmosis.[15] They found that the full weight-bearing resulted in a substantial lateral and posterior sagittal translation as well as external rotation of the distal fibula in relation to the incisura[15,16]

DEGREE OF ANKLE OSTEOARTHRITIS

The authors propose a four-degree classification AOA for WBCT (**Fig. 4**) The first degree of AOA includes joint space narrowing but not complete loss and osteophyte formation (see **Fig. 4A**). The second degree includes partial or complete loss of joint space (see **Fig. 4B,C**). The third degree includes additional subchondral cysts but remaining joint surface congruency (see **Fig. 4D**). The fourth degree includes additional joint surface destruction and incongruence (see **Fig. 4E,F**). This new classification combines the classical signs of osteoarthritis (joint space narrowing or loss, osteophyte formation, and subchondral cysts) with 3D visualization.

ASSESSMENT OF ALIGNMENT

Alignment is a paramount factor in the understanding of AOA, on which WBCT can shed significant new light. With regards to both the preoperative factors which lead

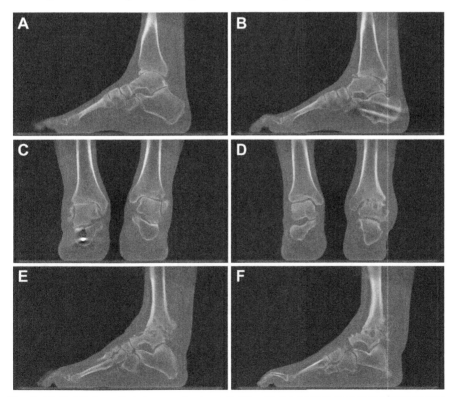

Fig. 4. (A–F). (A) show first degree of osteoarthritis with joint space narrowing but not complete loss and osteophyte formation. (B, C) show second degree of osteoarthritis with partial or complete loss of joint space. (D) shows third degree of osteoarthritis with additional subchondral cysts but remaining joint surface congruency. (E, F) show fourth degree of osteoarthritis with additional joint surface destruction and incongruence.

to the progressive degeneration of cartilage and the postoperative factors which may lead to surgical failure, 3D weight-bearing imaging using cone-beam technology has recently improved our level of understanding with higher quality evidence.[17–20]The classification of arthritic joint line degeneration based on the thickness of radiolucent cartilage, is complexified by being in 3D and necessitates the development of computerized algorithm such as distance mapping (DM) to provide accurate analysis and quantifiable data.[20,21] One of the 2 main reasons for this difficulty is our education as surgeons, based on 2D weight-bearing radiographs for measurements and 3D non–weight-bearing CT for details. The new modality of WBCT now replaces both (**Fig. 5**).

To improve this, several methods have been proposed to:

1 Adapt 2D alignment to the new 3D environment by defining reliable 3D landmarks.
   In this case, the measurement's plane is described based on reliable anatomic landmarks such as the lowest point on the calcaneus tuberosity and the longitudinal tibia axis, or the vertical axis for the coronal and transverse planes (**Fig. 6**)[22–24]
2 Identify the true 3D angles using computerized methods such as segmentation.
   In this case, a specialized software is required to perform segmentation (identification of individual bones) of the anatomy (**Fig. 7**), and 3D measurements.[23,25]
3 Propose a foot ankle offset, which requires identifying 3 landmarks on the weight-bearing plane (foot tripod) and the center of the ankle joint (**Fig. 8**).[26–29]

In daily practice, WBCT allows to evaluate alignment in a myriad way. First, a "skin" 3D rendering is possible, combined with digital podoscopy (**Fig. 9**), allowing for virtual clinical evaluation of hindfoot, ankle orientation, and arch type.[30] Second, most WBCT machines provide built in capacity to perform, or reconstruct conventional radiographs (or DRR, standing for digitally reconstructed radiographs) (**Fig. 10**). Third, the 3 methods listed above may be applied to the 3D dataset, using multiplanar viewing software (**Fig. 11**).

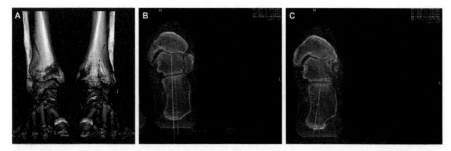

Fig. 5. (*A*) shows the 3D rendering view of the case. In our experience, this advantageously corresponds to a "snapshot" view which allows to have a general overview of the bony architecture before switching to Multi Planar View. In (*B*), the hindfoot alignment angle was measured while the antero-posterior axis of the scanner was set as the sagittal plane. A 1.4° varus was found. In (*C*), the axis of the second metatarsal was used as the sagittal reference plane. An 8.8° varus was found. We need to stress here that this does not mean that WBCT is not reliable in terms of measurement: on the contrary, it means that 2D angles which need to be set in a particular plane are not adapted to WBCT because of the choice of this plane, which is not reliable. Angles and distances are not compatible with 3D: they belong to the 2D world.

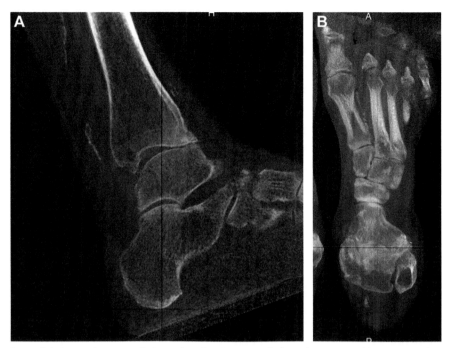

Fig. 6. (*A*) shows the sagittal view whereby the coronal plane (represented by the *blue line*) passes through the lowest point of the calcaneus and the center of the ankle joint. In (*B*), we are looking at the axial view whereby the sagittal plane (represented by the *green lines*) is set along the 2nd metatarsal.

WBCT AND FOOT AND ANKLE OFFSET (FAO) IN THE ASSESSMENT OF THE VALGUS ARTHRITIC ANKLE AS PART OF PROGRESSIVE COLLAPSING FOOT DEFORMITY.

Similarly, WBCT and semiautomatic biometric measurements such as the FAO can also be used in the preoperative and postoperative assessment of the arthritic valgus ankle, providing an idea in regard to the contribution of the ankle and hindfoot malalignment in the overall deformity.[29,31] WBCT is recommended in the assessment of this complex deformity, and allow proper assessment of the ankle and hindfoot components of the PCFD. Increased preoperative FAO measurements in patients undergoing patients with total ankle replacement (TAR) were found to significantly predict the number of additional realignment procedures, such as calcaneal osteotomies, that were needed to balance the foot and ankle, once the ankle deformity was corrected (**Figs. 12** and **13**)[29,32,33]

THREE-DIMENSIONAL MEASUREMENTS IN ANKLE OSTEOARTHRITIS USING WEIGHT-BEARING CONE-BEAM COMPUTED TOMOGRAPHY

Deformity is a critical contributor to the development and progression of ankle OA.[19,34,35] Two pivotal publications have examined the role of a WBCT specifically in ankle OA using 2-dimensional measurements.[1,19,34,36–41] Kim and colleagues quantified the rotation of the talus within the mortice of patients with varus ankle OA.[42] They found a higher internal rotation of the talus than the control group, which altered according to the severity of ankle OA. Krähenbühl and colleagues used a weight-

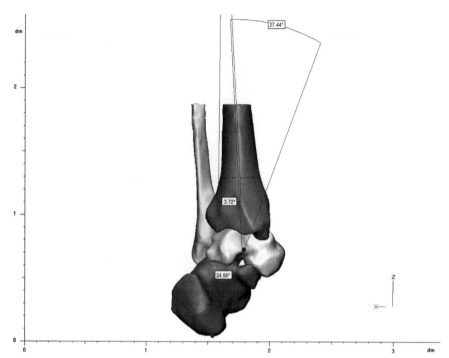

Fig. 7. Shows an example of 3D angles being measured directly using a 3D model created from a patient dataset using manual segmentation (contouring of the bones on each slice).

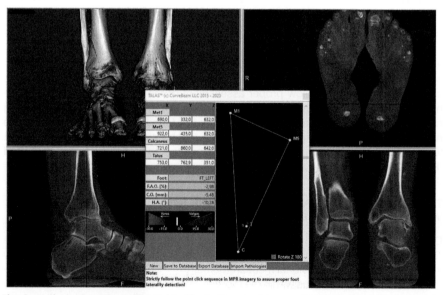

Fig. 8. In the same case as **Fig. 7**, hindfoot alignment is measured using the 3D biometric FAO, via semiautomatic software.

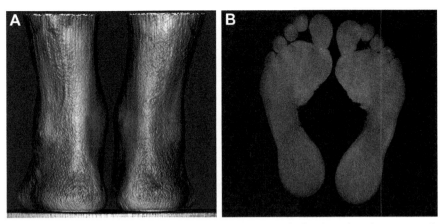

Fig. 9. (A) shows the 3D rendering of the skin view. In (B), the digital podoscopy can be observed.

bearing CT to assess the orientation of the subtalar joint in ankle varus and valgus OA.[43] They could demonstrate the compensation of the subtalar joint in varus—but not in valgus ankle OA. The aforementioned studies contained a first characterization of the structural configuration of hindfoot deformities in the presence of physiologic without superposition but remained limited by a 2-dimensional assessment of 3-dimensional deformities. Fortunately, recent software modalities are able to generate 3-dimensional model from weight-bearing CT images. Three studies focused specifically on techniques to translate former 2-dimensional measurements to their

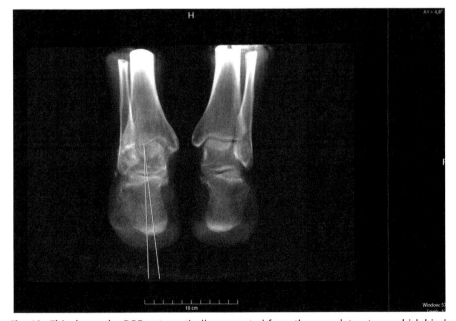

Fig. 10. This shows the DRR automatically generated from the case dataset, on which hindfoot alignment has been manually measured at 4.8° varus.

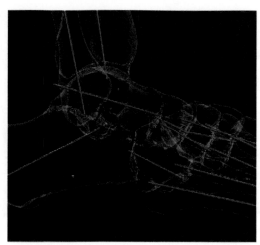

Fig. 11. An example of automatic segmentation of bones and recognition of the principal longitudinal axes.

3-dimensional equivalents using weight-bearing CT (see **Figs. 5** and **6; Fig. 14**).[25,40,44] One of the main advantages of these techniques is the ability of the software to compute different landmarks and axes based on the volumetric properties of the bone models. Geometric functions allow or the centroid for example, of the talus, which is used to calculate the measurements by the software. This overcomes the

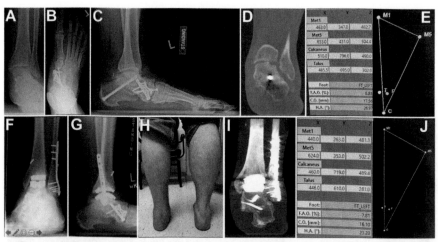

Fig. 12. (A–J) 58-year-old male patient with history of rigid PCFD and prior triple fusion, presenting with symptomatic end-stage ankle arthritis, fixed mild valgus ankle deformity. Preoperative conventional weight-bearing radiographic assessment with Mortise ankle (A), anteroposterior (B) and lateral foot incidences (C) and preoperative WBCT assessment demonstrating mild coronal plane ankle valgus deformity (D) and an FAO of 8.83% (E). Postoperative 6-month conventional weight-bearing radiographic assessment demonstrating well-aligned TAR implants on Mortise (F) and lateral ankle views (G), but with a clinically mild residual asymmetric left hindfoot valgus (H) and WBCT images confirming the residual deformity (I) and still increased FAO of 7.81% (J).

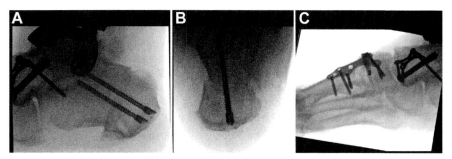

Fig. 13. *A–C*). Intraoperative fluoroscopic images demonstrating additional surgical realignment procedure in the same patient with a medial displacement calcaneal osteotomy (*A, B*) and plantarflexion fusion of the first tarsometatarsal joint (*C*), to realign the foot tripod underneath the ankle.

measurement errors caused by former manual acquisition of the axes or landmarks and is reflected in the higher reliability coefficients associated with 3-dimensional measurements compared with 2-dimensional measurements.[24] Moreover, the application of these measurements has demonstrated their relevance in the pre and

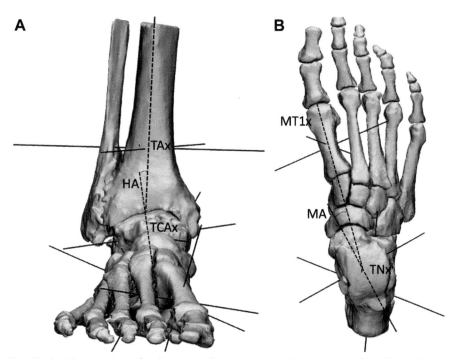

Fig. 14. (*A, B*). Overview of 3-dimensional measurements in a patient with AOA and varus deformity of the hindfoot. Computed measurements allow to calculate the best fitted axis of the tibia (TAx) and talocalcaneal axis (TCAx) by connecting the calculated most inferior point of the calcaneus and centroid of the talus. The hindfoot angle (HA) in the coronal plane is calculated based on the intersection of the TAx and TCAx (*A*). The software calculates the best fitted longitudinal axis of the first metatarsal (MT1x) and of the talar neck (TNx). The intersection of the MT1x and TNx constitutes the Méary angle (MA) in the axial plane (*B*).

postoperative assessment of both valgus and varus hindfoot deformities.[23,24,45] On the contrary, one of the main disadvantages remains the time consummation to segment each CT-slide separately to generate these models. This remains the main obstacle for their routine use in clinical practice at present. However, advances in the software modalities allow for automatic segmentations of the bony structures, which enabled the first applications of automated measurements.[46] It is expected that these automated measurements will facilitate the application of 3-dimensional measurement in clinical practice, but future research is still mandatory to confirm the initial promising findings (see **Fig. 14**).

Deformity Correction with Patient-Specific Guides

Supramalleolar osteotomies are an established treatment option to correct valgus or varus deformity in patients presenting with AOA, most frequently by an opening or closing of osteotomy.[16,43,47,48] This results in pain relief and improvement of function both on the mid- and long-term follow-up in patients with mild to moderate AOA.[12,48] This can be attributed to a shift in the weight-bearing axis, which redistributes and mitigates the peak concentration of stress within the ankle.[49,50] One biomechanical

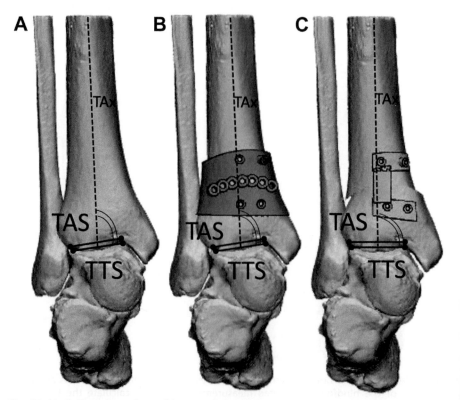

Fig. 15. (A–C). Overview of an ankle varus deformity correction using patient specific guides designed on weightbearing CT imaging. Pre-operative three-dimensional reconstruction of an ankle varus deformity (A) Fitting of the patient specific dome shaped osteotomy guide (B) A second patient specific guide is applied to hold the dome shaped correction of the distal tibia in place prior to a plate and screw osteosynthesis (C). Image courtesy of dr Kris Buedts

disadvantage of the closing or opening wedge osteotomy, is a medialized or lateralized center of the talus.[43] This shortcoming can be overcome in congruent ankle varus or valgus deformities by using a dome-shaped supramalleolar osteotomy, which keeps the talus centered under mechanical axis.[51] However, this procedure remains technically demanding to perform free-hand. This technical drawback can be overcome by the use of a patient-specific guide, which has shown to improve the accuracy of corrective osteotomies.[19] Even though the templates were first planned based on conventional CT, the advantages of implementing WBCT imaging to generate patient-specific guides are twofold. First, the correct level of the osteotomy can be determined based on the fit of the guide containing different sleeves to perform the multiple drill hole technique described by Wagner and colleagues[52] Second, the preoperative alignment can be determined using the aforementioned 3-dimensional measurements and a virtual correction can be performed until the desired position is achieved (**Fig. 15**A, B).

On this corrected model a second guide can be designed using the contours of the tibia proximal and distal of the osteotomy (**Fig. 15**C). During surgery, this second guide indicates the correct amount of rotation after a dome shape osteotomy based on the fit of the tibia proximal and distal of the osteotomy.

The preliminary results of this technique demonstrated a good clinical outcome and accuracy within the 2° of the planned correction. A similar approach can be used in other types of supramalleolar osteotomies, but the potential benefits should be confirmed in long-term and comparative prospective studies.

EFFECT OF ANKLE INSTABILITY

Krähenbühl and colleagues[53] established a cadaveric syndesmosis instability model by sectioning of anterior inferior tibiofibular ligament versus deltoid transection.[43]

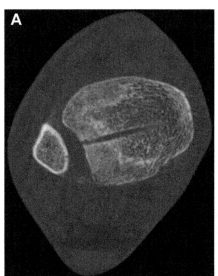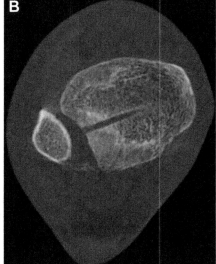

Fig. 16. Preoperative axial weight-bearing CT demonstrating recurrent syndesmotic instability. (*A*) shows imaging in the neutral position without rotation demonstrates substantial widening of distal syndesmosis. (*B*) shows that internal rotation results in substantial increase of posterior tibiofibular distance and decrease of anterior tibiofibular distance.

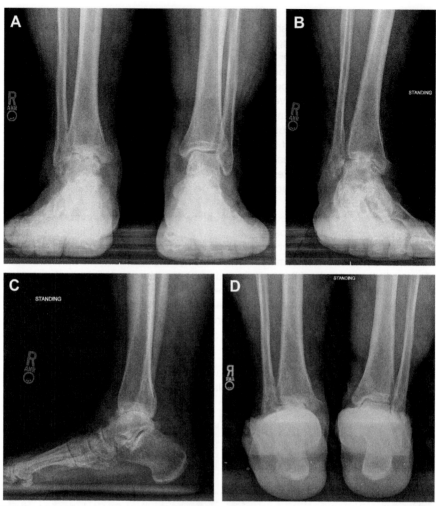

Fig. 17. (A–D) Preoperative (A) bilateral standing anteroposterior ankle (B) Mortise ankle (C) lateral ankle and (D) Saltzman radiographs demonstrating severe right bone-on-bone ankle joint osteoarthritis and bilateral varus deformities of the ankle, right greater than left.

There was no substantial difference in the radiographic assessment of ligamental syndesmosis instability between weight-bearing and non–weight-bearing conditions. However, torque application has a substantial impact on radiographic syndesmosis assessment using digitally reconstructive radiographs as well as axial WBCT scans (**Fig. 16**).[43] Del Rio and colleagues analyzed 2D syndesmosis area measurements on axial scans in both ankles of 39 patients with syndesmosis injury under weight-bearing versus non–weight-bearing conditions.[54] As expected, there were significant differences between healthy and injured ankles with 3.4 ± 6.7 mm^2 versus 16.6 ± 9.9 mm^2, respectively. Furthermore, injured ankles demonstrated a significantly higher increased in the measured surface between both conditions than noninjured ankles.[54] Bhimani and colleagues performed 3D volumetric measurements of the distal tibiofibular syndesmosis in 12 patients with unilateral syndesmotic instability.[55] The volumes were measured 3, 5, and 10 cm above the tibial plafond. At all

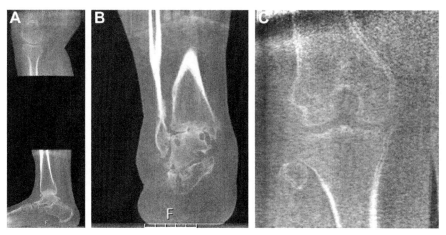

Fig. 18. Preoperative weight-bearing CT scan performed with Prophecy (Wright Medical Group, Memphis, TN, USA) protocol to define anatomic and mechanical axes of the ankle is shown. On the sagittal view (*A*), severe arthritis is noted at the level of the ankle and the corresponding slices of the knee joint are visualized. On the coronal views, the ankle and knee are not seen in the same view, but taken together (*B*) the severe arthritis of the ankle is noted and (*C*) the center of the knee joint can be visualized to establish the same axes.

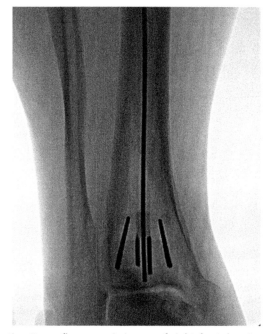

Fig. 19. Intraoperative C-arm fluoroscopic image of right foot showing placement of wire through the prophecy guide (not visible) along the mechanical axis of the tibia.

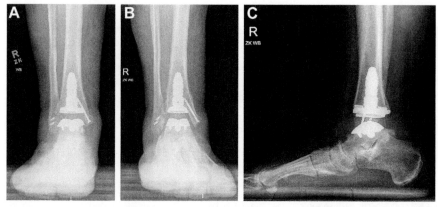

Fig. 20. Postoperative (*A*) anteroposterior (*B*) Mortise (*C*) lateral radiographs of the right ankle demonstrating implantation of INBONE Total Ankle System. A medial malleolus screw has been placed to prophylactically protect the bone and 2 anchors in the fibula have been placed to perform lateral ligament tightening/repair.

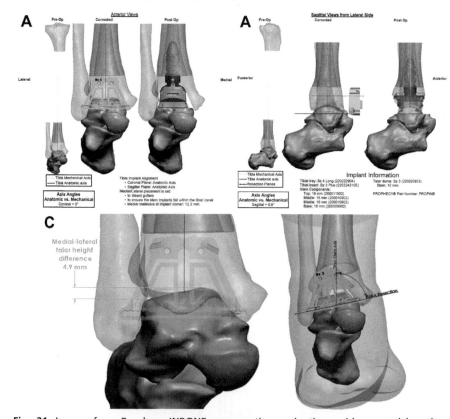

Fig. 21. Images from Prophecy INBONE preoperative navigation guide created based on weight-bearing CT imaging. Anterior view of the guide describing expected tibia implant alignment and medial/lateral placement, as well as angles for anatomic versus mechanical axes (*A*). Sagittal view from the lateral side describing expected implant sizing, as well as angles for anatomic versus mechanical axes (*B*). Preoperative medial-lateral talar height difference of 4.9 mm is described (*C*). The talus resection guide is shown relative to the talar bone and the planned tibia alignment axis, demonstrating expected correction from varus with resections.

3 levels, the measured volume was significantly higher with observed difference of 1.8 ± 1.4 cm^3, 5.9 ± 1.9 cm^3, and 9.5 ± 2.5 cm^3, respectively.[55]

Planning Total Ankle Replacement

WBCT can not only be used to assess hindfoot and ankle alignment and pathology in the setting of ankle arthritis, but it can couple with other developing technology to assist in the surgical planning and performance of total ankle replacement (**Figs. 17–21**). Now that WBCT can be performed up to the level of the knee or higher, it can be used to identify the anatomic and mechanical axis of the tibia, among other parameters, that can allow the surgeon to place an implant with accurate alignment.

CLINICS CARE POINTS

- Technology of WBCT allows for 3D imaging with weightbearing with low radiation dose
- Evidence of WBCT is high for accuracy and lower for clinical benefit
- Assessment of ankle OA in WBCT provides important information about degree of OA and alignment

DISCLOSURE

M. Richter is a consultant of Curvebeam, Ossio, Geistlich and Intercus, and proprietor of R-Innovation. F. Lintz is consultant of Curvebeam, Follow and Newclip Technics and proprietor of L-Innov. C. de Cesar Netto is a consultant for Curvebeam, Ossio and Paragon 28. A. Barg is a consultant of Medartis, A. Burssens is a consultant of Curvebeam. S. Ellis is a consultant for Paragon 28 and Wright Medical, and currently serves as the President of the AOFAS Foundation. All authors are board member of the International WBCT Society. The International WBCT Society is financially supported by Curvebeam, Carestream, Paragon 28 and Footinnovate.

REFERENCES

1. Richter M, Seidl B, Zech S, et al. PedCAT for 3D-Imaging in Standing Position Allows for More Accurate Bone Position (Angle) Measurement than Radiographs or CT. Foot Ankle Surg 2014;20:201–7.
2. Richter MZS, Hahn S. PedCAT for Radiographic 3D-Imaging in Standing Position. Fuss Sprungg 2015;13:85–102.
3. Richter M, Lintz F, Cesar de Netto C, et al. Weight bering cone beam computed tomography (WBCT) in the foot and ankle. A scientific, technical and clinical guide. Cham (Switzerland): Springer Nature Switzerland AG; 2020.
4. Ferri M, Scharfenberger AV, Goplen G, et al. Weightbearing CT scan of severe flexible pes planus deformities. Foot Ankle Int 2008;29(2):199–204.
5. Johnson JE, Lamdan R, Granberry WF, et al. Hindfoot coronal alignment: a modified radiographic method. Foot Ankle Int 1999;20(12):818–25.
6. Richter M. Computer aided surgery in foot and ankle: applications and perspectives. Int Orthop 2013;37(9):1737–45.
7. Richter M. Computer Based Systems in Foot and Ankle Surgery at the Beginning of the 21st Century. Fuss Sprungg 2006;4(1):59–71.
8. Kido M, Ikoma K, Imai K, et al. Load response of the tarsal bones in patients with flatfoot deformity: in vivo 3D study. Foot Ankle Int 2011;32(11):1017–22.

9. Richter M, Geerling J, Zech S, et al. Intraoperative three-dimensional imaging with a motorized mobile C-arm (SIREMOBIL ISO-C-3D) in foot and ankle trauma care: a preliminary report. J Orthop Trauma 2005;19(4):259–66.

10. Richter M, Lintz F, Zech S, et al. Combination of PedCAT Weightbearing CT With Pedography Assessment of the Relationship Between Anatomy-Based Foot Center and Force/Pressure-Based Center of Gravity. Foot Ankle Int 2018;39(3):361–8.

11. Richter M, Zech S, Hahn S, et al. Combination of pedCAT for 3D imaging in standing position with pedography shows no statistical correlation of bone position with force/pressure distribution. J Foot Ankle Surg 2016;55(2):240–6.

12. Colin F, Horn Lang T, Zwicky L, et al. Subtalar joint configuration on weightbearing CT scan. Foot Ankle Int 2014;35(10):1057–62.

13. Lepojarvi S, Niinimaki J, Pakarinen H, et al. Rotational Dynamics of the Normal Distal Tibiofibular Joint With Weight-Bearing Computed Tomography. Foot Ankle Int 2016;37(6):627–35.

14. Hagemeijer NC, Chang SH, Abdelaziz ME, et al. Range of Normal and Abnormal Syndesmotic Measurements Using Weightbearing CT. Foot Ankle Int 2019; 40(12):1430–7.

15. Malhotra K, Welck M, Cullen N, et al. The effects of weight bearing on the distal tibiofibular syndesmosis: A study comparing weight bearing-CT with conventional CT. Foot Ankle Surg 2019;25(4):511–6.

16. Krähenbühl N, Akkaya M, Dodd AE, et al. Impact of the rotational position of the hindfoot on measurements assessing the integrity of the distal tibio-fibular syndesmosis. Foot Ankle Surg 2020;26(7):810–7.

17. Lintz F, Bernasconi A, Baschet L, et al. Relationship Between Chronic Lateral Ankle Instability and Hindfoot Varus Using Weight-Bearing Cone Beam Computed Tomography. Foot Ankle Int 2019;40(10):1175–81.

18. Lintz F, Mast J, Bernasconi A, et al. 3D, Weightbearing Topographical Study of Periprosthetic Cysts and Alignment in Total Ankle Replacement. Foot Ankle Int 2020;41(1):1–9.

19. Barg A, Bailey T, Richter M, et al. Weightbearing Computed Tomography of the Foot and Ankle: Emerging Technology Topical Review. Foot Ankle Int 2018; 39(3):376–86.

20. Lintz F, Jepsen M, De Cesar Netto C, et al. Distance mapping of the foot and ankle joints using weightbearing CT: The cavovarus configuration. Foot Ankle Surg 2020;27(4):412–20.

21. Siegler S, Konow T, Belvedere C, et al. Analysis of surface-to-surface distance mapping during three-dimensional motion at the ankle and subtalar joints. J Biomech 2018;76:204–11.

22. Burssens A, Peeters J, Buedts K, et al. Measuring hindfoot alignment in weight bearing CT: A novel clinical relevant measurement method. Foot Ankle Surg 2016;22(4):233–8.

23. Burssens A, Peeters J, Peiffer M, et al. Reliability and correlation analysis of computed methods to convert conventional 2D radiological hindfoot measurements to a 3D setting using weightbearing CT. Int J Comput Assist Radiol Surg 2018;13(12):1999–2008.

24. Burssens A, Van Herzele E, Leenders T, et al. Weightbearing CT in normal hindfoot alignment - Presence of a constitutional valgus? Foot Ankle Surg 2018;24(3): 213–8.

25. Burssens A, Vermue H, Barg A, et al. Templating of syndesmotic ankle lesions by use of 3D analysis in weightbearing and nonweightbearing CT. Foot Ankle Int 2018;39(12):1487–96.

26. Lintz F, Barton T, Millet M, et al. Ground reaction force calcaneal offset: a new measurement of hindfoot alignment. Foot Ankle Surg 2012;18(1):9–14.

27. Lintz F, Welck M, Bernasconi A, et al. 3D biometrics for hindfoot alignment using weightbearing CT. Foot Ankle Int 2017;38(6):684–9.

28. Zhang JZ, Lintz F, Bernasconi A, et al. 3D Biometrics for Hindfoot Alignment Using Weightbearing Computed Tomography. Foot Ankle Int 2019;684–9.

29. de Cesar Netto C, Bang K, Mansur NS, et al. Multiplanar semiautomatic assessment of foot and ankle offset in adult acquired flatfoot deformity. Foot Ankle Int 2020;41(7):839–48.

30. de Cesar Netto C, Kunas GC, Soukup D, et al. Correlation of clinical evaluation and radiographic hindfoot alignment in Stage II adult-acquired flatfoot deformity. Foot Ankle Int 2018;39(7):771–9.

31. Bluman EM, Title CI, Myerson MS. Posterior tibial tendon rupture: a refined classification system. Foot Ankle Clin 2007;12(2):233–49, v.

32. de Cesar Netto C, Godoy-Santos AL, Saito GH, et al. Subluxation of the middle facet of the subtalar joint as a marker of peritalar subluxation in adult acquired flatfoot deformity: a case-control study. J Bone Joint Surg Am 2019;101(20): 1838–44.

33. de Cesar Netto C, Bernasconi A, Roberts L, et al. Foot alignment in symptomatic national basketball association players using weightbearing cone beam computed tomography. Orthopaedic J Sports Med 2019;7(2). https://doi.org/10.1177/2325967119826081.

34. Saltzman CL, Hagy ML, Zimmerman B, et al. How effective is intensive nonoperative initial treatment of patients with diabetes and Charcot arthropathy of the feet? Clin Orthop Relat Res 2005;435:185–90.

35. Valderrabano V, Leumann A, Rasch H, et al. Knee-to-ankle mosaicplasty for the treatment of osteochondral lesions of the ankle joint. Am J Sports Med 2009; 37(Suppl 1):105S–11S.

36. Hintermann B, Nigg BM. Influence of arthrodeses on kinematics of the axially loaded ankle complex during dorsiflexion/plantarflexion. Foot Ankle Int 1995; 16(10):633–6.

37. Knupp M, Schuh R, Stufkens SA, et al. Subtalar and talonavicular arthrodesis through a single medial approach for the correction of severe planovalgus deformity. J Bone Joint Surg Br 2009;91(5):612–5.

38. Hayashi K, Tanaka Y, Kumai T, et al. Correlation of compensatory alignment of the subtalar joint to the progression of primary osteoarthritis of the ankle. Foot Ankle Int 2008;29(4):400–6.

39. Steel MW 3rd, Johnson KA, DeWitz MA, et al. Radiographic measurements of the normal adult foot. Foot Ankle 1980;1(3):151–8.

40. Carrara C, Belvedere C, Caravaggi P, et al. Techniques for 3D foot bone orientation angles in weight-bearing from cone-beam computed tomography. Foot Ankle Surg 2020;27(2):168–74.

41. Lintz F, de Cesar Netto C, Burssens A, et al. The value of axial loading three dimensional (3D) CT as a substitute for full weightbearing (standing) 3D CT: Comparison of reproducibility according to degree of load. Foot Ankle Surg 2018; 24(6):553–4.

42. Kim JB, Yi Y, Kim JY, et al. Weight-bearing computed tomography findings in varus ankle osteoarthritis: abnormal internal rotation of the talus in the axial plane. Skeletal Radiol 2017;46(8):1071–80.

43. Krahenbuhl N, Siegler L, Deforth M, et al. Subtalar joint alignment in ankle osteoarthritis. Foot Ankle Surg 2019;25(2):143–9.

44. Lintz F, Welck M, Bernasconi A, et al. 3D Biometrics for Hindfoot Alignment Using Weightbearing CT. Foot Ankle Int 2017;38(6):684–9.
45. Cody EA, Williamson ER, Burket JC, et al. Correlation of Talar Anatomy and Subtalar Joint Alignment on Weightbearing Computed Tomography With Radiographic Flatfoot Parameters. Foot Ankle Int 2016;37(8):874–81.
46. Kvarda P, Heisler L, Krähenbühl N, et al. 3D Assessment in Posttraumatic Ankle Osteoarthritis. Foot Ankle Int 2020;42(2):200–14.
47. Pagenstert GI, Hintermann B, Barg A, et al. Realignment surgery as alternative treatment of varus and valgus ankle osteoarthritis. Clin orthopaedics Relat Res 2007;462:156–68.
48. Krähenbühl N, Horn-Lang T, Hintermann B, et al. The subtalar joint: A complex mechanism. EFORT Open'C Rev 2017;2(7):309–16.
49. Tanaka T, Takeda H, Izumi T, et al. Age-related changes in postural control associated with location of the center of gravity and foot pressure. Phys Occup Ther Geriatr 1997;15(2):1–14.
50. Lee DC, de Cesar Netto C, Staggers JR, et al. Clinical and radiographic outcomes of the Kramer osteotomy in the treatment of bunionette deformity. Foot Ankle Surg 2018;24(6):530–4.
51. Wagner P, Colin F, Hintermann B. Distal Tibia Dome Osteotomy. Techn Foot Ankle Surg 2014;13(2):103–7.
52. Wagner UA, Sangeorzan BJ, Harrington RM, et al. Contact characteristics of the subtalar joint: load distribution between the anterior and posterior facets. J Orthop Res 1992;10(4):535–43.
53. Krähenbühl N, Lenz AL, Lisonbee RJ, et al. Morphologic analysis of the subtalar joint using statistical shape modeling. J Orthop Res 2020;38(12):2625–33.
54. Del Rio A, Bewsher SM, Roshan-Zamir S, et al. Weightbearing Cone-Beam Computed Tomography of Acute Ankle Syndesmosis Injuries. J Foot Ankle Surg 2020;59(2):258–63.
55. Bhimani R, Ashkani-Esfahani S, Lubberts B, et al. Utility of Volumetric Measurement via Weight-Bearing Computed Tomography Scan to Diagnose Syndesmotic Instability. Foot Ankle Int 2020;41(7):859–65.
56. Kim Y, Kim JS, Young KW, et al. A new measure of tibial sesamoid position in hallux valgus in relation to the coronal rotation of the first metatarsal in CT Scans. Foot Ankle Int 2015;36(8):944–52.
57. Collan L, Kankare JA, Mattila K. The biomechanics of the first metatarsal bone in hallux valgus: a preliminary study utilizing a weight bearing extremity CT. Foot Ankle Surg 2013;19(3):155–61.
58. Mahmoud K, Metikala S, Mehta SD, et al. The role of weightbearing computed tomography scan in hallux valgus. Foot Ankle Int 2020;42(3):287–93.
59. Kimura T, Kubota M, Suzuki N, et al. Weightbearing computed tomography and 3-Dimensional analysis of mobility changes of the first ray after proximal oblique osteotomy for hallux valgus. Foot Ankle Int 2020;42(3):333–9.
60. Richter M, Zech S, Hahn S. PedCAT for radiographic 3D-imaging in standing position. Fuss Sprungg 2015;13(2):85–102.
61. Hirschmann A, Pfirrmann CW, Klammer G, et al. Upright cone CT of the hindfoot: comparison of the non-weight-bearing with the upright weight-bearing position. Eur Radiol 2014;24(3):553–8.
62. Krahenbuhl N, Tschuck M, Bolliger L, et al. Orientation of the subtalar joint: measurement and reliability using weightbearing CT scans. Foot Ankle Int 2016;37(1):109–14.

Joint Preservation Strategies for Managing Varus Ankle Deformities

Beat Hintermann, MD*, Roxa Ruiz, MD

KEYWORDS

• Varus ankle • Deformity • Ankle osteoarthritis • Joint preserving strategies

KEY POINTS

- A meticulous analysis of the varus deformity and thorough understanding of underlying causes is mandatory for success in joint preserving surgery
- A supramalleolar osteotomy (SMOT) cannot restore parallel joint lines between the tibial plafond and talar dome in ankles in most asymmetric varus osteoarthritic (OA) ankles
- Additional measures such as calcaneal osteotomies and dorsiflexion osteotomies of first ray and soft tissue procedures are necessary in most cases
- A better understanding of the 3-dimensional structural changes in the ankle mortise and the talus may be essential for further improvement of joint-preserving surgery

INTRODUCTION

Because of its posttraumatic origin, ankle osteoarthritis (OA) generally affects younger patients.[1,2] Ankle arthrodesis may relieve pain and thus be beneficial in the short-term; however, the outcome at midterm to long-term is often dissatisfying.[3,4] Though ankle replacement has become a viable alternative in the last years, the long-term outcome is still uncertain.[5–7] Therefore, reconstructive surgery including osteotomies and soft tissue balancing procedures have gained interest for the treatment of asymmetric ankle OA.[8–22] This is particularly true for varus ankle OA in younger patients, where long-standing untreated lateral ligament instability may result in unbalanced loading of the medial joint space, painful asymmetric ankle OA, and varus deformity of the foot and ankle.[12,23]

The focal static and a dynamic overload within the ankle joint leads to a medialization of the center of force.[18,24,25] Furthermore, the force within the joint is amplified by the activation of the triceps surae, which becomes an invertor and applies an

Center of Excellence for Foot and Ankle Surgery, Clinic of Orthopaedics and Traumatology, Kantonsspital Baselland, Rheinstrasse 26, Liestal CH-4410, Switzerland
* Corresponding author.
E-mail address: beat.hintermann@ksbl.ch

Foot Ankle Clin N Am 27 (2022) 37–56
https://doi.org/10.1016/j.fcl.2021.11.002
1083-7515/22/© 2021 Elsevier Inc. All rights reserved.

additional deforming force on the hindfoot.[11] A further additional deforming force may be created by the posterior tibial (PT) muscle when it exceeds the eversion force of the peroneus brevis (PB) muscle.[26] The goal of surgical measures is to balance the ankle to normalize the joint load, thus preserving the ankle joint from further deterioration.[11,21]

The goal of this article is to provide basic information on varus ankle deformities, to understand their pathology, and elaborate a rationale for joint preserving strategies to successfully treat this deformity and to postpone OA of the ankle joint.

BACKGROUND

Ankles with pathologic varus deformities suffer from medial joint overload with associated subsequent medial tibiotalar joint degeneration. This in turn causes further medial load shift resulting in a vicious cycle of ever-increasing mechanical malalignment.[25] The ability of the foot and ankle to tolerate created varus malalignment depends, to a significant extent, on the flexibility of the foot to secondarily accommodate and compensate for this deformity. With a proximal varus deformity, the subtalar joint must evert to maintain a plantigrade foot.[27] Most recently, in a cadaveric study on 8 ankles, Zhu and colleagues[28] found a lateral shift of the center of force and lateral stress concentration for mild tibial varus. However, as the tibial varus continued to progress, the center of force shifted medially, and the lateral stress concentration decreased. This phenomenon might be explained by the valgus inclination of the subtalar joint in compensation for the varus tibial malalignment. However, regardless of the ability of the subtalar joint to compensate for the deformity, the mechanics of the ankle joint remain abnormal and, ultimately, irreversible articular damage occurs.

MORPHOLOGY AND CLASSIFICATION OF VARUS DEFORMITY OF THE ANKLE

To assess the varus deformity of the ankle, the angle of distal tibial articular surface[29] (TAS; α, normal value 91°–93°) and the tibiotalar angle 22 (TT; β, normal value 91.5° ± 1.2°) are used (**Fig. 1**). The degree of the talar tilt (TT) in the ankle mortise can then be calculated as the difference between TAS and TT. When, according to earlier findings, the cut-off for clinically relevant ankle tilting is set at 4°,[30] 2 types of ankle joints can be differentiated: the congruent joint (tilt ≤4°) and the incongruent joint (tilt >4°) (**Fig. 2**).

According to Takakura and colleagues 1995,[21] varus-type OA of the ankle is classified into the following 4 stages: (1) no narrowing of the joint space, but early sclerosis and formation of osteophytes; (2) narrowing of the medial joint space; (3) obliteration of this space with subchondral bone contact; and (4) obliteration of the whole joint space with complete bone contact. An additional type of varus ankle where the obliteration of the joint space is localized only in the medial gutter, whereas the tibiotalar joint space is preserved and classified by the authors as stage 3a.[21]

PRINCIPLES OF JOINT PRESERVING SURGERY

The specific aim of joint preserving surgery is to redistribute the mechanical axis to change the intraarticular load distribution, for example, in the varus malaligned ankle to move the center of load from medial to lateral.[9,11,13–15,17–20,31–37] In general, the joint preserving surgeries address the hindfoot deformity above the level of the ankle joint using supramalleolar osteotomies (SMOT) and soft tissue procedures[11,13,14,16,17,19,20,31–33,36–38] or below

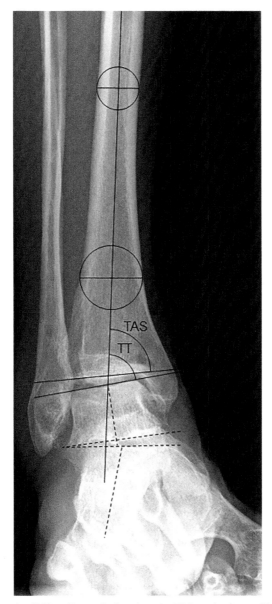

Fig. 1. Anteroposterior (AP) radiograph showing the TAS angle, formed between the longitudinal axis of the tibia and the distal articular surface of the tibia, and the talar tilt (TT) angle also measured with reference to the longitudinal axis of the tibia. The degree of the TT in the ankle mortise is calculated as the difference between TAS and TT. The compensatory valgus tilt of the subtalar joint can also be calculated with the help of measuring the calcaneal axis.

the ankle joint using calcaneal osteotomies and osteotomies of the first metatarsal or medial cuneiform.[26,39–42]

As a rule, the surgical procedure starts with supramalleolar correction, followed by soft tissue procedures. Once the ankle joint complex is balanced, a calcaneal

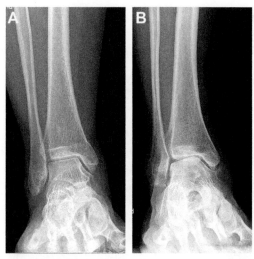

Fig. 2. Weight-bearing AP radiographs showing (*A*) a congruent varus deformity (Takakura. stage 0) and (*B*) an incongruent varus deformity (Takakura stage 2).

osteotomy may be considered in the case of a remaining heel malposition. Thereafter, remaining forefoot deformities are addressed, in particular correction of a plantar-flexed first ray.

SUPRAMALLEOLAR CORRECTING OSTEOTOMIES

Realignment surgeries include correcting osteotomies above the ankle (eg, SMOT), below the ankle (eg, inframalleolar osteotomies), and at the ankle (eg, intraarticular osteotomies).

As a principle, the correcting osteotomy is planned at the center of rotation of angulation (CORA). The closer the CORA is to the ankle joint, the greater is the effect on the ankle joint (greater lateral distal tibial angle).[20,43] Whereas, the closer the CORA is to the knee, the greater is the effect on the knee joint (greater medial proximal tibial angle). Congenital deformities usually have a CORA at the level of the plafond, developmental deformities a CORA just proximal to the distal tibial physis, and postfracture deformities a CORA at various levels, depending on the level of the original fracture and the magnitude and direction of associated translational deformities.

For the correction of a varus deformity, either a medial opening wedge osteotomy (**Fig. 3**A) or a lateral closing wedge osteotomy (**Fig. 3**B) can be used. Most authors prefer an open wedge osteotomy, as it allows the surgeon not only to perform gradual correction using distraction, until the desired degree of correction is obtained,[11,15,17,20,22,32,36–38,44–46] but also simultaneous correction in the sagittal plane, if necessary, by applying the distraction force anteromedially to move the anatomic axis of the tibia closer to the center of rotation of the talus. This correction may be necessary for patients in whom the talus is translated anteriorly.[47] Others prefer a lateral closing wedge osteotomy especially in patients with compromised medial soft tissues and in patients who have a congruent deformity (ie, Takakura stage 0 and 1) with substantial supramalleolar deformity, such as a malunion of a distal tibial fracture.[10,11] It has been suggested that lateral closing wedge osteotomies are technically easier.[36] Advantages of a lateral closing wedge osteotomy include stability, the lack of

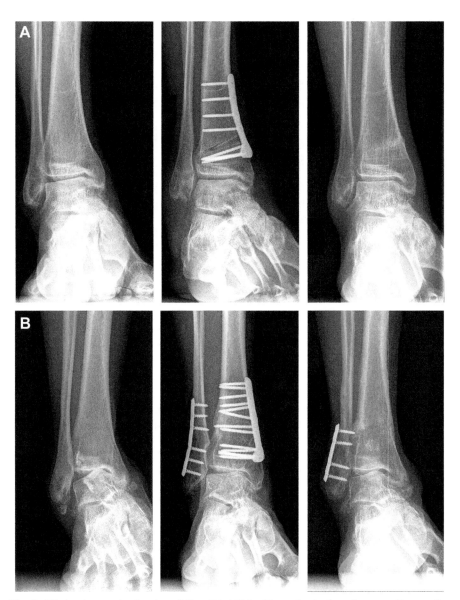

Fig. 3. Wedge-type osteotomies of the distal tibia. The extent of wedge resection or the quantity of bone graft needed to achieve the desired degree of correction can be calculated with equation $H = \tan \alpha 1 * W$, where H equals the height of the wedge to be resected or grafted, $\alpha 1$ is the magnitude of deformity plus the degrees of overcorrection, and W equals the width of the tibia at the level of the osteotomy.[8] (*A*) Open-wedge osteotomy of the distal tibia. A 51-year-old male patient with stage 3a OA. AP radiographs showing (a) pre-operative obliteration of the joint space only at the tip of the medial malleolus; (b) 8 weeks after surgery, a substantial improvement; and (c) 10 years after operation, an excellent clinical result with no pain. (*B*) Lateral closing wedge osteotomy. A 46-year-old male patient with stage 3b osteoarthritis. AP radiographs showing (a) preoperative obliteration of the

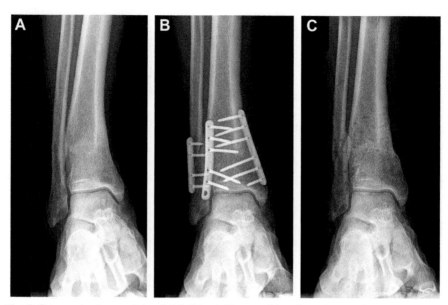

Fig. 4. Dome osteotomy of the distal tibia. A 63-year-old male patient with stage 2 OA. AP radiographs showing (*A*) preoperative narrowing of the joint space only in the medial gutter; (*B*) 8 weeks after surgery, a congruent joint; and (*C*) 5 years after surgery, an excellent clinical result with the patient sensing no pain.

a need for allograft, and the ability to perform a simultaneous fibular osteotomy through the same incision. Disadvantages include the inability to gradually determine the degree of correction and the need for a biplanar cut in patients with a coexisting sagittal plane deformity. Because the medial cortex of the distal tibia is weak and substantial soft-tissue contractures may be present, supplemental medial plate fixation may be necessary to avoid loss of correction. In addition, it has been suggested that a closing wedge osteotomy results in leg shortening and lateral compartment muscle weakening.[21] However, no differences regarding clinical outcome, radiographic outcome, or healing time of the osteotomy were reported in idiopathic ankle OA.[20,48]

In a patient with a varus deformity with a TAS angle of more than 6° to 8°, an opening wedge osteotomy would need a wide bone graft, which would significantly stretch the medial soft tissues, including the PT tendon. Thus, the authors prefer a dome osteotomy through an anterior exposure of the distal tibia (**Fig. 4**).[11,49,50] In most instances, a fibular osteotomy is needed through a separate lateral approach to achieve the wanted correction.[11,49–51] Similarly to the wedge osteotomy, the height of the dome osteotomy is determined such as to get the center of the tibiotalar joint slightly lateral to the anatomic axis of the tibia.

---

joint space at the medial corner in the roof of the dome of the talus of medial joint space and (b) 3.5 years and (c) after 5 years after correcting osteotomy of fibula an improved joint space. Even though there remained a talar tilt angle on weight-bearing of 12°, the patient was extremely satisfied.

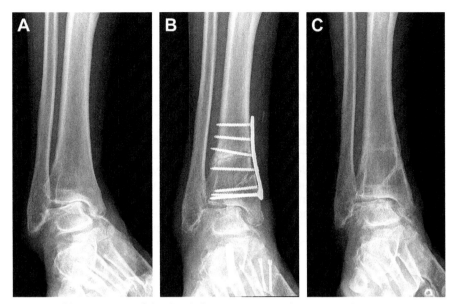

Fig. 5. Double osteotomy of the distal tibia. An intraarticular open-wedge osteotomy is performed to restore the distal articular surface, in addition to an open-wedge osteotomy to medialize the loading axis of the tibia. A 52-year-old male sports teacher with stage 3a OA. AP radiographs showing (*A*) preoperative obliteration of the joint space at the medial corner in the roof of the dome of the talus with impaction into the plafond and an angle of talar tilt on weight-bearing of 11°. (*B*) Four months after surgery, an improvement of talar tilt to 7° is seen, with remaining medial joint obliteration, and (*C*) 5 years postoperatively, no change can be seen. Despite this disappointing radiographical result, the patient was satisfied with the obtained result and was still able to perform his profession as a sports teacher.

If the TAS is impacted significantly, resulting in more than 5° of varus of the medial joint, an intraarticular osteotomy can be considered to restore congruency at the tibiotalar joint (**Fig. 5**).[31,52,53]

In the presence of a recurvatum deformity at the distal tibia and/or anterior extrusion of the talus, an additional antecurvatum correction is done following the same principles.[11,14,47,54]

After the osteotomy is performed, the distal tibial bloc is tilted posterior so that the elongation of the anatomic axis of the tibia, on the sagittal plane, meets the center of rotation of talus.[47]

In the incongruent varus OA ankle, where the talus has tilted into varus (Takakura stage 2–4), talar reduction can be hindered by medial soft tissue contracture (eg, deltoid ligament or PT contracture) and through bone formation in the lateral compartment of the ankle.[55]

To compensate for cartilage loss at the medial tibiotalar joint, a medial opening wedge osteotomy is aimed to obtain a TAS angle of 2° to 4° valgus. Once the amount of angular correction is determined, the height of the CORA for the osteotomy is determined so that the anatomic tibial axis at the tibiotalar joint is in its center or slightly lateral.[31]

ADDITIONAL PROCEDURES

Once supramalleolar correction is done, the achieved alignment is carefully assessed by visually inspecting the position of the heel to the axis of the calf. Fluoroscopy is used to check the achieved tibiotalar alignment (TAS angle) in the frontal plane and the achieved talocalcaneal alignment (talocalcaneal angle) in the horizontal plane. Also, lateral stability of the tibiotalar joint is checked by applying an inversion force.

- In the case of subtalar contracture, subtalar fusion is done for talocalcaneal realignment.[41,49,56]
- In the case of medial soft tissue contracture, a release of the PT tendon is done to restore talocalcaneal alignment.[57,58] In most instances, a release of the superficial deltoid ligament is also necessary.[16,57]
- Obtained correction is checked by fluoroscopy. If there is still a varus tilt of the talus that increases when applying inversion stress force, a lateral ligament reconstruction is considered usually as a Broström type repair.[16] If the remaining ligament structures are incompetent, reconstruction with the use of a free tendon graft or internal brace may be considered.[59]
- In the case of an incompetent PB tendon, a peroneus longus (PL) to PB tendon transfer is considered.[60,61] The base of the fifth metatarsal and the PL tendon are exposed. After dissection, the PL tendon is attached by a transosseous suture to the fifth metatarsal while the foot is held in dorsiflexion and eversion to get maximal tension to the transferred tendon.
- In the case of incompetent peroneal tendons (both) or nerve palsy, a transfer of the anterior tibial tendon[57,62] or PT tendon can be considered.[58,63]
- If thereafter, the heel is still in a varus position, a Z-osteotomy of the calcaneus is performed to tilt the heel into valgus and to slide it laterally (**Fig. 6**).[64] Alternatively, a lateral sliding osteotomy with or without a closing wedge[65] can be performed; however, the potential correcting effect is lower.
- If the forefoot evidences a pronation deformity due to a plantarflexed first ray, a dorsiflexion osteotomy is performed at the level of the first cuneiform or base of the first metatarsal (see **Fig. 6**).[57]

POTENTIAL COMPLICATIONS

All these techniques are often not sufficient to correct the talar position to normal or to fully restore joint congruency.[13,14,31] The underlying cause may be that the medial articular surface of the ankle joint is worn out, resulting in progressive joint incongruity with loss of intrinsic stability. This allows the talus to remain in a varus position. Furthermore, the medial malleolus can erode and become inclined medially instead of vertically, which further adds to the likelihood of a recurrent deformity. However, though the talus remains in varus, functional outcome and pain relief often significantly improve.[8–11,13–15,17,19–21,25,35]

DISCUSSION

Surgical realignment procedures can successfully restore normal joint function or halt further disease progression in ankles with asymmetric varus ankle OA.[13–15,19–22,32] Though progress has been made on indications and possibilities of joint preserving surgical treatment of the ankle with varus deformity and ongoing OA, the mechanism and the effect of the various measures are still not fully understood, and there are still some controversies.

SMOT in the varus ankle is designed to shift the weight-bearing axis to the lateral side of the ankle joint and unload the medial side, and, with this, it is expected to correct the often-existing TT.[11,31,49] Though joint space could not be restored to normal, SMOT was found to be successful in most cases.[8–11,13–17,19–21,25,35] Lee and

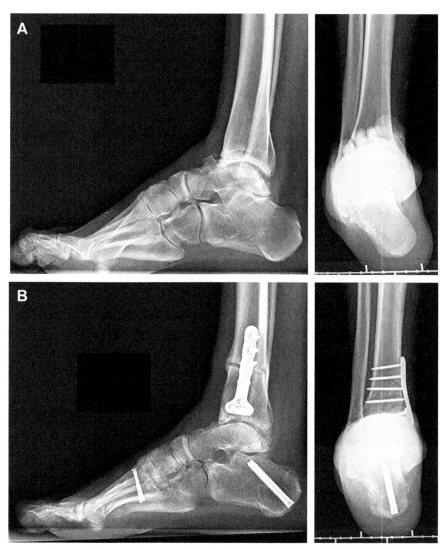

Fig. 6. Additional bony procedures Same patient as in **Fig. 5.** (*A*) Preoperatively, a severe. cavovarus deformity is seen with a heel varus and plantarflexed first ray. (a) lateral. view, (b) hindfoot alignment view. (*B*) Four months after surgery, the inframalleolar deformity has significantly been corrected after performing a z-osteotomy of the calcaneus with varus tilt and lateral slide, and a dorsiflexion osteotomy at the base of first metatarsal. (a) Lateral view, (b) hindfoot alignment view.

colleagues[35] reported that of 13 ankles with a preoperative Takakura stage 2 or 3A OA, only 4 improved to Takakura stage 1 after surgery. All 3 ankles with Takakura stage 3B, OA improved to stage 2 after surgery. In a series of 44 patients, Krähenbühl and colleagues[13] reported that ankles with a preoperative Takakura stage 2 or 3A showed a significantly higher survival rate at 5 years (88% [95% confidence interval (CI), 67–100] and 93% [95% CI, 80–100]) compared with ankles with a preoperative Takakura stage of 3B (47% [95% CI, 26–86], $P = .044$). In the same patient cohort, no higher failure rate was found in patients with Takakura stage 4.[66] Similar results were reported by Hongmou and colleagues[46] in a consecutive series of 41 patients of which a total of 22 cases (57%) achieved a lower Takakura stage, 13 (33%) had no change and 4 (10%) had an increased stage. The mean Takakura stage was significantly decreased (P = .008) postoperatively. These results were supported by others[8,9,11–15,17,19,35] who also reported that the preoperative OA stage did not correlate with the postoperative clinical findings. If an improvement to stage 1 is a requirement for a satisfactory result, as Tanaka and colleagues[22] had concluded, then SMOT should not have been considered effective. Therefore, the indication for SMOT cannot be dependent on the OA stage only, there must be other factors determining the outcome (**Fig. 7**).

One factor may be the TT angle. An excessive TT angle is often cited as one of the relative contraindications to SMOT. Some authors reported a significant decrease of the TT[9,31,32,54,66,67]; however, some did not.[19–21,35] Lee and colleagues[35] considered a TT angle exceeding 7.3° to be a negative factor, whereas Tanaka and colleagues[22] considered a TT angle exceeding 10° to be a negative factor for SMOT. A large TT angle implies disability of the lateral ligament complex or an erosion of the medial malleolar subchondral bone. However, no significant difference could be detected between the 5-year survival rate for patients with a preoperative tilt of the talus in the ankle mortise of 4° to 10° (85% [95% CI, 68–100]) and that for patients with a preoperative tilt of greater than 10° (65% [95% CI, 46–93], P = .117).[13] Obviously, preoperative TT angle should not be an over-estimated factor when SMOT is considered for the treatment of ankle OA.[38]

Overcorrection has been reported to lead to better results than undercorrection, particularly in advanced stages of OA.[55] The ideal amount of overcorrection is still a matter of debate. Tanaka and colleagues[22] aimed to achieve a TAS angle of 96° to 98° because overcorrection yielded better results in their patients. However, Lee and colleagues,[35] after having seen subsequent problems after performing major correction of up to 108°, such as subfibular pain, revised their strategy to an overcorrection of 3° to 5°, while adding a deltoid release and a calcaneal osteotomy instead. In general, there is agreement that the optimal correction with SMOT is a 2° to 4° slight overcorrection of the TAS angle or a correction in reference to the normal contralateral limb.[11,13,15,17,35,38,49] However, Harstall and colleagues[10] proposed a correction to neutral alignment of the tibial plafond only, to not decompensate the hindfoot into hypervalgus and to prevent creating a deformity that could compromise the results of a total ankle replacement, which might be necessary at a later time point.

With SMOT, the varus deformity can be effectively corrected proximal to the ankle joint, leading to restoration of the talar center on the axis of the tibia and dispersion of the stress on the ankle joint surface.[12,28,31,55,68] Traditional tibial correction based on the TAS angle leads to high variation in the locations of the postoperative mechanical ankle joint axis point.

Haragucchi and colleagues[55] found that if the crossing point of the tibial axis with articular surface of the tibial plafond was insufficiently moved to the lateral side, the clinical outcome was less satisfactory. They advocated that modification of the procedure to shift the mechanical axis more laterally is required for these ankles. This is supported by the findings of Hintermann and colleagues,[31] who reported better outcome after intraarticular plafond plasty combined with an additional medial open wedge osteotomy of the distal tibia to move the mechanical axis more lateral, than Mann and colleagues[53] had done with a singular intraarticular correction.

The necessity for adding a fibular osteotomy is still controversial. Some authors proposed to combine SMOT with a fibular osteotomy in all the cases,[10,20–22,35,55] some suggested the fibula should always be preserved,[32,44,53,67] and some decide to

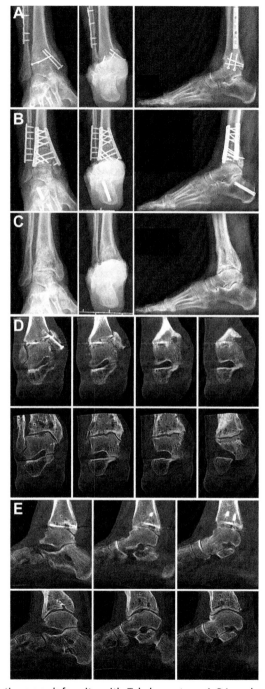

Fig. 7. Posttraumatic varus deformity with Takakura stage 4 OA and a nonunited medial malleolus. A 43-year-old trail runner who sustained a complex ankle fracture was advised by several doctors to go for an ankle fusion. (*A*) Two years and 3 months after internal fixation of the fracture, standard radiographs show a varus malunited ankle (TAS 12°) with

perform it depending on each case (**Fig. 8**).[9,11,12,19,46] As a rule, if the angle between the tibial axis and the line given by the tip of medial and lateral malleolus is more than 5° higher than the nonaffected site when compared (which indicates a longer fibula or varus shift, or the fibula has a rotational deformity, or interferes in the reduction of tibial plafond and talus), a fibular osteotomy is indicated through a lateral approach at the same level or higher than the tibial osteotomy.[46,50] When, after SMOT, a residual talar varus tilt is observed, a shortening and valgus osteotomy may be considered.[48] Stufkens and colleagues,[69] in a cadaveric study, found that creating a supramalleolar valgus deformity did not cause a shift in contact stress toward the lateral side of the tibiotalar joint, and the restricting role of the fibula was revealed by carrying out an osteotomy. Therefore, solely correcting the angle of the distal tibia on its own may not redistribute the intraarticular forces enough, an additional correction of the position and length of the fibula should be considered in every single case. In medial opening-wedge SMOT, a fibular osteotomy may be considered to minimize the increase of pressure in the talofibular joint, especially when the osteotomy gap is large.[70]

A high heel moment arm (HMA)[71] in varus ankle OA indicates a varus deformity of the distal tibia, a decrease in the height of the medial half of the talus, or abnormal alignment of the talus and calcaneus.[38] In rare cases, a high HMA is also associated with varus deformity of the calcaneus body, which sometimes requires a lateral sliding calcaneus osteotomy with[65] or without[15,64] a closing wedge. Although the HMA is usually seen to be significantly improved, it often does not reach the normal range (1.6–3.2 mm),[71] which may be related to the coexistence of hidden subtalar joint varus or the uncorrected varus deformity of the calcaneus body.[38] Several studies showed little change to the stress in the ankle joint stress alignment,[72,73] whereas in feet with a cavovarus deformity, a significant lateralization of the center of force, as well as a significant peak pressure reduction at the ankle joint, was found.[74,75] In analogous biomechanical studies, an SMOT provided equally good redistribution of elevated ankle joint contact forces[70,75]; the effect was higher in SMOT combined with a fibular osteotomy, however.[70]

When the talus is tilted into varus, the calcaneus may compensate in the opposite direction, resulting in a z-shaped deformity.[56,76] Such contradictory movement of the calcaneus may often result in a clinical appearance of a well-aligned hindfoot. As its height has decreased, the surrounding soft tissue structures do typically demonstrate additional loss of tension with clinical appearance of a "floppy hindfoot." A lateral sliding osteotomy will increase the varus tilt of the talus and the medial overload of the tibiotalar joint; therefore, a medial sliding osteotomy in association to soft tissue reconstruction or a subtalar fusion might be considered to reorientate the talus within the ankle mortise (**Fig. 9**).

The stability of the talus depends on the finely matched bone structure and the healthy soft tissue around the talus, including the lateral collateral ligaments, the ligaments between the talus and calcaneus, and the extrinsic tendons (ie, the created

complete obliteration of the tibiotalar joint space. (*B*) Postoperative situation after performing a dome osteotomy, fibular osteotomy, and medial sliding osteotomy of the calcaneus. (*C*) Nine years after correcting the osteotomy, the patient is still pain-free and very satisfied to be able to run. The radiographs show some incongruency and narrowing of the joint space, according to a Takakura OA stage 2. The recovery of the articular surfaces can be better seen in the weight-bearing CT scans: (*D*) coronal plane view; (*E*) sagittal plane view.

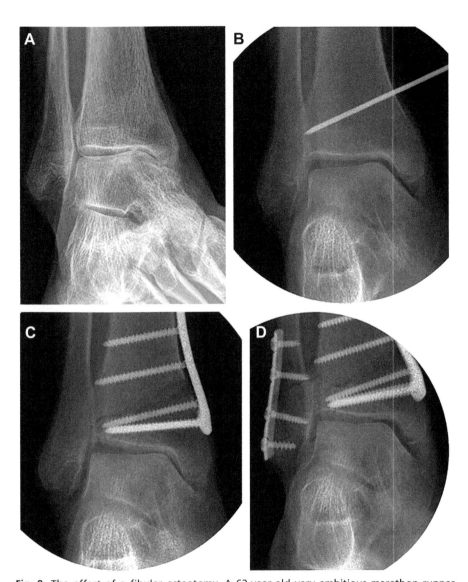

Fig. 8. The effect of a fibular osteotomy. A 62-year-old very ambitious marathon runner who is suffering from progressive medial ankle pain after having sustained several ankle sprains in the adolescence. (*A*) The AP radiograph shows a narrowing of the joint space at the medial corner in the roof of the dome of the talus and an obliteration only at the tip of medial malleolus preoperatively with an angle of talar tilt on weight-bearing of 6°. (*B*) Intraoperative fluoroscopy of the nonloaded ankle with a Kirschner wire placed where the medial open wedge osteotomy is planned. (*C*) After having performed the correcting osteotomy of the distal tibia, the talar tilt angle increased to 11° despite of a Broström type reconstruction of the lateral ankle ligaments. (*D*) A shortening osteotomy of the fibula with some valgus angulation was needed to achieve a congruent ankle joint.

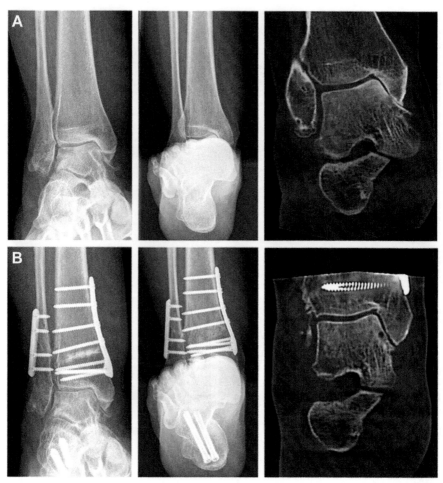

Fig. 9. Varus-valgus deformity in a 46-year-old female suffering from severe medial ankle pain. (*A*) The preoperative AP radiograph shows a narrowing of the joint space at the medial corner in the roof of the dome of the talus and an obliteration only at the tip of the medial malleolus with a talar tilt on weight-bearing of 7°. The hindfoot alignment view shows a valgus malalignment of the heel with a HMA of 6 mm. The obliteration of the medial gutter with subchondral sclerosis and beginning erosion can be best seen in the weight-bearing CT scan. (*B*) One year after performing a medial open wedge osteotomy of the distal tibia, correcting osteotomy of the fibula and a medial sliding osteotomy of the calcaneus, the joint incongruency persists with a talar tilt angle of 3°; the medial gutter is again open and subchondral sclerosis has significantly disappeared, which can be seen in the weight-bearing CT scan. Notice the big amount of medial translation of calcaneal tuberosity that was necessary to balance the ankle. Postoperatively, the medial ankle pain completely disappeared.

forces by their muscles) of the foot. Instability of the talus can be caused by abnormal bone structure, or dysfunction of related ligaments and tendons. In different stages, these abnormalities can exist alone or simultaneously and affect each other. Although lateral ligament reconstruction is considered in general as an important step of treatment for medial ankle OA,[2,16,45,53] some authors suggest that treatment of chronic lateral ankle instability is not important for the result of realignment surgery and believe that chronic instability disappears after shifting the weight-bearing load to the lateral aspect of the ankle.[21,22]

It has been suggested that besides insufficient lateral ankle ligaments, the altered morphologic characteristics of the bony, articular and periarticular anatomy, as well as muscular dynamics play an important role in the etiology of varus ankle deformity, especially of cavovarus deformity where the talus is typically seen to dislocate ante-rolaterally out of the ankle mortise.[26,41,61,77,78] Hyperactivation of PL and PT muscles may explain why cavovarus deformity often is accompanied by a plantarflexed first ray.[26,61,78] During the push-off phase of the gait cycle, the hindfoot is forced into su-pination creating varus malalignment. Plantarflexion of the first ray by the PL occurs in patients with spastic cerebral palsy.[79] Under such conditions, plantarflexion of the first ray in the sagittal plane is increased, provoking a supination force at the hindfoot in the push-off phase. As a result, the transmission of axial forces through the ankle joint is altered, and the Achilles tendon serves as an inverter of the hindfoot, enhancing the varus stress. Therefore, deforming forces should be transferred to obtain normal movement and function.[26,57,58,60–64,80] In addition, a correcting osteotomy to dorsiflex the first ray should be considered.[57,80] However, to date, little is known about the ef-fect of all these measures in joint preserving surgery of the OA varus ankle. Most re-ports have focused on how to balance the ankle in total ankle replacement surgery.[80–84]

SUMMARY

Careful clinical and radiographic assessment of the talar position in all 3 planes is mandatory for success in the treatment of asymmetric OA varus ankles. Because articular surfaces may be worn out, isolated ligament reconstruction on the lateral side of the ankle joint may not restore proper position of the talus within the ankle mortise. Osseous balancing with osteotomies above or below the ankle, or subtalar fusion, may thus be the main step for successful restoration of talar position within the ankle mortise. Overall, the key for the success of joint preserving surgery is to un-derstand the underlying causes that have contributed to the varus OA in each case, and to use all treatment modalities necessary to restore the appropriate alignment of the hindfoot complex. Although SMOT is suggested to have the main effect on restoring ankle joint function, additional procedures might be necessary for proper correction of varus deformity and thus to achieve long-term success. Overall, joint preserving surgery has evolved to a successful option in early and midstage medial ankle OA caused and slowing of the degenerative process.

CLINICS CARE POINTS

- A varus ankle deformity can be successfully addressed by osteotomies and soft tissues procedures.
- Osteotomies must aim to correct the deformity at its origin (supramalleolar, intramallelar and/or intraarticular).
- Additional soft tissue procedures might be necessary to stabilize the ankle and to eliminate the deforming forces.
- Though joint congruity cannot be fully restored in most cases, joint preserving prcedures were shown to significantly reduce pain and to delay the ongoing degenerative process.

- While the radiographic result may not meet the surgeon's expectation, the clinical result and patient's satisfaction is often higher.

DISCLOSURE

The authors have nothing to declare.

REFERENCES

1. Saltzman CL, Salamon ML, Blanchard GM, et al. Epidemiology of ankle arthritis: report of a consecutive series of 639 patients from a tertiary orthopaedic center. Iowa Orthop J 2005;25:44–6.
2. Valderrabano V, Hintermann B, Horisberger M, Fung TS. Ligamentous posttraumatic ankle osteoarthritis. Am J Sports Med 2006;34(4):612–20.
3. Fuentes-Sanz A, Moya-Angeler J, Lopez-Oliva F, Forriol F. Clinical outcome and gait analysis of ankle arthrodesis. Foot Ankle Int 2012;33(10):819–27.
4. Hendrickx RP, Stufkens SA, de Bruijn EE, Sierevelt IN, van Dijk CN, Kerkhoffs GM. Medium- to long-term outcome of ankle arthrodesis. Foot Ankle Int 2011;32(10): 940–7.
5. Jastifer JR, Coughlin MJ. Long-term follow-up of mobile bearing total ankle arthroplasty in the United States. Foot Ankle Int 2015;36(2):143–50.
6. Krishnapillai S, Joling B, Sierevelt IN, Kerkhoffs G, Haverkamp D, Hoornenborg D. Long-term Follow-up Results of Buechel-Pappas Ankle Arthroplasty. Foot Ankle Int 2019;40(5):553–61.
7. Mann JA, Mann RA, Horton E. STAR ankle: long-term results. Foot Ankle Int 2011; 32(5):S473–84.
8. Barg A, Pagenstert GI, Horisberger M, et al. Supramalleolar osteotomies for degenerative joint disease of the ankle joint: indication, technique and results. Int Orthop 2013;37(9):1683–95.
9. Colin F, Bolliger L, Horn Lang T, Knupp M, Hintermann B. Effect of supramalleolar osteotomy and total ankle replacement on talar position in the varus osteoarthritic ankle: a comparative study. Foot Ankle Int 2014;35(5):445–52.
10. Harstall R, Lehmann O, Krause F, Weber M. Supramalleolar lateral closing wedge osteotomy for the treatment of varus ankle arthrosis. Foot Ankle Int 2007;28(5): 542–8.
11. Hintermann B, Knupp M, Barg A. Supramalleolar Osteotomies for the Treatment of Ankle Arthritis. J Am Acad Orthop Surg 2016;24(7):424–32.
12. Knupp M, Stufkens SA, Bolliger L, Barg A, Hintermann B. Classification and treatment of supramalleolar deformities. Foot Ankle Int 2011;32(11):1023–31.
13. Krahenbuhl N, Akkaya M, Deforth M, Zwicky L, Barg A, Hintermann B. Extraarticular Supramalleolar Osteotomy in Asymmetric Varus Ankle Osteoarthritis. Foot Ankle Int 2019;40(8):936–47.
14. Knupp M, Hintermann B. Treatment of asymmetric arthritis of the ankle joint with supramalleolar osteotomies. Foot Ankle Int 2012;33(3):250–2.
15. Lee KB, Cho YJ. Oblique supramalleolar opening wedge osteotomy without fibular osteotomy for varus deformity of the ankle. Foot Ankle Int 2009;30(6): 565–7.
16. Lee HS, Wapner KL, Park SS, Kim JS, Lee DH, Sohn DW. Ligament reconstruction and calcaneal osteotomy for osteoarthritis of the ankle. Foot Ankle Int 2009;30(6): 475–80.

17. Lee WC. Extraarticular Supramalleolar Osteotomy for Managing Varus Ankle Osteoarthritis, Alternatives for Osteotomy: How and Why? Foot Ankle Clin 2016; 21(1):27–35.
18. Nuesch C, Huber C, Paul J, et al. Mid- to Long-term Clinical Outcome and Gait Biomechanics After Realignment Surgery in Asymmetric Ankle Osteoarthritis. Foot Ankle Int 2015;36(8):908–18.
19. Pagenstert GI, Hintermann B, Barg A, Leumann A, Valderrabano V. Realignment surgery as alternative treatment of varus and valgus ankle osteoarthritis. Clin Orthop Relat Res 2007;462:156–68.
20. Stamatis ED, Cooper PS, Myerson MS. Supramalleolar osteotomy for the treatment of distal tibial angular deformities and arthritis of the ankle joint. Foot Ankle Int 2003;24(10):754–64.
21. Takakura Y, Tanaka Y, Kumai T, Tamai S. Low tibial osteotomy for osteoarthritis of the ankle. Results of a new operation in 18 patients. J Bone Joint Surg Br 1995; 77(1):50–4.
22. Tanaka Y, Takakura Y, Hayashi K, Taniguchi A, Kumai T, Sugimoto K. Low tibial osteotomy for varus-type osteoarthritis of the ankle. J Bone Joint Surg Br 2006; 88(7):909–13.
23. Barg A, Pagenstert GI, Hugle T, et al. Ankle osteoarthritis: etiology, diagnostics, and classification. Foot Ankle Clin 2013;18(3):411–26.
24. Davitt JS, Beals TC, Bachus KN. The effects of medial and lateral displacement calcaneal osteotomies on ankle and subtalar joint pressure distribution. Foot Ankle Int 2001;22(11):885–9.
25. Knupp M, Stufkens SA, van Bergen CJ, et al. Effect of supramalleolar varus and valgus deformities on the tibiotalar joint: a cadaveric study. Foot Ankle Int 2011; 32(6):609–15.
26. Ortiz C, Wagner E. Tendon transfers in cavovarus foot. Foot Ankle Clin 2014; 19(1):49–58.
27. Wang BSCL, Chalayon O, Barg A. Does the Subtalar Joint Compensate for Ankle Malalignment in End-stage Ankle Arthritis? Clin Orthop Relat Res 2015;473(1): 318–25.
28. Zhu Y, Li X, Xu X. Ankle joint pressure change in varus malalignment of the tibia. BMC Musculoskelet Disord 2020;21(1):148.
29. Stiehl JB. Inman's joints of the ankle. Baltimore, Maryland: Williams & Wilkins; 1991.
30. Cox JS, Hewes TF. Normal" talar tilt angle. Clin Orthop Relat Res 1979;140:37–41.
31. Hintermann B, Ruiz R, Barg A. Novel Double Osteotomy Technique of Distal Tibia for Correction of Asymmetric Varus Osteoarthritic Ankle. Foot Ankle Int 2017; 38(9):970–81.
32. Kim YS, Park EH, Koh YG, Lee JW. Supramalleolar Osteotomy With Bone Marrow Stimulation for Varus Ankle Osteoarthritis: Clinical Results and Second-Look Arthroscopic Evaluation. Am J Sports Med 2014;42(7):1558–66.
33. Knupp MSSA, Pagenstert GI, Hintermann B, Valderrabano V. Supramalleolar Osteotomy for Tibiotalar Varus Malalignment. Tech Foot Ankle Surg 2009;8(1):17–23.
34. Kroon M, Faber FW, van der Linden M. Joint preservation surgery for correction of flexible pes cavovarus in adults. Foot Ankle Int 2010;31(1):24–9.
35. Lee WC, Moon JS, Lee K, Byun WJ, Lee SH. Indications for supramalleolar osteotomy in patients with ankle osteoarthritis and varus deformity. J Bone Joint Surg Am 2011;93(13):1243–8.
36. Myerson MS, Zide JR. Management of varus ankle osteoarthritis with joint- preserving osteotomy. Foot Ankle Clin 2013;18(3):471–80.

37. Takakura Y, Takaoka T, Tanaka Y, Yajima H, Tamai S. Results of opening-wedge osteotomy for the treatment of a post-traumatic varus deformity of the ankle. J Bone Joint Surg Am 1998;80(2):213–8.

38. Qu W, Xin D, Dong S, Li W, Zheng Y. Supramalleolar osteotomy combined with lateral ligament reconstruction and talofibular immobilization for varus ankle osteoarthritis with excessive talar tilt angle. J Orthop Surg Res 2019;14(1):402.

39. Kraus JC, Fischer MT, McCormick JJ, Klein SE, Johnson JE. Geometry of the lateral sliding, closing wedge calcaneal osteotomy: review of the two methods and technical tip to minimize shortening. Foot Ankle Int 2014;35(3):238–42.

40. Maskill MP, Maskill JD, Pomeroy GC. Surgical management and treatment algorithm for the subtle cavovarus foot. Foot Ankle Int 2010;31(12):1057–63.

41. Ortiz C, Wagner E, Keller A. Cavovarus foot reconstruction. Foot Ankle Clin 2009; 14(3):471–87.

42. Tennant JN, Carmont M, Phisitkul P. Calcaneus osteotomy. Curr Rev Musculoskelet Med 2014;7(4):271–6.

43. Horn DM, Fragomen AT, Rozbruch SR. Supramalleolar osteotomy using circular external fixation with six-axis deformity correction of the distal tibia. Foot Ankle Int 2011;32(10):986–93.

44. Ahn TK, Yi Y, Cho JH, Lee WC. A cohort study of patients undergoing distal tibial osteotomy without fibular osteotomy for medial ankle arthritis with mortise widening. J Bone Joint Surg Am 2015;97(5):381–8.

45. DeCarbo WT, Granata AM, Berlet GC, Hyer CF, Philbin TM. Salvage of severe ankle varus deformity with soft tissue and bone rebalancing. Foot Ankle Spec 2011;4(2):82–5.

46. Hongmou Z, Xiaojun L, Yi L, Hongliang L, Junhu W, Cheng L. Supramalleolar Osteotomy With or Without Fibular Osteotomy for Varus Ankle Arthritis. Foot Ankle Int 2016;37(9):1001–7.

47. Scheidegger P, Horn Lang T, Schweizer C, Zwicky L, Hintermann B. A flexion osteotomy for correction of a distal tibial recurvatum deformity: a retrospective case series. Bone Joint J 2019;101-B(6):682–90.

48. Krause F, Veljkovic A, Schmid T. Supramalleolar Osteotomies for Posttraumatic Malalignment of the Distal Tibia. Foot Ankle Clin 2016;21(1):1–14.

49. Knupp M. The Use of Osteotomies in the Treatment of Asymmetric Ankle Joint Arthritis. Foot Ankle Int 2017;38(2):220–9.

50. Wagner PCF, Hintermann B. Distal Tibia Dome Osteotomy. Tech Foot Ankle Surg 2014;13(2):103–7.

51. Siddiqui NA, Herzenberg JE, Lamm BM. Supramalleolar osteotomy for realignment of the ankle joint. Clin Podiatr Med Surg 2012;29(4):465–82.

52. Al-Nammari SS, Myerson MS. The Use of Tibial Osteotomy (Ankle Plafondplasty) for Joint Preservation of Ankle Deformity and Early Arthritis. Foot Ankle Clin 2016; 21(1):15–26.

53. Mann HA, Filippi J, Myerson MS. Intra-articular opening medial tibial wedge osteotomy (plafond-plasty) for the treatment of intra-articular varus ankle arthritis and instability. Foot Ankle Int 2012;33(4):255–61.

54. Cheng YM, Huang PJ, Hong SH, et al. Low tibial osteotomy for moderate ankle arthritis. Arch Orthop Trauma Surg 2001;121(6):355–8.

55. Haraguchi N, Ota K, Tsunoda N, Seike K, Kanetake Y, Tsutaya A. Weight-bearing-line analysis in supramalleolar osteotomy for varus-type osteoarthritis of the ankle. J Bone Joint Surg Am 2015;97(4):333–9.

56. Hintermann B, Knupp M, Barg A. Joint-preserving surgery of asymmetric ankle osteoarthritis with peritalar instability. Foot Ankle Clin 2013;18(3):503–16.

57. Chen ZY, Wu ZY, An YH, Dong LF, He J, Chen R. Soft tissue release combined with joint-sparing osteotomy for treatment of cavovarus foot deformity in older children: Analysis of 21 cases. World J Clin Cases 2019;7(20):3208–16.
58. Dreher T, Beckmann NA, Wenz W. Surgical Treatment of Severe Cavovarus Foot Deformity in Charcot-Marie-Tooth Disease. JBJS Essent Surg Tech 2015;5(2):e11.
59. Hintermann B, Ruiz R. Foot and ankle instability. Springer International Publishing; 2021.
60. Kilger RKM, Hintermann B. Peroneus Longus to Peroneus Brevis Tendon Transfer. Tech Foot Ankle Surg 2009;8(3):146–9.
61. Krause FG, Henning J, Pfander G, Weber M. Cavovarus foot realignment to treat anteromedial ankle arthrosis. Foot Ankle Int 2013;34(1):54–64.
62. Krause FG, Pohl MJ, Penner MJ, Younger AS. Tibial nerve palsy associated with lateralizing calcaneal osteotomy: case reviews and technical tip. Foot Ankle Int 2009;30(3):258–61.
63. Kagaya H, Yamada S, Nagasawa T, Ishihara Y, Kodama H, Endoh H. Split posterior tibial tendon transfer for varus deformity of hindfoot. Clin Orthop Relat Res 1996;(323):254–60.
64. Knupp MHM, Hintermann B. A New Z-Shaped Calcaneal Osteotomy for 3-Plane Correction of Severe Varus Deformity of the Hindfoot. Tech Foot Ankle Surg 2008; 7(2):90–5.
65. Dwyer FC. Osteotomy of the calcaneum for pes cavus. J Bone Joint Surg Br 1959;41-B(1):80–6.
66. Krahenbuhl N, Zwicky L, Bolliger L, Schadelin S, Hintermann B, Knupp M. Mid- to Long-term Results of Supramalleolar Osteotomy. Foot Ankle Int 2017;38(2): 124–32.
67. Kobayashi H, Kageyama Y, Shido Y. Treatment of Varus Ankle Osteoarthritis and Instability With a Novel Mortise-Plasty Osteotomy Procedure. J Foot Ankle Surg 2016;55(1):60–7.
68. Tanaka Y. The concept of ankle joint preserving surgery: why does supramalleolar osteotomy work and how to decide when to do an osteotomy or joint replacement. Foot Ankle Clin 2012;17(4):545–53.
69. Stufkens SA, van Bergen CJ, Blankevoort L, van Dijk CN, Hintermann B, Knupp M. The role of the fibula in varus and valgus deformity of the tibia: a biomechanical study. J Bone Joint Surg Br 2011;93(9):1232–9.
70. Choi GW, Lee SH, Nha KW, Lee SJ, Kim WH, Uhm CS. Effect of Combined Fibular Osteotomy on the Pressure of the Tibiotalar and Talofibular Joints in Supramalleolar Osteotomy of the Ankle: A Cadaveric Study. J Foot Ankle Surg 2017;56(1): 59–64.
71. Saltzman CL, el-Khoury GY. The hindfoot alignment view. Foot Ankle Int 1995; 16(9):572–6.
72. Michelson JD, Mizel M, Jay P, Schmidt G. Effect of medial displacement calcaneal osteotomy on ankle kinematics in a cadaver model. Foot Ankle Int 1998; 19(3):132–6.
73. Steffensmeier SJ, Saltzman CL, Berbaum KS, Brown TD. Effects of medial and lateral displacement calcaneal osteotomies on tibiotalar joint contact stresses. J Orthop Res 1996;14(6):980–5.
74. Krause FG, Sutter D, Waehnert D, Windolf M, Schwieger K, Weber M. Ankle joint pressure changes in a pes cavovarus model after lateralizing calcaneal osteotomies. Foot Ankle Int 2010;31(9):741–6.

75. Schmid T, Zurbriggen S, Zderic I, Gueorguiev B, Weber M, Krause FG. Ankle joint pressure changes in a pes cavovarus model: supramalleolar valgus osteotomy versus lateralizing calcaneal osteotomy. Foot Ankle Int 2013;34(9):1190–7.
76. Hintermann B, Knupp M, Barg A. Peritalar instability. Foot Ankle Int 2012;33(5): 450–4.
77. Vienne P, Schoniger R, Helmy N, Espinosa N. Hindfoot instability in cavovarus deformity: static and dynamic balancing. Foot Ankle Int 2007;28(1):96–102.
78. Younger AS, Hansen ST Jr. Adult cavovarus foot. J Am Acad Orthop Surg 2005; 13(5):302–15.
79. Aleksic M, Bascarevic Z, Stevanovic V, Rakocevic J, Baljozovic A, Cobeljic G. Modified split tendon transfer of posterior tibialis muscle in the treatment of spastic equinovarus foot deformity: long-term results and comparison with the standard procedure. Int Orthop 2020;44(1):155–60.
80. Hintermann B, Ruiz R. Total replacement of varus ankle: three-component prosthesis design. Foot Ankle Clin 2019;24(2):305–24.
81. Choi WJ, Kim BS, Lee JW. Preoperative planning and surgical technique: how do I balance my ankle? Foot Ankle Int 2012;33(3):244–9.
82. Daniels TR. Surgical technique for total ankle arthroplasty in ankles with preoperative coronal plane varus deformity of 10 degrees or greater. JBJS Essent Surg Tech 2014;3(4):e22.
83. Roukis TS. Tibialis posterior recession for balancing varus ankle contracture during total ankle replacement. J Foot Ankle Surg 2013;52(5):686–9.
84. Roukis TS, Elliott AD. Use of soft-tissue procedures for managing varus and valgus malalignment with total ankle replacement. Clin Podiatr Med Surg 2015; 32(4):517–28.

Joint Preserving Surgery for Valgus Ankle Osteoarthritis

Ahmad Alajlan, MD[a,b], Victor Valderrabano, MD, PhD[a,*]

KEYWORDS

- Joint-preserving surgery • Valgus ankle osteoarthritis
- Supramalleolar osteotomy of the tibia (SMOT)

KEY POINTS

- Valgus ankle osteoarthritis (OA) is a complex deformity with multiple etiologies.
- Joint-preserving surgery (JPS) of ankle OA avoids sacrificing reconstructions of the ankle joint.
- Medial closing-wedge supramalleolar osteotomy of the tibia (SMOT) is the primary procedure in JPS for valgus ankle OA.

INTRODUCTION

Valgus ankle osteoarthritis (OA) is a complex deformity with numerous etiologies that can be classified as posttraumatic, degenerative, congenital, and neurologic. Posttraumatic entities are considered the most common causes of ankle OA.[1] However, the degenerative factor via chronic posterior tibial tendon (PTT)/muscle dysfunction remains the most common cause of valgus ankle deformity.[2,3] Patients with valgus ankle OA typically present with different symptoms and signs depending on the causative factor, chronicity level, and the number of etiology entities existing in a particular case. These etiologies often begin with lateral ankle pain, calcaneofibular impingement, medial ankle pain with instability, restricted range of motion (ROM), and joint and limb dysfunction. The early identification of valgus ankle OA pathology provides surgeons with a window of opportunity to avoid joint-sacrificing surgeries (eg, total ankle arthroplasty and ankle arthrodesis) and allows them to use joint-preserving surgery (JPS) that equally distributes the load within the ankle joint, reduces pain, and restores function—especially in the younger population.

Valderrabano and colleagues defined JPS for their group by changing the load axis from the osteoarthritic side to the healthy side of the joint, thereby restoring the parallelism of the joint in the frontal plane and providing stability.[4] In JPS, it is very important to appropriately analyze the etiology and biomechanics of the case since neglecting or

[a] SWISS ORTHO CENTER, Schmerzklinik Basel, Swiss Medical Network, Hirschgässlein 15, Basel 4010, Switzerland; [b] Orthopaedic Department, Security Forces Hospital, Riyadh, Saudi Arabia
* Corresponding author.
E-mail address: vvalderrabano@swissmedical.net

Foot Ankle Clin N Am 27 (2022) 57–72
https://doi.org/10.1016/j.fcl.2021.11.003
1083-7515/22/© 2021 Elsevier Inc. All rights reserved.

not recognizing all pathobiomechanical issues might deteriorate the condition and lead to end-stage ankle OA in the long-term.[4,5]

ETIOLOGY OF VALGUS ANKLE OA

Valgus ankle OA can be classified based on the clinical etiology, level of deformity, severity, and tissue initiating the deformity (eg, bone, ligament, muscle, or combined).[2,3,6] Regarding the clinical etiology grouping, the most common cause of ankle OA is posttraumatic (80% of cases) and often due to lower leg fractures. Although grade IV PTT/muscle insufficiency is the most common cause of degenerative valgus ankle OA, primary ankle OA may also start with valgus ankle OA.[3,7] To simplify the etiology, we attempt to classify valgus ankle OA as posttraumatic, degenerative, congenital, or neurologic (**Box 1**). Furthermore, a classification of ankle OA based on the level of the deformity is also presented in **Box 1**.

Biomechanics of Valgus Ankle Osteoarthritis

A valgus ankle/hindfoot OA shows typically a valgus hindfoot, lateralized mechanical lower leg axis, reduced contact area in the joint with subsequent increased joint reaction forces, lateral joint overuse with increased peak forces, medial ligament ankle complex deficiency, and fibulotalar/calcaneal impingement.

Box 1
Etiologies of Valgus Ankle Osteoarthritis

Posttraumatic Etiologies
  Fibular malunion (shortening, external rotation)
  Valgus malunion of tibial shaft fractures
  Valgus malunion of tibial plafond fractures
  Valgus malunion of talus and calcaneus fractures
  Chronic medial ankle ligament insufficiency (after acute deltoid ligament injury or part of rotational chronic ankle instability (lateral and medial ankle instability))
  Chronic syndesmotic injury
  Avascular necrosis of talus

Degenerative Etiologies
  Posterior tibial tendon dysfunction (grade IV)
  Primary ankle osteoarthritis
  Rheumatoid osteoarthritis
  Charcot osteoarthropathy

Congenital Etiologies
  Tarsal coalition
  Excessive tibial external rotation
  Fibular hemimelia

Neurologic Etiologies
  Stroke
  Central and peripheral nerve disorders
  Hereditary motor sensory neuropathy
  Spina bifida
  Cerebral palsy

Deformity Levels of Valgus Ankle Osteoarthritis
  Supramalleolar deformity: mDTAA $\geq$ 92° and CORA supramalleolar
  Intraarticular deformity: mTTA $\geq$ 4° and CORA intraarticular
  Inframalleolar deformity: mDTAA and mTTA normal, but HAA greater than 10°

Altering the mechanical axis of the lower leg or hindfoot leads to an unequal distribution of load in the ankle joint (ie, an overload of the lateral compartment of the tibiotalar joint) and an overloading of the medial ankle ligaments with consecutive medial ligament complex deficiency, resulting in a vicious circle.[2] In a cadaver study by Knupp and colleagues, incongruent valgus ankle malalignment shifted the pressure to the posterolateral ankle compartment.[8,9] This aspect was also proven by a radiological study using single-photon emission computed tomography (SPECT-CT) in patients with valgus ankle OA. In the SPECT-CT images, the valgus malaligned ankles showed significantly greater uptake in the lateral areas than in the medial ankle regions.[10]

In the area of in vivo biomechanics, Nüesch and colleagues found the following kinematic and kinetic changes in patients with asymmetric ankle OA when compared to a healthy control: at least 25% lower sagittal ankle ROM, at least 15% lower peak dorsiflexion movement, at least 40% lower ankle power, and less gastrocnemius medialis and soleus muscle activity in electromyogram around push-off.[11]

Furthermore, as per fractures with bone loss, alterations of the contact surface area in the ankle joint increase pathologic joint reaction forces.[12] Pathologic changes in subchondral density and mineralization that occur in the asymmetric arthritic ankle area as a compensatory effect to the chronic load can be reversed by corrective supramalleolar osteotomy, as proven by Egloff and colleagues in a study using CT-osteoabsorptiometry (CT-OAM).[13] However, calcaneal osteotomy alone has only a minor effect on the pressure distribution of the ankle joint.[14] The effect of the fibula in controlling ankle stability should not be neglected as the shortening and the external rotation might play a major role in disrupting the contact area in the tibiotalar joint.[15]

Clinical Assessment

A good clinical assessment starts with a meticulous history evaluation that includes the history of trauma or ankle instability, past treatment and surgical history, and comorbidities such as neurologic disorders, diabetes mellitus, or any inflammatory disease. A proper history and physical examination are crucial to analyze the etiology of valgus ankle OA.

Standing examination: The evaluation of shoes and insoles is important to obtain indirect information regarding the amount of hindfoot/ankle deformity and the quality of the conservative treatment performed. Hindfoot/ankle alignment, old scars, and muscle atrophy are assessed with the patient standing via inspection of the whole leg, lower leg, hindfoot, and foot from all sides (ie, front, back, and side). Evaluation of limb length discrepancy should also be performed. Assessment of the gait and hindfoot/ankle with painful asymmetric limping, possible arch collapse, ligament ankle instability, and neuromuscular dysbalance is also part of good documentation. Furthermore, a thorough evaluation of the signs of PTT insufficiency is important to confirm or rule out this entity (eg, the "too many toes" sign, single and double heel raise test). The reverse Coleman block test is important to rule out forefoot-driven deformity and assess the flexibility of the deformity.[16,17]

Sitting examination: While the patient is sitting, the following examination points should be addressed: evaluation of skin condition; documentation of all tenderness points; measurement of active and passive ROM of the ankle joint, subtalar joint, and Chopart joint; assessment of lateral and medial ankle instability; evaluation of muscle power around the ankle (ie, posterior tibial muscle, peroneal muscle, anterior tibial muscle, gastrocnemius/soleus muscles). Furthermore, the Silfverskiöld test is important to evaluate a possible triceps surae contracture that may need to be addressed at the time of surgery.

Finally, a neurovascular examination is also a crucial part of the orthopedic assessment.

IMAGING

Conventional Weight-bearing Radiography is the basic level of imaging in valgus ankle OA. In our institution, the following weight-bearing x-rays are defined as the standard radiological status: standing anteroposterior (AP) view of the ankle joint (mortise view), standing hindfoot view (Saltzman view), lateral view of the foot, and dorsoplantar view of the foot. In severe lower leg, knee, and leg deformities, lower limb radiography of both legs is advisable to accurately define the center of rotation and angulation (CORA).

In valgus ankle OA, the *AP ankle view/mortise* allows the confirmation of a reduction in joint space of the lateral ankle joint, reduction of space in the lateral gutter with a talofibular impingement,[3,18] and a medial increase in clear space, which suggests the involvement of the deltoid ligament.[3]

In the AP ankle view/mortise view, these angles can be measured. The medial distal tibial articular angle (mDTAA) is normally 92.4° ± 3.1 (range, 88–100), whereas an mDTAA value of greater than 92° is considered a valgus ankle OA with supramalleolar deformity.[19] In the mortise view, the midline tibiotalar angle (MTTA) can also be measured. An average normal MTTA value is 88.7° ± 5.1 (range, 77–104), whereas greater than 90° is considered a valgus ankle OA.[20] Furthermore, in the mortise view, the medial talar tilt angle (mTTA) can clarify the congruency status of the tibiotalar joint (incongruent >4°, suggesting instability of the ankle joint[21]).

Syndesmotic integrity can be measured (1 cm above the tibial plafond) in the AP view using the following variables: The width of the tibiofibular clear space with a normal range of less than 6 mm; tibiofibular overlap with a normal value of greater than 1 mm in the mortise view and greater than 6 mm in the AP view.[22]

Fibular length is also evaluated in the mortise view based on disruption of the parallelism of the tibiotalar line (talar tilt), disruption of Shenton's line, and disruption of the dime sign/Weber circle at the tip of the fibula/lateral talar process.[23–25]

In the *hindfoot alignment view* (Saltzman view), an inframalleolar deformity can be detected. In this view, the hindfoot valgus angle (HVA) can be measured as the angle between the anatomic axis of the tibia and the axis of the calcaneus. A physiologic HVA has a value of 0 to 5°valgus. Pathologic HVAs are greater than 10°.[26]

In the weight-bearing *AP foot view*, an important angle is the talonavicular coverage angle, which should be smaller than 7° in a plantigrade foot.[27] Furthermore, the AP talar-first metatarsal angle also describes a medial collapse in a flatfoot deformity (normally 7.7° ± 8.2).[28]

The weight-bearing *lateral foot views* are valuable in assessing the sagittal deformity of the ankle as well as the hindfoot and midfoot involvement of the deformity. The tibia lateral surface angle has a normal value of 81° to 82°.[29] The lateral talar-first metatarsal angle depicts the amount of flatfoot deformity. Notably, an angle greater than 4° convex downward is considered pes planus.[30]

MRI represents the second line of imaging for the evaluation of the cartilage, ligaments, syndesmosis, tendons, and soft tissues in the ankle joint and hindfoot. In addition, weight-bearing MRI can provide further information to improve diagnostic accuracy.[31,32]

CT scan helps to better evaluate the bone condition of the lower leg, ankle, and hindfoot—especially in fracture-related cases. Weight-bearing CT (WBCT) scans of the foot and ankle have improved the understanding of deformities and the real orientation of the bone and the joint, which provides a better understanding of the pathology, especially in complex cases.[33,34]

The authors performed *SPECT-CT* to evaluate the extent of degenerative changes and the biological activity of valgus ankle OA to localize hot spots, which is very important for the planning of JPS.[10,35] Knupp and colleagues used weight-bearing radiographs, conventional CT, bone scintigraphy, and SPECT-CT in patients with valgus or varus ankle OA.[10] In SPECT-CT images, the valgus ankles showed significantly greater uptake in the lateral areas than in the medial regions. The results of the present study showed that SPECT-CT is a unique radiographic tool that allows the simultaneous analysis of the structure and metabolism of degenerative changes of the tibiotalar joint.[10] Besides information about the ankle joint, SPECT-CT can provide diagnostic information about additional co-entities such as other OA in the foot joints, stress fractures, and tarsal coalitions.[32,36]

TREATMENT
Conservative Treatment

Classic conservative treatment aims to achieve pain reduction and increase of function. This type of treatment consists of adaptation of physical activity, painkillers, viscosupplementation (orally or by joint infiltration), platelet-rich plasma (PRP), physiotherapy, and orthotics (eg, insoles, stabilizing shoes). Conservative treatment should be attempted for 3 to 6 months before a possible surgery. Physiotherapy programs typically involve stretching the foot evertors and strengthening the invertors and contracted calf muscles. In addition, orthosis plays a major role in conservative treatment. Notably, it is important to adjust solid insoles with a well-padded medial arch support to appropriately varisate the hindfoot and ankle.

The use of oral glucosamine sulfate has been expanded to cover ankle OA because it is a safe chondroprotective agent.[37] Moreover, intraarticular injection with hyaluronic acid might help to reduce ankle pain and is one of the treatment options for ankle OA.[38] Effectiveness and improvement were observed using multiple rating scales, including that of the American Orthopedic Foot and Ankle Society (AOFAS; 50.7 ± 13.8–79.9 ± 13.8) and visual analog scales (VAS; 5.7 ± 1.2–2.7 ± 1.6).[39]

PRP injection should not be neglected—especially in valgus ankle OA—because of its multiple effects as an anti-inflammatory and analgesic agent, which help to delay the destruction process.[40,41] Notably, physicians must support nonoperative management. However, conservative treatment does not increase the deformity and degenerative changes because a process delay reduces the opportunity for and outcome of JPS. Increasing pain severity and instability is an alarming sign that suggests the need to accelerate surgical intervention (if indicated).

Joint Preserving Surgery (JPS)

JPS represents a variety of surgical methods used to retain the natural joint and extend its survivorship by improving its biomechanics and biology (eg, a partial arthritic joint can be transformed from a pathobiomechanical to an almost normal biomechanical joint). The most important factor for JPS in valgus ankle OA is that the tibiotalar cartilage must be intact in more than half of the intraarticular area. The goal is to restore the anatomic alignment, de-load the osteoarthritic area, improve joint congruency, and achieve joint ankle stability to reach a pain-free ankle with a plantigrade, flexible, functional ankle/hindfoot/foot and postpone or avoid end-stage full-ankle OA. In the ankle OA timeline, the window of opportunity to perform JPS is narrow. Therefore, early patient presentation and timely surgery can avoid the rapid progression to full ankle OA, thereby avoiding a total ankle arthroplasty or ankle arthrodesis.

Technically, JPS may have the following surgical content: osteotomies (supramalleolar, hindfoot/calcaneal, malleolar, mid-/forefoot), ankle ligament surgery (lateral, medial, syndesmosis), tendon surgery (PTT, peroneal, etc.), and osteo-/chondral surgery.

The indications for JPS for valgus ankle OA include painful asymmetrical lateral ankle OA with preserved medial half of tibiotalar cartilage, conserved ankle motion (>20° ROM), and patient age less than 60 years (relative indication).

The JPS contraindications generally include poor patient health conditions such as the presence of multiple comorbidities, severe vascular deficiency or neurologic disability, and severe systemic disorders. In addition, factors that could affect compliance and postoperative rehabilitation should be considered. Caution should also be exercised in patients with noncompliance, vitamin D3 insufficiency, immunosuppression, and tobacco use.[2,6,42] These factors can lead to complications such as infections, malunions/nonunions of the bony corrections, and failed JPS surgery.

Radiological Preoperative Planning

Many x-ray measurement guidelines for angles around the ankle joint are available in the literature. The purpose of these guidelines is to facilitate a proper diagnosis to identify and localize the deformity level and augment the clinical diagnosis (see the Imaging section in this article). Measuring these angles will help surgeons in preoperative assessment, surgical planning, and postoperative evaluation. Good preoperative planning of the JPS is crucial for good surgical outcomes (**Box 2**).

Ankle Arthroscopy

Diagnostic and therapeutic ankle joint arthroscopy is part of ankle JPS and helps at the beginning of JPS to intraoperatively assess the valgus ankle OA intraarticularly and judge chronic ankle instability (medial, lateral, and syndesmotic) as well as bony ankle impingement.[43,44] As we shift the load to the medial part of the ankle in JPS, evaluating the joint condition before the osteotomy is crucial. A simple and common classification used to judge the cartilage is the Outerbridge classification: grade 0, no cartilage damage; grade 1, cartilage softening; grade 2, cartilage damage with the stripping of superficial cartilage layers; grade 3, deep cartilage ulceration without visible subchondral bone; grade 4, visible subchondral bone.[45]

The therapeutic use of ankle arthroscopy before JPS might help to remove possible loose bodies, shave osteophytes anteriorly, or perform arthroscopic cartilage repair techniques.

Box 2
Rules for optimizing the surgical intervention of joint preserving surgery for valgus ankle osteoarthritis

1. Perform a solid preoperative analysis and define the primary cause of osteoarthritis
2. Correct the alignment with slight overcorrection (2°–5°) to substantially de-load the osteoarthritic ankle area
3. Correct the largest deformity entity first, then address any proximal deformity before any distal one
4. First address the bony deformities, then the soft tissue pathologies

Supramalleolar Osteotomy of the Tibia (SMOT)

The goals of the supramalleolar osteotomy of the tibia (SMOT) procedure are to realign the ankle/hindfoot and restore the mechanical axis to avoid or delay a possible joint-sacrificing procedure. Proven by multiple studies, asymmetric ankle OA can be improved by the SMOT procedure.[46–48] This is in addition to the clinical and radiological outcomes showing a promising result.[49] The SMOT is a powerful tool that optimizes the lower limb alignment in the presence of coronal, sagittal, and rotational deformity of the tibia.[50] In this type of osteotomy, the goal is to reduce pain and improve function. Even in the case of a suboptimal outcome, the patient and surgeon would not have caused harm by realigning the lower leg/ankle/hindfoot for possible future joint-sacrificing surgery (eg, total ankle arthroplasty, ankle arthrodesis). For the treatment of lateral valgus ankle OA, a medial closing-wedge SMOT is indicated, especially for cases with tibial plafond lateral damage, intraarticular ankle valgus OA, pathologic mDTAA >92°, or a supramalleolar tibia CORA deformity. Furthermore, a medial closing-wedge SMOT is part of the treatment for a valgus ankle OA with post-traumatic shortened fibula after fibular fracture malunion/nonunion or a valgus ankle OA with a chronic syndesmotic instability or chronic medial ankle instability.

Medial Closing-Wedge SMOT Technique

The patient is placed in a supine position with a thigh tourniquet for homeostasis and heel flush with the end of the operation table. A 15-cm incision is performed on the medial distal tibia. As the structures at risk include the saphenous vein and nerve, they must be identified and gently retracted. A sharp incision of the medial distal tibia periosteum is performed. Hohmann retractors are inserted around the tibia to protect the soft tissue structures anteriorly and posteriorly. For intraoperative osteotomy guidance, two K-wires are placed under fluoroscan guidance from the medial side to represent the wedge to be medially resected. The required amount of correction/angular degrees, which is preoperatively calculated from weight-bearing x-rays, can be roughly used as millimeters in the medial tibial wedge resection. In AP views, the surgical goal is to overcorrect the medial distal tibial joint surface angle by 2° to 5° over the physiologic normal average angle.[21] The formula proposed by Warnock (tanα = h/W) facilitates preoperative planning for the possible medial closing tibial wedge size calculation, where α is the angle to be corrected, H is the wedge height in millimeters, and W is the tibial width.[51] Regarding the K-wires, it is important to place the tip of both K-wires laterally proximal to the incisura fibularis because, distal of it, the SMOT could endanger syndesmotic stability. Approximately, the proximal K-wire is more or less perpendicular to the tibia, whereas the distal K-wire is more or less parallel to the joint line or talus surface, depending on the case. Using an oscillating saw and continuous irrigation to avoid thermal injury, the medial closing-wedge osteotomy is performed. The lateral part of the osteotomy is gently weakened by using an osteotome. The preservation of the lateral tibial cortex and periosteum is important because this helps the healing process of the osteotomy and enhances osteotomy stability.[4,5,52] With compressive K-wire-forceps (or by hand), the osteotomy can be gently closed and compressed on acceptable level. We recommend using a robust anatomic angular stable medial tibia plate with compression options (as oblong eccentric holes) to compress the osteotomy on a micro level (Anatomic APTUS Medial Supramalleolar Tibia Osteotomy Plate, Medartis, Switzerland; **Figs. 1** and **2**). If the osteotomy breaks on the lateral cortex, this can be left unaddressed if the medial tibial plate is of good quality and the patient is compliant. If the lateral osteotomy tibia cortex breaks with a significant shift, we recommend augmenting the SMOT fixation with a second additional ventral or lateral tibia plate. During the SMOT procedure, it is

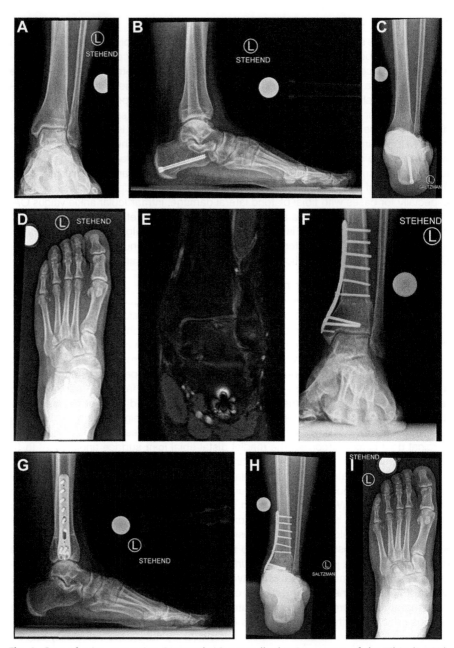

Fig. 1. Case of Joint preserving Surgery by Supramalleolar Osteotomy of the Tibia (SMOT) for Valgus Ankle Osteoarthritis with a Lateral Talar Osteochondral Lesion. A 28-year-old male with chronic painful asymmetric posttraumatic lateral ankle osteoarthritis with a multicystic osteochondral lesion (OCL) on the lateral talus (A–E). Preoperative angles: mDTAA 97°, TTSA 96°, mTTA 1°, and HAA 8°. Previous surgeries: St. after ankle arthroscopy and retrograde drilling of the lateral OCL talus 2 years ago; St. after ankle arthroscopy, medial-sliding-calcaneus-osteotomy, and AMIC lateral talus OCL 1 year ago. We performed a medial closing-wedge supramalleolar tibial osteotomy SMOT (Anatomic APTUS Medial

important to control the rotational and sagittal plane of the distal fragment. If simultaneous correction occurs in the sagittal plane, one should consider anterior or posterior wedge cutting (depending on the deformity on the sagittal plane) for the required amount to achieve the optimum sagittal alignment required, while also considering the downsizing of the recurvatum and antecurvatum to reduce the anterior or posterior impingement of the ankle joint and allow an optimal pressure distribution in the ankle joint.[53,54] After the final intraoperative x-rays, the medial tibial soft tissues are closed with drainage to avoid a possible lower leg hematoma.

Possible additional surgeries include:

- *Fibular osteotomy*: An additional fibular osteotomy is required in cases with a shortened or external malrotated fibula (eg, after a fibular or lower leg fracture). Furthermore, an unreduced talus after restoring the mDTAA angle could indicate the need for fibular lengthening osteotomy.[21] After SMOT, the optimal fibular length adds value to the ankle joint by supporting, inverting, and medially shifting the talus, which provides strain reduction on the deltoid.
- *Ankle ligament reconstruction*: Medial ankle ligament complex reconstruction (ie, deltoid, spring ligament): In cases with medial ankle instability, medial ankle ligament complex reconstruction via the shortening or enhancement of the deltoid/spring ligament is required. If this entity is unclear preoperatively, the medial ligament complex can be judged manually or under fluoroscopic evaluation (stress view) after SMOT plate fixation by balance testing the medial and lateral ligaments. In some cases, lateral ligament reconstruction must also be performed (rotational ankle instability: medial and lateral ankle ligament instability combined).
- *Posterior tibial tendon reconstruction*: In PTT insufficiency, a PTT surgery that involves shortening or augmentation of the PTT via an FDL-tendon transfer must be added to the SMOT.
- *Calcaneal osteotomy*: In cases of remaining hindfoot valgus (inframalleolar deformity), a calcaneus osteotomy or varisating subtalar arthrodesis of the arthritic subtalar joint is required. In the case of a calcaneal osteotomy, the surgeon must differentiate between a medial sliding calcaneal osteotomy or lateral lengthening calcaneal osteotomy—especially the latter if a forefoot abductus is present.
- *Cotton osteotomy*: If valgus ankle OA is combined with a medial arch/midfoot collapse, a cotton osteotomy at the medial cuneiform must be added.
- *Gastrocnemius recession/Strayer procedure*: This procedure is indicated for patients with a tightness of the calf muscle as a cause of their hindfoot valgus and equinus contracture.
- *Osteochondral reconstructive ankle surgery*: Only osteochondral defects need to be addressed (eg, with arthroscopic procedures or an Autologous Matrix Induced Chrondrogenesis [AMIC]-Membrane technique), whereas chondral lesions can be healed by the simple deloading effect of the SMOT.

Supramalleolar Tibia Osteotomy Plate, Medartis, Switzerland), re-do of AMIC cartilage reconstruction of the lateral talus (debridement OCL, spongiosaplasty from ipsilateral tibia; Chondro-Gide Membrane, Geistlich Surgery, Switzerland), and lateral ankle ligament reconstruction. Six months after final SMOT surgery, the patient is pain-free and x-rays show a healed osteotomy and a physiologic position of the ankle joint with an mDTAA of 88° (*F–I*).

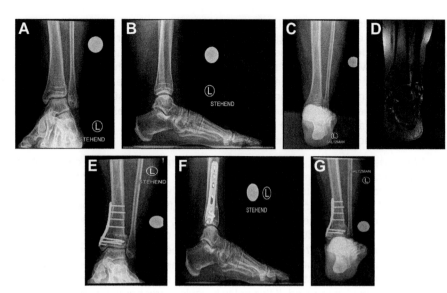

Fig. 2. Case of Joint Preserving Surgery (JPS) by Supramalleolar Osteotomy of the Tibia (SMOT) for Valgus Ankle Osteoarthritis. Preoperative weight-bearing AP (*A*) and lateral (*B*) radiographs of the ankle and Saltzman view (*C*) demonstrating valgus ankle deformity, posttraumatic chronic painful lateral ankle cartilage degeneration (*D*) with a lateral osteochondral lesion (OCL) of the talus with medial and lateral chronic ankle instability and pes valgus. Postoperative weight-bearing AP (*E*) and lateral (*F*) radiographs of the ankle and Saltzman view (*G*) after the following surgeries: diagnostic ankle arthroscopy, debridement and abrasion of the lateral talus OCL, supramalleolar medial closing tibial osteotomy SMOT (Anatomic APTUS Medial Supramalleolar Tibia Osteotomy Plate, Medartis, Switzerland), medial ankle ligament surgery, and lateral ankle ligament surgery with an ipsilateral semitendinosus tendon graft.

Post-treatment of the medial closing-wedge SMOT: The patient must be immobilized and maintain a 15 kg partial weight-bearing for 8 weeks (eg, using a lower leg/ankle/foot walker). We recommend immediately performing postoperative physiotherapy to improve ankle motion and reduce the swelling of the soft tissues via lymphatic drain massage. Practically, full weight bearing is only allowed if the SMOT is radiologically healed.

Fibular Osteotomy

Valgus ankle OA possibly requires fibular osteotomy, the goal of which is to restore anatomic ankle alignment, improve joint congruency at the tibia plafond of the ankle, and reduce the risk of chronic medial ankle instability. Notably, fibular osteotomy restores the fibular length and talus position in the mortise view.[55,56] In a cadaver study, Stufkens and colleagues clarified the augmentation and restriction effects of fibular osteotomy above the syndesmosis on the SMOT.[8] They showed that adding a fibular osteotomy to the SMOT directly above the syndesmosis was helpful for reaching the desired load, which reveals the restriction and augmentation effect of the fibula.

The evaluation of fibular length is performed preoperatively in the weight-bearing mortise view or WBCT by disrupting the parallelism of the tibiotalar line (talar tilt), Shenton's line, or dime sign/Weber circle at the tip of the fibula/lateral talar.[23–25,57]

Although multiple types of fibular osteotomies have been described in the literature, there is no consensus in the literature regarding the realignment osteotomy for the malunited fibula.[58] We prefer the Z-shaped fibular osteotomy with or without fibular rotational wedge resection unless the rotation deformity is less than 10°; if the malrotation is over 10°, an oblique osteotomy is preferred.[25,57]

Fibular-lengthening Osteotomy Surgical Technique: Z-shaped fibular osteotomy is performed using an oscillating saw under Hohmann protection. It is important to perform the z-part with sufficient length to have a good bridge area after fibular elongation. After restoring the desired length, wedge removal osteotomy in the horizontal part of the osteotomy is performed for external rotation correction. The osteotomy is then fixed by an angular stable plate with an AP screw in the z-bridging area.

It is important to perform the osteotomy above the level of the syndesmotic ligament to avoid iatrogenic instability of the ankle joint. A cadaver study showed that sectioning of the anterior inferior tibiofibular ligament alone increases the tibiofibular space by up to 10 mm and 20° of varus tilt and 40° of rotational instability if the osteotomy is performed below the level of syndesmosis.[23,59] Furthermore, the laxity of the syndesmotic ligament should be evaluated before and after osteotomy. On the other hand, scarring in the syndesmotic should be removed to restore the correct fibular length.[24] It is recommended to fill the gap with bone grafts if the gap is too large.

DISCUSSION

Ankle OA does not always involve full tibiotalar degeneration. Malaligned valgus or varus ankle OA is quite often.[1] Valgus ankle OA has a typical etiologic profile: posttraumatic, degenerative, congenital, or neurologic and can be supramalleolar, intraarticular, or inframalleolar (see **Box 1**). The treatment of valgus ankle OA should follow the same treatment pathway as ankle OA in general: conservative treatment, JPS, total ankle arthroplasty, and ankle arthrodesis. After a solid conservative treatment for 3 to 6 months, JPS might be required to avoid a total ankle arthroplasty or even an ankle arthrodesis. Deloading the osteoarthritic joint area while simultaneously optimizing the joint load is a crucial part of JPS. The content of JPS depends on the underlying etiology of the valgus ankle OA: osteotomies, ligament reconstruction, tendon surgery, and osteochondral surgery. The most powerful osteotomy for valgus ankle OA is SMOT, which is performed as a varisating medial closing-wedge osteotomy. If the deformity is not only intraarticular or supramalleolar, a calcaneal or midfoot bony surgery might be required as an inframalleolar correction.

Stamatis and colleagues showed a satisfactory result in 12 patients with SMOT: improvement of AOFAS score from 53.8 to 87 and no progression in ankle OA over 2 years.[60] Furthermore, Knupp and colleagues reported the effect of SMOT on 92 patients with asymmetric ankle OA with a mean follow-up of 3.6 years. None of the patients suffered nonunion and the healing period did not exceed 12 weeks. In addition, the AOFAS hindfoot and VAS scores improved significantly.[61] Moreover, Pagenstert and colleagues proved that JPS for valgus ankle OA has a good outcome. In their study, pain visual analog scale scores decreased from 6.6 ± 1.5 preoperatively to 2.4 ± 1.6 points after treatment ($P<.0001$). In addition, the AOFAS hindfoot score increased from 43 points (range, 16–67) preoperatively to 84 points (range, 63–100; $P<.0001$).[5] The literature also suggests that JPS improves the ability to perform sports by reducing pain and increasing the function of the ankle joint.[62] In an *in vivo* biomechanics study, Nüesch and colleagues showed that JPS improved the function of patients through a 25% average increase in AOFAS score in addition to a 50% reduction in pain. Moreover, there were no significant differences in muscle activation in the long-term when compared with the control group. This is especially valuable for younger patients because the improvement of function and pain reduces the need for (or could delay) joint-sacrificing ankle procedures.[11] In addition to pain reduction and functional outcomes, Ayyawsawmy reported significant improvements to radiological parameters including the tibial articular surface ankle and talar tilt angle (TT).[63]

In cases where the JPS result was suboptimal or did not provide the desired pain relief, the JPS served as a good presurgery for the next step in the timeline-treatment/pathway of ankle OA, which is total ankle arthroplasty. Wood and colleagues found that the failure rate for total ankle arthroplasty was lower in ankles that were well aligned than in ankles with over 15° preoperative valgus or varus deformity.[64]

Notably, complications from supramalleolar osteotomies are possible. Wound healing complications and infections have a reported incidence of up to 22%, whereas malunion or nonunion occurred in up to 22% of cases.[65] OA progression is one of the most common complications after JPS for ankle OA.[4,5,62] In a series of 22 patients who underwent SMOT for valgus ankle OA with a mean follow-up of 4.5 years, 2 patients (9%) developed progressive OA.[5] In a more recent report of 56 patients who underwent SMOT for valgus ankle OA, 4 patients (7%) had to undergo a secondary TAA or ankle fusion because of the progression of ankle OA. This is in addition to 4% who had delayed union and another 4% who had delayed wound healing.[49] Undercorrection of the varisation osteotomy is considered one of the risk factors for ankle OA progression.[5,6] Espinosa and colleagues considered the persistence of pain beyond 12 months after the surgery as an indication of failure and categorized the failure factors into surgery-related failures, global OA of the joint (progression), and infection.[66]

SUMMARY

Valgus ankle OA is a complex problem with multiple etiologies that can either be isolated or superimposed on top of other medical or musculoskeletal disorders. Proper medical history, physical, and preoperative radiological examinations are crucial in deciding on surgery and planning the surgical approach. JPS, especially the varisating medial closing-wedge SMOT with solid plate fixation, has been consistently associated with good outcomes for patients with valgus ankle OA. To further improve JPS for valgus ankle OA, further clinical and biomechanical studies are required to address the long-term clinical and functional outcomes and complications.

DISCLOSURE

Victor Valderrabano: Consultant of: Medartis, Geistlich Surgery.

REFERENCES

1. Valderrabano V, Horisberger M, Russell I, et al. Etiology of Ankle Osteoarthritis. Clin Orthop Relat Res 2009;467(7). https://doi.org/10.1007/s11999-008-0543-6.
2. Valderrabano V, Paul J, Monika H, et al. Joint-preserving surgery of valgus ankle osteoarthritis. Foot Ankle Clin 2013;18(3):481–502.
3. Gibson V, Prieskorn D. The Valgus Ankle. Foot Ankle Clin 2007;12(1):15–27.
4. Pagenstert GI, Hintermann B, Barg A, et al. Realignment Surgery as Alternative Treatment of Varus and Valgus Ankle Osteoarthritis. Clin Orthop Relat Res 2007;462. https://doi.org/10.1097/BLO.0b013e318124a462.
5. Pagenstert G, Knupp M, Valderrabano V, et al. Realignment surgery for valgus ankle osteoarthritis. Oper Orthop Traumatol 2009;21(1):77–87.
6. Barg A, Pagenstert GI, Leumann AG, et al. Treatment of the Arthritic Valgus Ankle. Foot Ankle Clin 2012;17(4). https://doi.org/10.1016/j.fcl.2012.08.007.

7. Barg A, Pagenstert GI, Hügle T, et al. Ankle osteoarthritis: Etiology, diagnostics, and classification. Foot Ankle Clin 2013;18(3):411–26.
8. Stufkens SA, Van Bergen CJ, Blankevoort L, et al. The role of the fibula in varus and valgus deformity of the tibia: A biomechanical study. J Bone Joint Surg Br 2011;93 B(9):1232–9.
9. Knupp M, Stufkens SAS, Van Bergen CJ, et al. Effect of supramalleolar varus and valgus deformities on the tibiotalar joint: A cadaveric study. Foot Ankle Int 2011; 32(6):609–15.
10. Knupp M, Pagenstert GI, Barg A, et al. SPECT-CT compared with conventional imaging modalities for the assessment of the varus and valgus malaligned hindfoot. J Orthop Res 2009;27(11):1461–6.
11. Nüesch C, Valderrabano V, Huber C, et al. Effects of supramalleolar osteotomies for ankle osteoarthritis on foot kinematics and lower leg muscle activation during walking. Clin Biomech 2014;29(3). https://doi.org/10.1016/j.clinbiomech.2013.12.015.
12. Delco ML, Kennedy JG, Bonassar LJ, et al. Post-traumatic osteoarthritis of the ankle: A distinct clinical entity requiring new research approaches. J Orthop Res 2017;35(3). https://doi.org/10.1002/jor.23462.
13. Egloff C, Paul J, Pagenstert G, et al. Changes of density distribution of the subchondral bone plate after supramalleolar osteotomy for valgus ankle osteoarthritis. J Orthop Res 2014;32(10). https://doi.org/10.1002/jor.22683.
14. Davitt JS, Beals TC, Bachus KN. The effects of medial and lateral displacement calcaneal osteotomies on ankle and subtalar joint pressure distribution. Foot Ankle Int 2001;22(11):885–9.
15. Curtis MJ, Michelson JD, Urquhart MW, et al. Tibiotalar contact and fibular malunion in ankle fractures A cadaver study. Acta Orthop Scand 1992;63(3). https://doi.org/10.3109/17453679209154793.
16. Coleman SS, Chesnut WJ. A simple test for hindfoot flexibility in the cavovarus foot. Clin Orthop Relat Res 1977;123:60–2.
17. Wood EV, Syed A, Geary NP. Clinical Tip: The Reverse Coleman Block Test Radiograph. Foot Ankle Int 2009;30(7). https://doi.org/10.3113/FAI.2009.0708.
18. Klammer G, Espinosa N, Iselin LD. Coalitions of the Tarsal Bones. Foot Ankle Clin 2018;23(3). https://doi.org/10.1016/j.fcl.2018.04.011.
19. Barg A, Harris MD, Henninger HB, et al. Medial Distal Tibial Angle: Comparison between Weightbearing Mortise View and Hindfoot Alignment View. Foot Ankle Int 2012;33(8). https://doi.org/10.3113/FAI.2012.0655.
20. Najefi A-A, Buraimoh O, Goldberg A. Should the Tibiotalar Angle Be Measured Using an AP or Mortise X-ray? Foot Ankle Orthop 2018;3(3). https://doi.org/10.1177/2473011418S00364.
21. Hintermann B, Knupp M, Barg A. Supramalleolar Osteotomies for the Treatment of Ankle Arthritis. J Am Acad Orthop Surg 2016;24(7). https://doi.org/10.5435/JAAOS-D-12-00124.
22. Kellett JJ, Lovell GA, Eriksen DA, et al. Diagnostic imaging of ankle syndesmosis injuries: A general review. J Med Imaging Radiat Oncol 2018;62(2). https://doi.org/10.1111/1754-9485.12708.
23. Davis JL, Giacopelli JA. Transfibular osteotomy in the correction of ankle joint incongruity. J Foot Ankle Surg 1995;34(4). https://doi.org/10.1016/S1067-2516(09)80010-0.
24. van Wensen RJA, van den Bekerom MPJ, Marti RK, et al. Reconstructive osteotomy of fibular malunion: review of the literature. Strateg Trauma Limb Reconstr 2011;6(2). https://doi.org/10.1007/s11751-011-0107-2.

25. Weber BG. Lengthening osteotomy of the fibula to correct a widened mortice of the ankle after fracture. Int Orthop 1981;4(4):289–93.

26. Buck FM, Hoffmann A, Mamisch-Saupe N, et al. Hindfoot Alignment Measurements: Rotation-Stability of Measurement Techniques on Hindfoot Alignment View and Long Axial View Radiographs. Am J Roentgenol 2011;197(3). https://doi.org/10.2214/AJR.10.5728.

27. Chi TD, Toolan BC, Sangeorzan BJ, et al. The Lateral Column Lengthening and Medial Column Stabilization Procedures. Clin Orthop Relat Res 1999;365. https://doi.org/10.1097/00003086-199908000-00011.

28. Younger AS, Sawatzky B, Dryden P. Radiographic Assessment of Adult Flatfoot. Foot Ankle Int 2005;26(10). https://doi.org/10.1177/107110070502601006.

29. Tanaka Y, Takakura Y, Hayashi K, et al. Low tibial osteotomy for varus-type osteoarthritis of the ankle. J Bone Joint Surg Br 2006;88-B(7). https://doi.org/10.1302/0301-620X.88B7.17325.

30. Gould N. Graphing the adult foot and ankle. Foot Ankle 1982;2(4):213–9.

31. Bruno F, Arrigoni F, Palumbo P, et al. Weight-bearing MR Imaging of Knee, Ankle and Foot. Semin Musculoskelet Radiol 2019;23(06). https://doi.org/10.1055/s-0039-1697940.

32. Huang J, Servaes S, Zhuang H. Os trigonum syndrome on bone SPECT/CT. Clin Nucl Med 2014;39(8):752–4.

33. Conti MS, Ellis SJ. Weight-bearing CT Scans in Foot and Ankle Surgery. J Am Acad Orthop Surg 2020;28(14). https://doi.org/10.5435/JAAOS-D-19-00700.

34. Barg A, Bailey T, Richter M, et al. Weightbearing Computed Tomography of the Foot and Ankle: Emerging Technology Topical Review. Foot Ankle Int 2018; 39(3). https://doi.org/10.1177/1071100717740330.

35. Gougoulias N, O'Flaherty M, Sakellariou A. Taking Out the Tarsal Coalition Was Easy. Foot Ankle Clin 2014;19(3). https://doi.org/10.1016/j.fcl.2014.06.011.

36. Chicklore S, Gnanasegaran G, Vijayanathan S, et al. Potential role of multislice SPECT/CT in impingement syndrome and soft-tissue pathology of the ankle and foot. Nucl Med Commun 2013;34(2):130–9.

37. Bloch B, Srinivasan S, Mangwani J. Current Concepts in the Management of Ankle Osteoarthritis: A Systematic Review. J Foot Ankle Surg 2015;54(5). https://doi.org/10.1053/j.jfas.2014.12.042.

38. Vannabouathong C, Del Fabbro G, Sales B, et al. Intra-articular Injections in the Treatment of Symptoms from Ankle Arthritis: A Systematic Review. Foot Ankle Int 2018;39(10):1141–50.

39. Hwang YG, Lee JW, Park KH, et al. Intra-articular Injections of Hyaluronic Acid on Osteochondral Lesions of the Talus After Failed Arthroscopic Bone Marrow Stimulation. Foot Ankle Int 2020;41(11):1376–82.

40. Zhu Y, Yuan M, Meng HY, et al. Basic science and clinical application of platelet-rich plasma forcartilage defects and osteoarthritis: A review. Osteoarthr Cartil 2013;21(11):1627–37.

41. Meheux CJ, McCulloch PC, Lintner DM, et al. Efficacy of Intra-articular Platelet-Rich Plasma Injections in Knee Osteoarthritis: A Systematic Review. Arthroscopy 2016;32(3):495–505.

42. Lee JJ, Patel R, Biermann JS, et al. The Musculoskeletal Effects of Cigarette Smoking. J Bone Joint Surg Am 2013;95(9). https://doi.org/10.2106/JBJS.L.00375.

43. Hintermann B, Boss A, Schäfer D. Arthroscopic findings in patients with chronic ankle instability. Am J Sports Med 2002;30(3):402–9.

44. Tol JL, Verheyen CPPM, Van Dijk CN. Arthroscopic treatment of anterior impingement in the ankle. J Bone Joint Surg Am 2001;83(1). https://doi.org/10.1302/0301-620X.83B1.10571.

45. Outerbridge RE. THE ETIOLOGY OF CHONDROMALACIA PATELLAE. J Bone Joint Surg Br 1961;43-B(4). https://doi.org/10.1302/0301-620X.43B4.752.

46. Knupp M, Hintermann B. Treatment of asymmetric arthritis of the ankle joint with supramalleolar osteotomies. Foot Ankle Int 2012;33(3):250–2. https://doi.org/10.3113/FAI.2012.0250.

47. Takakura Y, Takaoka T, Tanaka Y, et al. Results of opening-wedge osteotomy for the treatment of a post-traumatic varus deformity of the ankle. J Bone Joint Surg Am 1998;80(2):213–8.

48. Lee WC, Moon JS, Lee K, et al. Indications for supramalleolar osteotomy in patients with ankle osteoarthritis and varus deformity. J Bone Joint Surg Am 2011;93(13):1243–8.

49. Krähenbühl N, Susdorf R, Barg A, et al. Supramalleolar osteotomy in post-traumatic valgus ankle osteoarthritis. Int Orthop 2020;44(3). https://doi.org/10.1007/s00264-019-04476-x.

50. Takakura Y, Tanaka Y, Kumai T, et al. Low tibial osteotomy for osteoarthritis of the ankle. Results of a new operation in 18 patients. J Bone Joint Surg Br 1995;77(1):50–4.

51. Warnock KM, Johnson BD, Wright JB, et al. Calculation of the opening wedge for a low tibial osteotomy. Foot Ankle Int 2004;25(11):778–82.

52. Goshima K, Sawaguchi T, Shigemoto K, et al. Large opening gaps, unstable hinge fractures, and osteotomy line below the safe zone cause delayed bone healing after open-wedge high tibial osteotomy. Knee Surg Sports Traumatol Arthrosc 2019;27(4). https://doi.org/10.1007/s00167-018-5334-3.

53. Knupp M. The Use of Osteotomies in the Treatment of Asymmetric Ankle Joint Arthritis. Foot Ankle Int 2017;38(2). https://doi.org/10.1177/1071100716679190.

54. Lamm BM, Paley D. Deformity correction planning for hindfoot, ankle, and lower limb. Clin Podiatr Med Surg 2004;21(3). https://doi.org/10.1016/j.cpm.2004.04.004.

55. Yablon IG, Leach RE. Reconstruction of malunited fractures of the lateral malleolus. J Bone Joint Surg Am 1989;71(4):521–7.

56. Marti R, Raaymakers E, Nolte P. Malunited ankle fractures. The late results of reconstruction. J Bone Joint Surg Br 1990;72-B(4). https://doi.org/10.1302/0301-620X.72B4.2116416.

57. Weber BG, Simpson LA. Corrective lengthening osteotomy of the fibula. Clin Orthop Relat Res 1985;199:61–7.

58. Chu A, Weiner L. Distal Fibula Malunions. J Am Acad Orthop Surg 2009;17(4). https://doi.org/10.5435/00124635-200904000-00003.

59. Menelaus MB. INJURIES OF THE ANTERIOR INFERIOR TIBIO-FIBULAR LIGAMENT. ANZ J Surg 1961;30(4). https://doi.org/10.1111/j.1445-2197.1961.tb03125.x.

60. Stamatis ED, Cooper PS, Myerson MS. Supramalleolar Osteotomy for the Treatment of Distal Tibial Angular Deformities and Arthritis of the Ankle Joint. Foot Ankle Int 2003;24(10). https://doi.org/10.1177/107110070302401004.

61. Knupp M, Stufkens SAS, Bolliger L, et al. Classification and Treatment of Supramalleolar Deformities. Foot Ankle Int 2011;32(11). https://doi.org/10.3113/FAI.2011.1023.

62. Pagenstert G, Leumann A, Hintermann B, et al. Sports and Recreation Activity of Varus and Valgus Ankle Osteoarthritis before and after Realignment Surgery. Foot Ankle Int 2008;29(10). https://doi.org/10.3113/FAI.2008.0985.
63. Ayyaswamy B, Jain N, Limaye R. Functional and radiological medium term outcome following supramalleolar osteotomy for asymmetric ankle arthritis- A case series of 33 patients. J Orthop 2020;21:500–6.
64. Wood PLR, Clough TM, Smith R. The present state of ankle arthroplasty. Foot Ankle Surg 2008;14(3). https://doi.org/10.1016/j.fas.2008.05.008.
65. Chopra V, Stone P, Ng A. Supramalleolar Osteotomies. Clin Podiatr Med Surg 2017;34(4):445–60.
66. Espinosa N. What Leads to Failure of Joint-preserving Surgery for Ankle Osteoarthritis? Foot Ankle Clin 2013;18(3). https://doi.org/10.1016/j.fcl.2013.06.014.

Joint Preservation for Posttraumatic Ankle Arthritis After Tibial Plafond Fracture

Xingchen Li, MD, Xiangyang Xu, MD, PhD*

KEYWORDS

- Malunited ankle fracture • Malunited tibial pilon • Posttraumatic ankle osteoarthritis
- Pathophysiology • Distal tibial plafond-plasty • Joint-preserving surgery

KEY POINTS

- Management of posttraumatic ankle arthritis due to tibial plafond fracture is technically demanding. Distal tibial plafond-plasty could be an alternative to preserve the ankle joint for young patients with limited ankle arthritis.
- The surgical principles are to realign the mechanical axis, reconstruct the articular surface of the distal tibial plafond, and achieve a congruent and stable ankle joint.
- In addition to the anteroposterior view of the ankle joint, the lateral view was also paramount for surgeons to fully evaluate the reduction quality intraoperatively and postoperatively.
- The revision procedures can be divided into 4 steps: osteotomy for exposure, articular surface reconstruction, bone grafting, and osteotomy fixation.

INTRODUCTION

Ankle osteoarthritis (OA), a debilitating disease that causes ankle pain and limitations in activities of daily living, is one of the most common reasons for visits at foot and ankle clinics. Unlike knee OA, trauma is the most common etiology for ankle OA, accounting for approximately 80%.[1] Malleolar fracture and tibial pilon fracture are typical intra-articular fractures, and open reduction and internal fixation are the gold standard and indicated for those with displaced fractures.

Although the development of ankle OA after fractures is the result of a combination of different etiologies, including fracture energy, fracture pattern, time between injury and initial operation, surgeon experience, reduction quality, patient age, and so forth,[2] residual articular step-off is the most common reason for posttraumatic ankle OA.[1]

Department of Orthopaedics, Ruijin Hospital, Shanghai Jiaotong University School of Medicine, No. 999, Xiwang Road, Jiading District, Shanghai, China
* Corresponding author.
E-mail address: xu664531@126.com

Foot Ankle Clin N Am 27 (2022) 73–90
https://doi.org/10.1016/j.fcl.2021.11.005
1083-7515/22/© 2021 Elsevier Inc. All rights reserved.
foot.theclinics.com

Any imperfect reduction leads to joint incongruency and articular step-off, which further causes stress concentration within the ankle joint, damaging the cartilage upon weight-bearing.[3,4] Thus, surgical intervention is often indicated for patients with residual articular step-off, except for those with absolute contraindications. It is far more preferable to anatomically reconstruct the malunited ankle to a normal alignment than to allow weight-bearing on the incongruent ankle joint until joint sacrificing procedures are indicated.[5,6]

In this article, we focused on the discussion about malunited distal tibial plafond fractures and our clinical experience in managing these patients. Based on the major deformity that the patients presented, we classified them into the following 3 categories: varus deformity, valgus deformity, and anterior translation. We also introduced the major surgical principles and joint-preserving techniques in this article.

PATHOMECHANISM
Varus Deformity

According to the Lauge-Hansen Classification, patients with supination-adduction-type ankle fractures sustain an adduction force. Damage to the lateral ligaments and lateral malleolus may occur initially. If the force goes on, the vertical load can continue to invert the talus and cause impactions on the medial tibial plafond and generate a characteristic vertical medial malleolar fracture.[7,8] As the medial malleolar fracture line is vertical, the medial malleolar fragment has the potential to migrate proximally when screws are introduced at an angle because of the shear force. In addition, the impacted medial tibial plafond should also be reduced, and bone grafts are often needed to fill the gap. Upon failure to pay special attention to this injury mechanism, the potential shear force may lead to improper use of internal fixations, wrong placement of the malleolar screws, and inadequate reduction of the medial impaction, which can result in malunion of the medial malleolus and varus ankle deformity (**Fig. 1**).[9]

Valgus Deformity

Fibular malunion is the most common scenario for patients with malunited malleolar fractures.[10] At the emergency, when the initial x-rays show minor displacement of the ankle fracture, doctors or patients may choose conservative treatments with a short leg cast and pay little attention to their fractures. In China, some obstinate patients prefer to treat fractures with external applications of Chinese medicine and splints regardless of the significant displacement of the fractures. However, as bimalleolar or trimalleolar ankle fractures are very unstable, a short leg cast or splint is not reliable enough to stabilize the fractures and often results in significant ankle malunion. The lateral malleolus is often externally rotated and shortened, the talus is laterally shifted and tilted (**Fig. 2**), distal tibiofibular syndesmosis may be widened, the medial malleolus is also shifted laterally or the medial clear space is widened.[10–12] Because of osseous valgus configuration of the talus, despite the greater range of inversion at the subtalar joint, the valgus deformity at the ankle joint is poorly compensated through the subtalar motion.[13] Weight-bearing may even exacerbate valgus deformities, accelerating degenerative changes in the ankle joint. Prolonged weight-bearing may eventually cause erosion of the cartilage and impaction on the lateral distal tibial plafond.

Syndesmosis malreduction is also among the most common reasons for valgus deformity. This can be both the reason and the result of fibular malreduction. For patients with severe open fractures, Kirschner wires or external fixations are often used

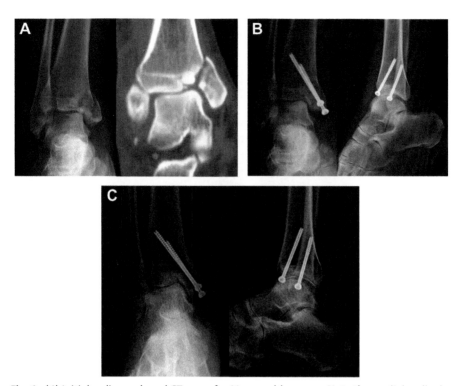

Fig. 1. (A) Initial radiograph and CT scan of a 41-year-old woman. Note the medial malleolar fracture with impaction on the medial tibial plafond. (B) Immediate radiographs after fracture fixation. Two oblique screws were used for fracture fixation. (C) Four months after initial operation. Weight-bearing radiographs showed varus ankle malalignment with medial tibial plafond impaction.

for temporary fixation of the fractures. The initial open reduction and internal fixation are often delayed because of soft tissue compromise. Inadequate exposure and debridement of the scar tissue at the syndesmosis lead to malreduction and diastasis. Syndesmotic screws, so-called position screws, should be inserted only when the syndesmosis is anatomically reduced,[14] and surgeons should never use syndesmotic screws as a reduction tool with the expectation that introduction of the screws can reduce distal tibiofibular diastasis. In addition, insertion of the screw through the hole may often cause malreduction of the diastasis. As the syndesmotic screws should be placed at 25° to 30° relative to the coronal plane, surgeons would find it very difficult to achieve this angle when introducing the syndesmotic screws through the holes on the fibular plate (**Fig. 10B**). The inappropriate direction of the syndesmotic screws leads to translation and rotation of the distal fibula, leading to syndesmosis malreduction.

Although osteochondral fragments or soft tissue incarcerations are rare in ankle fractures, it is important to remember that incarcerations could play a role in certain irreducible ankle fractures.[15] The incarcerations are often neglected during the initial open reduction and internal fixation. Patients often complain of significant pain and restriction of ankle motion after surgery, and equinus and claw toe deformities can occur for patients with posterior tibialis tendon incarceration.[16] Anatomic reduction of the ankle and malleolus is almost impossible, as the incarceration is not addressed.

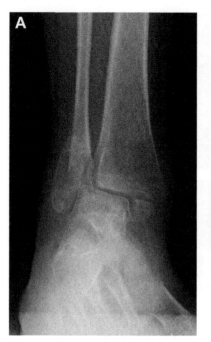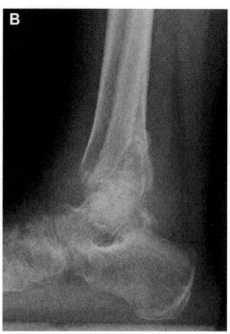

Fig. 2. Radiographs of a 31-year-old woman. (*A*) Weight-bearing anteroposterior view of the ankle joint. (*B*) Lateral view. She had a malunited Weber B ankle fracture. Note that the fibula was shortened and externally rotated, the talus was laterally shifted and tilted, and the medial malleolus was also shifted laterally.

In addition, the valgus fracture pattern of the distal tibial pilon can also result in valgus deformity of the ankle (**Fig. 3**). The lateral shoulder of the talus impacts the distal tibial plafond. As the tibial plafond fragments are impacted proximally, the talus remains in the valgus position within the ankle mortise. Any imperfect reduction of the impacted fragments leads to residual valgus deformity of the ankle.[17]

Anterior Translation Deformity of the Talus

Pilon fractures often involve high energy with metaphyseal comminution and significant displacement of articular fragments. The anterior distal tibial plafond provides stability for the ankle joint in the sagittal plane. The highly comminuted nature of pilon fractures and extensive stripping of periosteum causes bone healing problems and result in nonunion of these fragments.[18]

It is also critical to keep in mind that these fractures may need a much longer time to heal; thus, premature weight-bearing exercise after initial open reduction and internal fixation can lead to reduction loss of the impacted fragments (**Fig. 4**).

In addition, anterior translation is also seen in Weber type C ankle fractures. This particular type of ankle fracture is potentially very unstable and correlates with inferior clinical outcome.[19] Any inadequate reduction or fixation of syndesmosis, fibula, posterior or medial malleolus may result in residual anterior translation of the ankle.[20] These patients do not initially have anterior tibial plafond fractures; however, they develop impaction in this area postoperatively (see **Fig. 10**). We assume that the cyclic

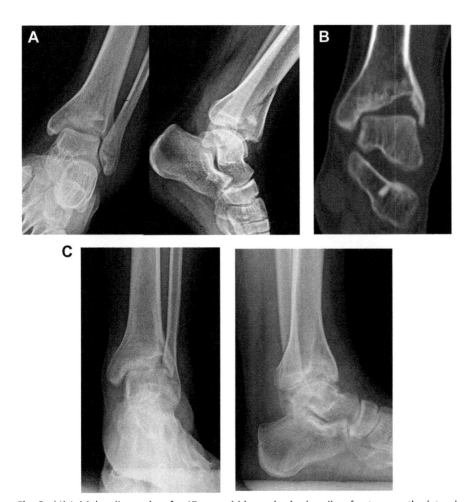

Fig. 3. (A) Initial radiographs of a 17-year-old boy who had a pilon fracture on the lateral tibial plafond. (B, C) He preferred conservative treatment with a short leg cast. At 9 months after the initial injury, the weight-bearing radiographs showed valgus ankle malalignment with articular impaction on the lateral tibial plafond.

loading of translated talus onto the anterior part of the distal tibial plafond may be the reason for developing impaction.

A lateral view of the ankle is often paramount for intraoperative reduction evaluation.[21] The surgeon would make an incorrect decision if he or she were satisfied with the anteroposterior (AP) view only. This view could be almost normal, whereas the anterior translation could be remarkable on the lateral view. Failure to recognize this pathology intraoperatively might predispose the patient to anterior translation after initial fracture fixation.

INDICATIONS AND CONTRAINDICATIONS

Age and the severity of posttraumatic ankle OA are 2 major factors that surgeons should consider when making decisions. Young and active patients (<55 years old), grade 1 to 3 OA according to the Kellgren-Lawrence classification,[22] and good

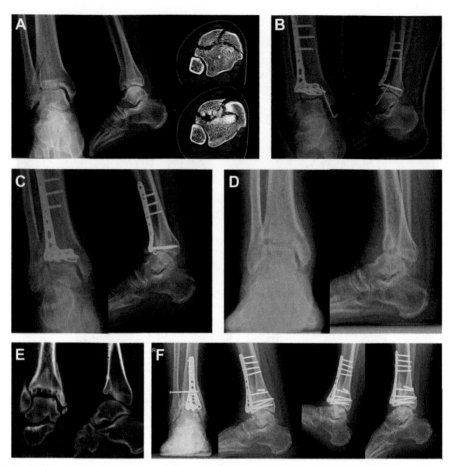

Fig. 4. (A) Initial radiographs and CT scans of a 35-year-old man. He had a pilon fracture on the anterior and anteromedial tibial plafond. (B) Immediate radiographs after fracture fixation. The ankle joint was normal. (C) Eight months after initial operation. The reduction failed, and the ankle was anteriorly translated. (D, E) Weight-bearing radiographs and CT scans 11 months after the initial operation. The hardware was removed 10 months after fracture fixation. Noting the anterior translation of the talus with impaction on the anterior tibial plafond. (F) Sixteen months after revision operation. Although osteoarthritis did exist, the ankle was normally aligned with a good range of motion.

bone quality are indications for joint-preserving surgery. Contraindications include elderly patients (>55 years old), end-stage OA (grade 4), osteoporosis, and other comorbidities, such as diabetes, peripheral vascular disorders, and smoking.

PREOPERATIVE PLANNING

Patients' history of their initial injury is essential to evaluate the energy that is involved. We normally require the patients to provide their radiological films as much as possible, especially the initial x-rays or computed tomography (CT) scans at the emergency. Initial radiographs are paramount to analyze the injury mechanism and develop thoughtful treatment protocols.

Physical examination should include the patient's soft tissue and alignment. A poor soft tissue envelope is often anticipated for patients with initial polytrauma or open fractures. The initial surgical incisions should be well recorded. Normally, we make previous incisions for our revision operations; however, when the initial incision cannot meet the demand for adequate exposure during the operation, new surgical incisions should be thoughtfully designed with respect to the initial incisions and the soft tissue envelope.

Weight-bearing x-rays, including the AP, mortise, lateral, and Saltzman's views, are obtained for each individual for the assessment of mechanical alignment. CT scans with axial, sagittal, coronal views, and 3-dimensional reconstruction are paramount for decision-making about the surgical approach. The fracture pattern and die punch fragments can be well identified and evaluated by analyzing different planes of CT scans. The selection of the surgical approach mainly depends on the location of major fragments.

In addition, preoperative communication with the patients and their major family members is crucial. They should be fully informed about their current health conditions, our surgical philosophy, and the possibility to develop end-stage ankle OA, which may end up with joint-sacrificing procedures. It is quite important to gain their trust and understanding before the operation.

SURGICAL TECHNIQUE
Principles

The aim of realignment surgery is to preserve the ankle joint. The major surgical principles are to realign the mechanical axis of the distal tibial plafond in both the coronal and sagittal planes, reconstruct the articular surface of the distal tibial plafond, and achieve a congruent and stable ankle joint. Although different approaches are used based on the major impaction location, revision surgery for malunited distal tibial plafond fractures can be summarized in the following 4 major steps:

Step 1: Osteotomy for exposure. Osteotomy is often mandatory for the further exposure of impacted articular fragments.

Step 2: Articular surface reconstruction. Once the impacted articular fragment is fully exposed, a second osteotomy is performed over the subchondral bone of the impacted area with small chisels to reduce the step-off until a congruent ankle joint is achieved.

Step 3: Bone graft. A structural bone graft is inserted into the osteotomy gap. Bone grafts are usually harvested from the iliac crest, or a structural allograft is used.

Step 4: Fixation. The distal tibial fragment is reduced and fixed with buttress plates or cannulated screws.

The incisions should be carefully designed before the revision operation. The initial incisions, soft tissue envelope, and location of major fragments are all factors that the surgeon should consider when making decisions about the surgical approach.[23] For most cases, we prefer to use initial incisions. However, for patients with anterior distal tibial plafond impactions, the initial incisions are mainly made on the medial and lateral sides of the ankle. In this situation, the new anterior incision is much more straightforward for exposure of the major fragments, and it is easier to place the buttress plate for further stabilization.

Extensive soft tissue release is often mandatory to anatomically reduce the ankle joint. Extensive scar formation and adhesion of soft tissue are often anticipated for patients with malunited ankle fractures. For patients with anterior translation of the talus, adequate posterior joint capsule release is often required. Achilles tendon lengthening may also be needed for prolonged equinus deformity.[24] For patients with malunited medial and lateral malleoli, the medial and lateral clear space should be explored and debrided extensively. Extensive debridement and release are often indicated for malreduced distal tibiofibular syndesmosis. For malunited pilon fractures with severe impaction on the distal tibial plafond, sometimes one-stage open reduction and internal fixation are impossible because of joint contracture. A staged treatment protocol is advocated by using external fixation for ankle distraction. Ankle distraction is used to make space for the subsequent anatomic reduction of the impacted distal tibial plafond.

The reduction should be carried out based on the reverse injury mechanism. Thus, it is extremely critical for surgeons to understand the patient's injury mechanism. Severe displacement and bone remodeling are anticipated for the same cases, and it is extremely difficult to determine the anatomic landmark for reduction. In this situation, we find it much easier to take anatomic restoration of the tibiotalar joint as the priority immediately following osteotomies of the initial fracture lines. For tibial pilon and malleolar fractures, the talar dome is often intact and should be anatomically reduced within the ankle mortise (see **Fig. 10**E). Then, the distal tibial fragments or the malleolus are reduced according to the contour of the talar dome until a congruent ankle joint is achieved.

Patient Positioning

The patient is placed in the supine position, and general anesthesia is routinely performed with a popliteal block to control pain after the operation. A pneumatic thigh tourniquet is routinely used to control bleeding.

The Medial Approach

A 10 cm longitudinal incision is made over the medial malleolus. The dissection continues down to the tibia, the anterior joint capsule is opened, and the posterior tibialis tendon is retracted posteriorly and protected. Medial malleolar osteotomy is performed to expose the medial impaction (**Fig. 5**). K-wires can be temporarily used for guidance of the osteotomy under fluoroscopy. The medial malleolus is turned distally to expose the impaction area. A second osteotomy is performed above the impaction, and the impacted articular fragment is reduced to achieve a congruent ankle joint under direct vision. A structural bone graft is inserted into the gap. If the patient does not have concomitant varus deformity of the distal tibial plafond, the medial malleolus is reduced anatomically and fixed with cannulated screws. A medial buttress plate is routinely used for final fixation. For patients with concomitant varus deformity of the distal tibial plafond, supramalleolar osteotomy is indicated to address varus malalignment. Supramalleolar osteotomy is routinely performed approximately 5 cm above the tip of the medial malleolus and directed to the lateral distal tibial plafond. A laminar spreader or K-wire spreader is used to open the osteotomy. A structural bone graft is inserted again to fill the gap. The width of the structural bone wedge is determined preoperatively according to the deformity. Finally, a medial buttress plate is used for the final fixation of the osteotomies.[9]

The Anterolateral Approach

The incision is made along the anterior crest of the fibula, extended distally to the joint level, and gently curved medially over the talus. The superficial peroneal nerve is identified and protected. Blunt dissection is carried over the anterolateral tibial plafond. Muscles and tendons of the anterior compartment together with the neurovascular bundle are retracted medially to access the Tillaux-Chaput fragment.[25,26] Osteotomy

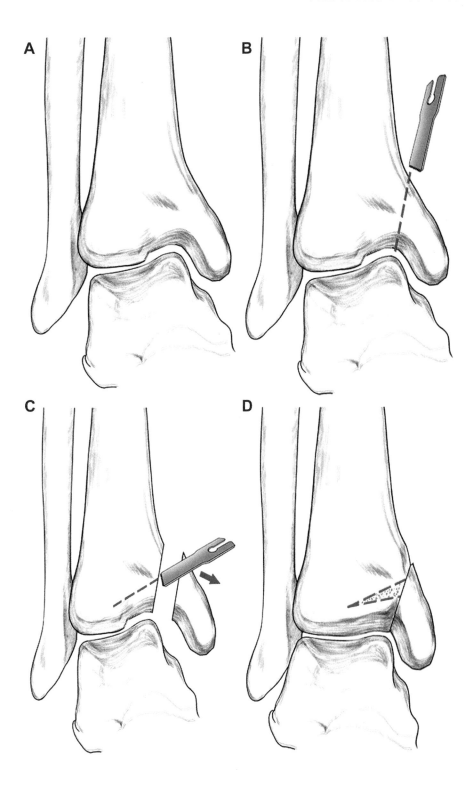

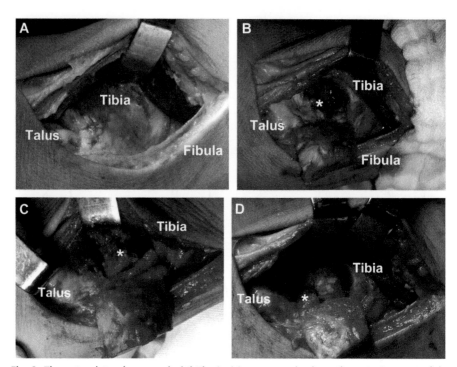

Fig. 6. The anterolateral approach. (*A*) The incision was made along the anterior crest of the fibula, went distally and gently curved medially over the talus. The muscles, tendons of the anterior compartment and the neurovascular bundle were retracted medially. (*B*) The osteotomy of the Tillaux-Chaput bone block was generated and turned laterally to expose the impacted articular fragment. The asterisk (*) indicated impacted articular fragment. (*C*) The articular surface was reconstructed under direct vision. (*D*) Bone graft was inserted into the osteotomy gap.

is carried out to generate the Tillaux-Chaput bone block using an oscillating saw.[27] The width, depth, and height of the bone block are determined according to the assessment of preoperative CT scans. Then, the Tillaux-Chaput bone block is turned laterally for exposure of the impacted articular surface. The articular surface is reduced, and a bone graft is inserted, as described previously (**Fig. 6**). Finally, the Tillaux-Chaput fragment is placed back to its anatomic position and fixed with cannulated screws or buttress plates.

The Transfibular Approach

The authors introduce the transfibular approach for the management of posterior malleolar malunion in this section. The posterior malleolus and the articular step-off can be

Fig. 5. Schematic drawing of the medial approach for distal tibial plafond-plasty. (*A*) Impaction was on the medial distal tibial plafond. (*B*) Medial malleolar osteotomy was performed as indicated by the red dashed line for the exposure of articular impaction. (*C*) A second osteotomy as indicated by the red dashed line was carried out, and the articular surface was reconstructed until a congruent ankle joint was achieved under direct vision. (*D*) A bone graft was inserted to fill the osteotomy gap, and the medial malleolus was reduced.

fully exposed when the distal fibula is retracted posteriorly.[28,29] A lateral incision is made along the fibular, and blunt dissection is continued down to the fibula. Most patients tend to have malunited posterolateral malleoli concomitant with lateral malleolar fracture. The former fibular fracture line is identified. If the fracture has already healed, osteotomy is often required. An oblique osteotomy is often used for Weber B fractures, whereas transverse osteotomy is used for Weber C fractures.[10] For oblique osteotomy, the posterolateral malleolus is exposed under direct vision when the distal fibula was retracted posteriorly. For malunited Weber C fractures, malreduction of the syndesmosis is always anticipated. Extensive soft tissue release at the syndesmosis is often mandatory for exposure of the posterior malleolus. After the identification of articular step-off of the posterolateral malleolus, osteotomy along the former fracture line is needed if the fragment has healed, which can be done under the guidance of fluoroscopy (**Fig. 7**). Then, a wide osteotomy is used to release the fragment, which is reduced under direct vision until a congruent joint surface is achieved. Cannulated screws or buttress plates are used for fixation of the posterolateral fragment (**Fig. 8**). Finally, the fibula is reconstructed and fixed with a plate. Syndesmotic screws are indicated for Weber C fractures.

The Anterior Approach

A 10 cm anterior incision is made lateral to the anterior tibialis tendon. The tendon sheath and the neurovascular bundle are carefully protected and retracted. The blunt dissection is performed immediately down to the anterior surface of the distal tibia. The anterior distal tibial plafond and talar dome are fully exposed by opening the anterior joint capsule.

For patients with prolonged anterior translation of the talus, adequate soft tissue release around the ankle is often mandatory to achieve anatomic reduction of the ankle joint (**Fig. 9**). Once the talus is reduced back to its anatomic position, K-wires are temporarily introduced to maintain the reduction. Another K-wire is used to indicate the direction of the osteotomy from the superior anterior to the apex of the

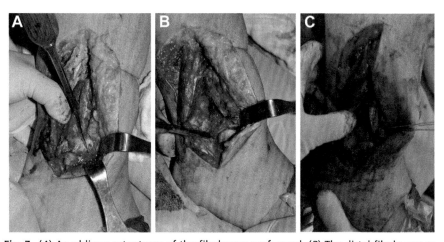

Fig. 7. (*A*) An oblique osteotomy of the fibula was performed. (*B*) The distal fibula was retracted posteriorly with excellent exposure of the lateral aspect of the distal tibial plafond. Noting the articular step-off of the tibial plafond. (*C*) Osteotomy of the posterior malleolus was carried out, and the articular surface was reconstructed and fixed with screws in the anteroposterior direction.

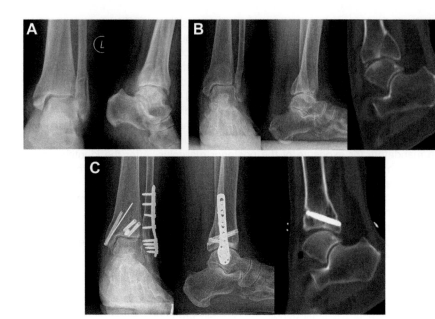

Fig. 8. (*A*) Initial radiographs of a 50-year-old woman. She had a trimalleolar fracture. (*B*) Weight-bearing radiographs and CT scan after 6 months of conservative treatment. Noting the articular step-off of the posterior malleolus. (*C*) Weight-bearing radiographs and CT scan at 16 months after revision operation.

impacted area under fluoroscopy. Anterior distal tibial osteotomy is performed with an oscillating saw. Sagittal cuts on the medial and lateral sides of the anterior distal tibia might be needed to separate the fragment. The distal fragment is turned distally to expose the impacted articular surface. After the identification of major impaction, the articular surface is reduced, and a bone graft is inserted, as described previously. The anterior distal tibial fragment is slid distally until a congruent ankle joint is achieved. This must be confirmed intraoperatively under fluoroscopy. An allograft is inserted into the osteotomy gap, and K-wires are used for temporary fixation. Excessive bone is resected to match the contour of the anterior tibial surface. Cannulated screws and anterior buttress plates are used to secure the osteotomy (**Fig. 10**).

The Use of External Fixators

For patients with severe impaction of the distal tibial plafond, reduction is impossible because of severe contracture of the ankle joint after impaction. In this circumstance, we prefer to treat the patient in a staged manner with external fixators. Ankle distraction is carried out with external fixators to make space for future reduction.

The external fixator system consists of 2 tibial rings, a proximal ring and a middle ring, a unilateral frame connecting the 2 tibial rings, a foot half-ring, 4 struts, and 2 hinges connecting the tibial ring and the foot half-ring. A temporary K-wire is introduced from the tip of the medial malleolus to the tip of the lateral malleolus to simulate the axis of ankle motion. Two pins are introduced into the calcaneus from the medial to lateral side, and another 2 pins are introduced into the midfoot and metatarsal bones. The middle ring and the foot half-ring are connected with 2 hinges to ensure that the rotation axis of the ankle is coordinated with the rotation axis of the hinges. Four struts are used to adjust the ankle to a neutralized position, 2 in front and the other 2 in back

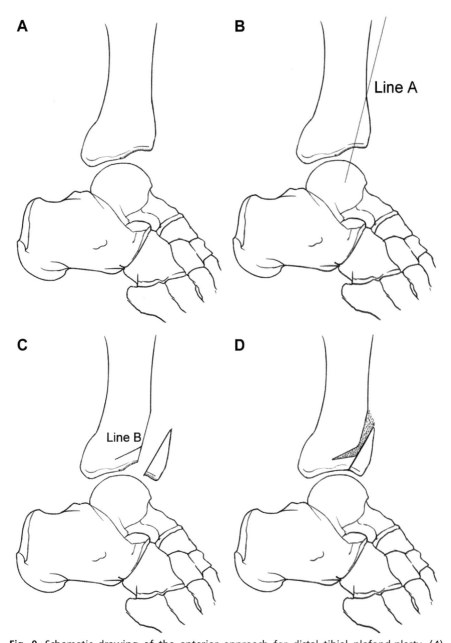

Fig. 9. Schematic drawing of the anterior approach for distal tibial plafond-plasty. (*A*) Impaction on the anterior distal tibial plafond was significant after the talus was reduced back to its anatomic position. (*B*) An anterior distal tibial osteotomy was carried out along line A for exposure of articular impaction. (*C*) A second osteotomy (*line* B) was performed, and the articular surface was reconstructed under direct vision. (*D*) The anterior distal tibial fragment was slid distally until a congruent ankle joint was achieved.

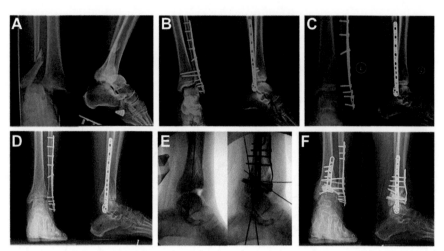

Fig. 10. (*A*) Initial radiographs of a 28-year-old man who had a Weber C ankle open fracture. The fracture was temporarily fixed with K-wires and calcaneal distraction. (*B*) Immediate radiographs after fracture fixation, which was carried out 12 days after initial injury because of soft tissue compromise. Noting the malreduction of the fibula and the ankle was anterior translated on the lateral view. The 2 syndesmotic screws were inserted through the fibular plate. (*C*) The syndesmotic screws were removed 40 days after fracture fixation. Noting the ankle remained anteriorly translated even though the syndesmotic screws were removed. The distal tibial plafond was normal at this point. (*D*) Weight-bearing radiographs at 10 months after fracture fixation. Noting the anterior distal tibial plafond became impacted, and the ankle was anteriorly translated. (*E*) Intraoperative fluoroscopy at the revision operation. The impaction was remarkable when the anteriorly translated talus was reduced back to its anatomic position. The articular surface was reconstructed by anterior distal tibial plafond-plasty. (*F*) Eighteen months after revision operation. The ankle was normally aligned.

(**Fig. 11**). Distraction is initiated 3 days after the operation with 1 mm of distraction per day. The distraction is evaluated under fluoroscopy. Based on our experience, we prefer to overdistract the ankle by approximately 5 mm, which makes the following procedures much easier. We prefer to maintain the external fixator for approximately 1 month. Definitive surgery is carried out immediately after the removal of external fixator, preventing recurrence of joint contracture. Thus, a circumspect planning of pin sites is of paramount importance. The authors do not use external fixators after revision operation. However, when the patient shows severe osteoporosis and the fragment fixations are not strong enough to maintain the reduction, the authors advocate the use of external fixators for another 4 to 6 weeks after revision to prevent reduction loss.

POSTOPERATIVE CARE

The ankle is immobilized in a neutral position with a well-padded, short leg splint. The wound is inspected on the second day after the operation, and the splint is replaced by a walking boot. Non–weight-bearing active range of motion exercise of the toes, ankle, and knee joint is encouraged as soon as the patient was tolerated. If the authors feel the ankle is not stable during the operation, 2 ankle-spanning K-wires are used to temporarily fix the ankle in the neutral position for 3 weeks. Partial weight-bearing exercises are initiated at 6 weeks after operation under the protection of walking boots

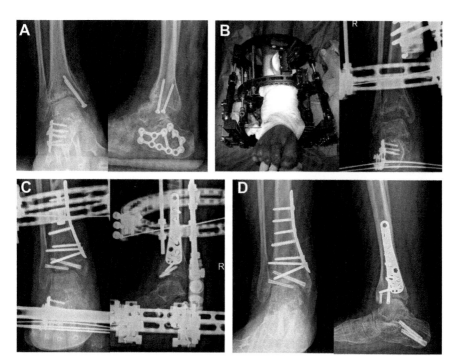

Fig. 11. Weight-bearing radiographs of a 15-year-old girl at 6 months after initial injury. (*A*) She had a malunited pilon fracture and calcaneal fracture. Noting the severe varus deformity and impaction on the distal tibial plafond. (*B*) External fixators were applied because of severe ankle contracture. The ankle was distracted to make adequate space for reduction. (*C*) Immediate radiographs after revision operation. The external fixators were applied again to decompress and maintain the reduction. (*D*) Weight-bearing radiographs at 2 years after revision operation.

and crutches or walking aids. Rehabilitation gradually progresses to full weight-bearing 3 months after the operation. For patients with highly comminuted fractures of the distal tibial plafond, the delayed union or nonunion rate is potentially high, and the authors advocate initiating weight-bearing exercise until 3 months after the operation.

CLINICAL RESULTS IN THE LITERATURE

In 2016, Weber and colleagues[30] published a detailed review about malunited malleolar fractures, and the authors concluded that midterm and long-term outcomes of joint-preserving osteotomies for malunited malleolar fractures are satisfactory, with good and very good results ranging from 67% to 91%. Rammelt and colleagues[6] also published important literature about joint-preserving osteotomies for malunited tibial pilons. The authors extensively introduced joint-preserving osteotomies for both extra-articular and intra-articular deformities after malunited tibial pilon. Fourteen patients were included with a mean follow-up duration of 5 years. The good and excellent rate was 71.4%.

In 2018, we reported a supramalleolar osteotomy combined with distal tibial plafond-plasty in the coronal plane,[9] and 24 patients were followed with a mean follow-up duration of 45.2 months. According to Weber's classification, 10 had type A fractures, and 14 had type B fractures. Both the radiological and ankle functional scores showed significant differences between the preoperative and follow-up assessments. One patient underwent ankle arthrodesis, and 1 patient received ankle joint distraction after the procedure. Most recently, we reported anterior distal tibial plafond-plasty in the sagittal plane.[31] A total of 21 patients were followed with a mean follow-up of 34 months. Sixteen patients had pilon fractures, whereas 5 patients had Weber type C ankle fractures. Of the 21 patients, 18 showed improvement in or no worsening of ankle OA on the sagittal plane, whereas 3 developed advanced ankle OA.

SUMMARY

Posttraumatic ankle arthritis after malunited distal tibial plafond fractures can be salvaged by distal tibial plafond-plasty. The principles for the joint-preserving operation are to realign the mechanical axis, reconstruct the articular surface, and achieve a congruent and stable ankle joint. The revision procedures can be divided into the following 4 steps: osteotomy for exposure, articular surface reconstruction, bone grafting, and osteotomy fixation.

CLINICS CARE POINT

- Management for posttraumatic ankle arthritis is clinically challenging, the best treatment is to prevent it at primary surgery. Weight-bearing AP and lateral radiographs, CT scans are often mandatory for the evaluation of deformity, key fragment identification and surgical approach selection. The principles for joint-preserving operation are to realign the mechanical axis, reconstruct the articular surface, and achieve a congruent and stable ankle joint. The revision procedures can be divided into the following 4 steps: osteotomy for exposure, articular surface reconstruction, bone grafting, and osteotomy fixation. Posttraumatic ankle arthritis after malunited distal tibial plafond fractures can be salvaged by distal tibial plafond-plasty for carefully selected patients.

DISCLOSURE

This study was supported by a grant from the National Natural Science Foundation of China (no. 81772372).

REFERENCES

1. Nwankwo EC Jr, Labaran LA, Athas V, et al. Pathogenesis of posttraumatic osteoarthritis of the ankle. Orthop Clin North Am 2019;50(4):529–37.
2. Horisberger M, Valderrabano V, Hintermann B. Posttraumatic ankle osteoarthritis after ankle-related fractures. J Orthop Trauma 2009;23(1):60–7.
3. Ramsey PL, Hamilton W. Changes in tibiotalar area of contact caused by lateral talar shift. J Bone Joint Surg Am 1976;58(3):356–7.
4. Berkes MB, Little MT, Lazaro LE, et al. Articular congruity is associated with short-term clinical outcomes of operatively treated SER IV ankle fractures. J Bone Joint Surg Am 2013;95(19):1769–75.
5. Branfoot T. Revision of malunited ankle fractures. Clin Podiatr Med Surg 2004; 21(3):385–391vii.

6. Rammelt S, Zwipp H. Intra-articular osteotomy for correction of malunions and nonunions of the tibial pilon. Foot Ankle Clin 2016;21(1):63–76.
7. Lauge-Hansen N. Fractures of the ankle. II. Combined experimental-surgical and experimental-roentgenologic investigations. Arch Surg 1950;60(5):957–85.
8. Haller JM, Ross H, Jacobson K, et al. Supination adduction ankle fractures: Ankle fracture or pilon variant? Injury 2020;51(3):759–63.
9. Guo C, Liu Z, Xu Y, et al. Supramalleolar osteotomy combined with an intra-articular osteotomy for the reconstruction of malunited medial impacted ankle fractures. Foot Ankle Int 2018;39(12):1457–63.
10. Egger AC, Berkowitz MJ. Operative treatment of the malunited fibula fracture. Foot Ankle Int 2018;39(10):1242–52.
11. Marti RK, Raaymakers EL, Nolte PA. Malunited ankle fractures. The late results of reconstruction. J Bone Joint Surg Br 1990;72(4):709–13.
12. Mosca M, Buda R, Ceccarelli F, et al. Ankle joint re-balancing in the management of ankle fracture malunion using fibular lengthening: prospective clinical-radiological results at mid-term follow-up. Int Orthop 2020;45(2):411–7.
13. Krahenbuhl N, Siegler L, Deforth M, et al. Subtalar joint alignment in ankle oste-oarthritis. Foot Ankle Surg 2019;25(2):143–9.
14. Solan MC, Davies MS, Sakellariou A. Syndesmosis stabilisation: screws versus flexible fixation. Foot Ankle Clin 2017;22(1):35–63.
15. Ermis MN, Yagmurlu MF, Kilinc AS, et al. Irreducible fracture dislocation of the ankle caused by tibialis posterior tendon interposition. J Foot Ankle Surg 2010; 49(2):166–71.
16. Anderson JG, Hansen ST. Fracture-dislocation of the ankle with posterior tibial tendon entrapment within the tibiofibular interosseous space: a case report of a late diagnosis. Foot Ankle Int 1996;17(2):114–8.
17. Zelle BA, Dang KH, Ornell SS. High-energy tibial pilon fractures: an instructional review. Int Orthop 2019;43(8):1939–50.
18. Cinats DJ, Stone T, Viskontas D, et al. Osteonecrosis of the distal tibia after pilon fractures. Foot Ankle Surg 2020;26(8):895–901.
19. Warner SJ, Schottel PC, Hinds RM, et al. Fracture-dislocations demonstrate poorer postoperative functional outcomes among pronation external rotation IV ankle fractures. Foot Ankle Int 2015;36(6):641–7.
20. Perera A, Myerson M. Surgical techniques for the reconstruction of malunited ankle fractures. Foot Ankle Clin 2008;13(4):737–751, ix.
21. Guo C, Zhu Y, Hu M, et al. Reliability of measurements on lateral ankle radio-graphs. BMC Musculoskelet Disord 2016;17:297.
22. Kellgren JH, Lawrence JS. Radiological assessment of osteo-arthrosis. Ann Rheum Dis 1957;16(4):494–502.
23. Assal M, Ray A, Stern R. Strategies for surgical approaches in open reduction in-ternal fixation of pilon fractures. J Orthop Trauma 2015;29(2):69–79.
24. Younger A, Veljkovic A. Current update in total ankle arthroplasty: salvage of the failed total ankle arthroplasty with anterior translation of the talus. Foot Ankle Clin 2017;22(2):301–9.
25. Hickerson LE, Verbeek DO, Klinger CE, et al. Anterolateral approach to the pilon. J Orthop Trauma 2016;30(Suppl 2):S39–40.
26. Kim GB, Shon OJ, Park CH. Treatment of AO/OTA Type C pilon fractures through the anterolateral approach combined with the medial MIPO technique. Foot Ankle Int 2018;39(4):426–32.

27. Gianakos AL, Hannon CP, Ross KA, et al. Anterolateral tibial osteotomy for accessing osteochondral lesions of the talus in autologous osteochondral transplantation: functional and t2 MRI analysis. Foot Ankle Int 2015;36(5):531–8.

28. Gonzalez TA, Watkins C, Drummond R, et al. Transfibular approach to posterior malleolus fracture fixation: technique tip. Foot Ankle Int 2016;37(4):440–5.

29. Tosun B, Selek O. Lateral transfibular approach to tibial pilon fractures: a case report. J Am Podiatr Med Assoc 2019;109(6):459–62.

30. Weber D, Weber M. Corrective osteotomies for malunited malleolar fractures. Foot Ankle Clin 2016;21(1):37–48.

31. Li X, Xu Y, Guo C, et al. Anterior distal tibial plafond-plasty for the treatment of posttraumatic ankle osteoarthritis with anterior translation of the talus. Sci Rep 2021;11(1):4381.

Correction of the Valgus Ankle with a Joint Sparing Supra-Malleolar Osteotomy
The Modified Wiltse Technique

Ignatius P.S. Terblanche, MBChB, FCS(Orth)SA[a,b,*],
Jacques du Toit, MBChB, MSc Clin Epi, FCS(Orth)SA, PhD[a]

KEYWORDS

- Orthopaedic surgery • Valgus ankle deformity • Joint-sparing surgical treatment
- Wiltse osteotomy

KEY POINTS

- The reconstitution of normal anatomy in the presence of a valgus ankle deformity is complicated by the position of the Center of Rotation and Angulation (CORA), soft tissue limitations, and complexities related to achieving stable distal fixation.
- The Wiltse osteotomy correctly uses "osteotomy rule two" to reconstitute normal angular- and maintaining mechanical alignment.
- The reproduction of the preplanned "Wiltse Triangle" on the distal tibia allows for highly accurate correction, inherent stability, and coronal plane adaptability.

INTRODUCTION AND HISTORICAL OVERVIEW

The valgus ankle is a common cause of pain, deformity, and disability in the pediatric, adult, and geriatric population due to impaired ankle and/or foot mechanics.[1-3] The "valgus ankle" could present as a relatively simple coronal plane deformity or as a more complex multiplanar deformity around the ankle joint. The deformity might be situated supramalleolar, within the ankle joint or even the hindfoot. Additional deformities, joint instability, contractures, muscular imbalance as well as loss of motion within the ankle joint and/or the foot could further complicate the management thereof.[4]

[a] Division of Orthopaedic Surgery, Faculty of Medicine and Health Sciences, Stellenbosch University, Francie van Zijl Drive, Tygerberg 7505, South Africa; [b] CapeFootSurgery, Louis Leipoldt Mediclinic, Room 2057, 7 Broadway Street, Bellville West, Cape Town 7530, South Africa
* Corresponding author. CapeFootSurgery, Louis Leipoldt Mediclinic, Room 2057, 7 Broadway Street, Bellville West, Cape Town 7530, South Africa.
E-mail address: naas@footsurgery.co.za

Foot Ankle Clin N Am 27 (2022) 91–113
https://doi.org/10.1016/j.fcl.2021.11.004
1083-7515/22/© 2021 Elsevier Inc. All rights reserved.
foot.theclinics.com

Longitudinal studies evaluating the long-term outcome and sequela of valgus ankle malalignment are lacking.[2,5] Confounding factors of existing evidence include patient selection bias, a multitude of causes, slow deformity progression, early utilization of treatment, as well as the added complexities of the ankle joint anatomy and biomechanical considerations.[2] Additionally, the ankle is situated in close proximity to the foot that can either cause ankle deformities or structurally and functionally adapt to a valgus ankle, thereby rendering subtalar joint malposition and/or stiffness.[6]

Although several retrospective studies imply that mild to moderate valgus malalignment around the tibiotalar joint does not cause significant ankle arthritis and/or other secondary long-term sequelae,[2,7–9] other authors recommend early surgical correction for valgus deformities as little as 5°.[2,10] However, basic science studies,[2,11,12] the profound effect of fibular malalignment on the ankle mortise,[2,13] the risk of progression of valgus angulation[13,14] support early, aggressive correction.[2,6] In addition, the secondary effect on foot mobility and deformities and the known advantages of joint-sparing procedures, combined with mechanical axis realignment further suggest that an early and customized approach to those patients is beneficial in the long term.[15]

Surgical correction of a predominant coronal plane valgus supra-malleolar deformity without inherent contraindications for joint-sparing osteotomies can be achieved by different types of varus angulating osteotomies.[3,14,15]

- Medial closing wedge osteotomies
- Lateral opening wedge osteotomies
- Focal dome osteotomies.
- Minimally invasive Gigli saw osteotomies (frame assisted correction)

Each osteotomy has distinct advantages and disadvantages to consider when planning which osteotomy to use[5,10,15,16] (**Table 1**).

A multitude of stabilizing and fixation methods after performing a supramalleolar varus angulating osteotomy are available and determined by various factors:

- Patient preference, anxieties, or tolerance especially when external frame application is considered
- The physiologic age, functional demands and etiology of the valgus ankle in individualized patients
- The quality of the soft tissue envelope, vascular compromise, and presence of previous or current infection
- The need to simultaneously address leg length discrepancies
- The severity of the deformity
- The inherent stability of the specific osteotomy
- The presence or absence of protective sensation, for example, children with myelomeningocele.

Stabilizing and Fixation techniques include[15]:

- Kirschner-wires: frequently used in the pediatric population due to the potential for accelerated union in inherently stable osteotomies
- External fixators: typically used in multiplanar deformities, poor soft tissue, and/or loss of length
- Plate fixation: gold standard of fixation in the adult population when using acute corrections

The Wiltse Osteotomy, a modification of the wedge resection osteotomy, is a viable alternative for the treatment of valgus coronal plane deformities in and around the

Table 1
Advantages and disadvantages of different osteotomies for the correction of ankle valgus deformities[5,10,15,16]

Approach	Advantages	Disadvantages
Opening wedge	Straightforward preoperative planning	Delayed union
	Simple intraoperative technique	Soft tissue compromise
	Adds length	Unintentional mechanical axis translation (osteotomy rule 3)
Closing wedge	Straightforward preoperative planning	Loss of length
	Simple intraoperative technique	Unintentional mechanical axis translation (osteotomy rule 3)
	Inherent stability	
	Soft tissue friendly	
Dome	Inherent stability	Moderate technical complexity
	Maintaining mechanical axis (osteotomy rule 2)	Inability to address multiplanar deformities
	Length neutral	
Wiltse	Accurate preoperative planning	Moderate technical complexity
	Inherent stability	Inability to address multiplanar deformities
	Length neutral	
	Maintaining mechanical axis (osteotomy rule 2)	
	Applicable to large deformities	

tibiotalar joint.[17] Leon Wiltse, in 1972, observed that a simple wedge resection osteotomy causes mechanical axial malalignment with secondary medial translation of the tibiotalar joint and a prominent medial malleolus. By the resection of a triangular bone segment combined with a rotation of the distal fragment, he achieved mechanical axis realignment and an ankle with a more "normal appearance."[17] He additionally performed an oblique fibula osteotomy that maintained the integrity of the syndesmosis and allowed rotation of the ankle complex when correction the deformity.[17]

While not explicitly stated, Wiltse achieved the compensatory and corrective translation when an osteotomy is performed a distance away from the center of rotation of angulation (CORA) thus successfully and correctly using rule 2 of osteotomies (compensatory translation within the osteotomy site) and preventing osteotomy rule 3 (**Figs. 1** and **2**).[15,18]

Frequently used osteotomies for the treatment of a valgus ankle include medial closing wedge or lateral opening wedge osteotomies, performed proximal to the center of rotation of angulation. Although angular correction is achieved, a compensatory medial mechanical axis deviation with a prominent medial malleolus occurs (**Fig. 3**).

The dome osteotomy adheres to rule 2 and can simultaneously achieve angular correction as well as maintaining mechanical axis alignment (**Fig. 4**).[15,18]

When the predominant coronal plane valgus deformity is situated close to the ankle joint and/or within the hindfoot or is of considerable magnitude, it is frequently not possible to perform your osteotomy at the CORA and stabilizing your osteotomy

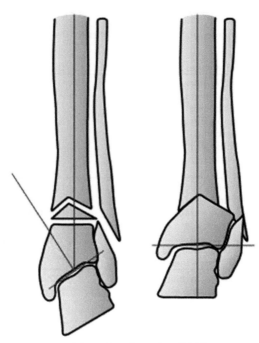

Fig. 1. The Wiltse osteotomy: excision of a triangular tibial bone segment and oblique osteotomy of the fibula. Rotation and translation of the distal tibial fragment within the apex of the triangle achieve normalization of the ankle. Correct utilization of rule 2 of osteotomies by the Wiltse technique corrects the valgus angulation as well as the mechanical axis of the ankle.

without compromising the tibiotalar joint or the physis in a child. The Wiltse osteotomy is an excellent alternative to achieve mechanical realignment (angulation and translation) even though the deformity is situated close to the ankle joint. Additional secondary advantages are inherent stability of the osteotomy, as well as early mobilization. The distal tibial and fibular physis is not compromised and the tibia-fibular relationship and syndesmoses remain unchanged. Additionally, the Wiltse osteotomy renders itself to allow accurate preoperative planning and templating and is adaptable to allow relative ease of intraoperative adjustment.

The goal of this article is to outline the indications/contraindications, preoperative and preprocedure planning, surgical technique, postoperative care, and surgical outcomes of the Wiltse Osteotomy.

INDICATIONS AND CONTRAINDICATIONS FOR THE WILTSE OSTEOTOMY

Indications:
- Developmental and congenital valgus deformities around the ankle
- Mild to moderate osteoarthritis and pain or local osteoarthritis predominantly situated in the lateral pillar of the ankle mortise
- Severe osteoarthritis combined with a large valgus deformity whereby mechanical realignment is indicated for preparation for a future total ankle arthroplasty
- Malunited distal tibial fractures around the supramalleolar area and/or extending intraarticular

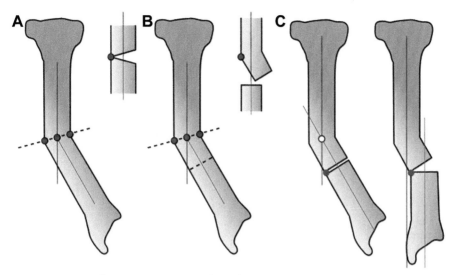

Fig. 2. The "rules of osteotomies" as popularized by Paley and colleagues (*A*) Osteotomy rule 1: The osteotomy is performed at the location of the center of rotation of angulation (CORA) and only requires angulation for reduction. (*B*) Osteotomy rule 2: The osteotomy is performed at a location other than the CORA, but the angulation correction axis (ACA) is located at the CORA, thus angulation around the site of the deformity and translation at the osteotomy is required for correct reduction of alignment. The Wiltse osteotomy frequently uses rule 2 to obtain a normal mechanical axis. (*C*) Osteotomy rule 3: The osteotomy is created away from both the CORA and ACA and will result in a secondary deformity – the ankle joint and the knee joint will be parallel, but a secondary translation deformity will be created.

- Malunited valgus ankle and/or subtalar arthrodesis
- Fixed abnormal valgus deformity of the subtalar joint and the surgery around the foot is contraindicated due to host, soft tissues, or certain congenital abnormalities

Contraindications:

- Multiplanar deformities in and around the ankle joint whereby the main deformity is in the sagittal plane
- Deformities less than 10° whereby the medial translation is neglectable (relative contraindication)
- Varus deformity

PREOPERATIVE PLANNING

A comprehensive clinical assessment, radiographic evaluation, and templating of a patient with an ankle valgus deformity is critical and is frequently complicated by the following factors and considerations:

Clinical Examination

- Etiology: The valgus ankle can be caused by developmental and congenital abnormalities, malunited distal tibia fractures, osteoarthritis, or postoperative sequelae of arthrodesis of the foot and/or ankle.[15] Host factors, for example, the skeletally immature patient with congenital abnormalities or poor local biology, needs to be carefully assessed

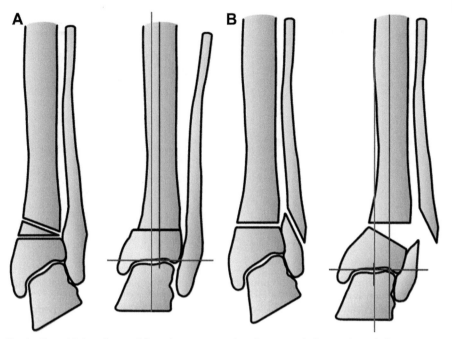

Fig. 3. Closed (*A*) and open (*B*) wedge osteotomies of a coronal plane valgus deformity in or around the ankle joint will result in a medial translational deformity, illustrating the concerns related to rule 3 of osteotomies.

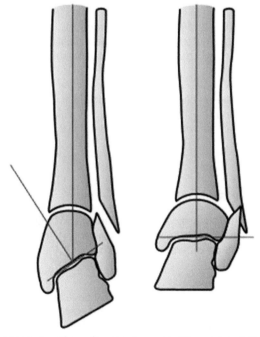

Fig. 4. The dome osteotomy allows for angular correction and maintains the mechanical axis.

- The future effect of growth on the deformity and the "at risk" anatomic position of the distal tibia and fibula physis
- Previous operations performed in and around the ankle and the affected lower limb
- Additional lower limb malalignment above or below the ankle. Severe rotational abnormalities should be clinically noted and measured as this will have a profound effect on the radiological evaluation and preoperative planning and templating.
- Poor mobility, contractures, and/or instability of the hip, knee, ankle, and/or subtalar joint. The range of movement of the ankle and the presence and type of Achilles tendon contracture should be assessed. The Silfverskiöld test should be performed to determine the need for a gastrocnemius slide (fractional lengthening of the gastroc-soleus complex)
- Muscular and tendinous imbalance due to congenital, traumatic, or degenerative causes
- A compromised soft tissue envelope in and around the ankle
- Previous surgical or posttraumatic scars that could compromise a standard surgical approach to the supramalleolar area.
- Neurovascular compromise
- Active or previous infection
- The magnitude and location of the deformity
- Presence or absence of compensating motion or deformity of adjacent joints, especially the subtalar joint. Should the subtalar joint be rigid and unable to accommodate the valgus correction, additional realignment foot osteotomy procedures may be required.

Preoperative Radiological Planning

Standardized radiological assessment is critical to enable the surgeon to detect and anticipate any additional deformities of the affected and unaffected lower limb via structured deformity analysis.[18] The presence of posttraumatic or procedural nonunions, previous hardware, and osteomyelitis or previous sequelae of septic arthritis needs to be noted. Radiographic evaluation of the ankle valgus deformity enables exact deformity location, the magnitude of the coronal, sagittal and axial deformity, and the integrity of the ankle joint and the fibular anatomy. Anatomically correct plain radiographs are also essential for preoperative templating and planning of the Wiltse Osteotomy.

Recommendations for radiographs depend on etiologic and host factors, with the typical workup including[18]:

- Full-length standing antero-posterior (AP) radiographs of both lower extremities
- AP radiograph of the ankle that includes the tibia (weight bearing)
- Lateral radiograph of the ankle that includes the tibia (weight bearing)
- AP, lateral, and mortise views of the ankle
- AP and lateral weight-bearing radiographs of the foot
- Hindfoot alignment views if clinically indicated

Magnetic resonance imaging (MRI) and/or computed tomography (CT) is usually not required but a CT scan for 3D printing of the deformity and a custom cutting block may be indicated.

Basic deformity analysis is conducted according to the method described by Paley and colleagues[19] to identify any additional malalignment deformities in the affected limb. Specifically exclude large sagittal plane deformities around the affected ankle that would contraindicate the use of a Wiltse Osteotomy.

Step 1: Basic Deformity Analysis of the Ankle Joint Using the AP Radiograph (Including the Distal Tibia)

- Insert the mid-diaphyseal longitudinal line to obtain the anatomic axis of the tibia **(Fig. 5)**
- Insert the ankle joint orientation line along the flat subchondral line of the tibial plafond and identify the ankle joint center (mid-width of the located talus or mid-width of the tibia and fibula) **(Fig. 6)**
- Draw and measure the normal LDTA angle (use the contralateral normal side or the accepted norm of ± 89°) (see **Fig. 6**)
- The abnormal joint orientation angle of the ankle (lateral distal tibial angle - LDTA) is measured (in this case identifying the magnitude of the valgus coronal plane deformity) **(Fig. 7)**
- The site of the valgus deformity is represented by the point whereby the anatomic axis line of the tibia and the longitudinal line of the normal LDTA transect. This may be located proximal, within, or distal to the ankle joint. The magnitude of the deformity that needs to be corrected to restore the normal LDTA is measured (see **Fig. 7**).

Step 2: Osteotomy Planning and Templating

- The Wiltse osteotomy planning is based on constructing a scalene "Wiltse Triangle". This triangle in which all 3 sides have different lengths and all 3 angles differ is influenced by the magnitude of the valgus deformity.
- The overarching aim for constructing the "Wiltse Triangle" is to determine the site of the osteotomy, to incorporate the deformity angle, and to define the correct placement of the apex of the triangle, thus predetermining the correct translation and restoring the mechanical axis. The base of the triangle is the leg perpendicular to the mechanical axis of the tibia **(Fig. 8)** By convention we place this base

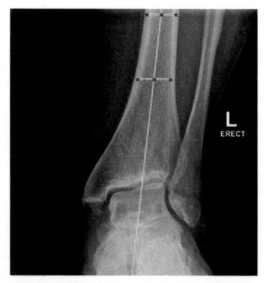

Fig. 5. Step 1 of preoperative templating: the mid-diaphyseal longitudinal line to obtain the anatomic axis of the tibia is inserted.

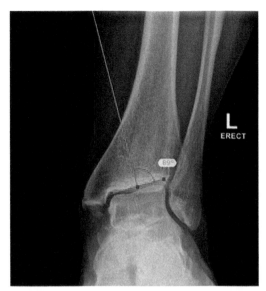

Fig. 6. The normal lateral distal tibial angle (LDTA) – 89°.

line just above the syndesmosis but as closely as possible to the articular surface to maintain and protect the integrity of the ankle mortise.
- The lateral base angle (LBA) is equal to the magnitude of the measured deformity in degrees, enabling correction of the angular deformity (**Fig. 9**).

Step 3: The Calculation of the Medial Base Angle

- The medial flare angle (MFA) is calculated by drawing a line parallel to the anatomic axis and traversing the base osteotomy line at the medial cortex. An additional angle line is drawn along the medial flare toward the area whereby the base osteotomy line crosses the aforementioned parallel line (**Fig. 10**)
- Calculation of the MBA - Accurate measurement of this angle allows the medial flare of the medial distal tibia to fit snugly on the superior medial leg of the osteotomy, thus replicating normal medial ankle anatomy.

$90° - (MFA + LBA) = MBA$ of the Wiltse triangle (**Fig. 11**)

The MBA line and the LBA line are extended to form the apex of the triangle. This angle's value is not important but the position within the tibia is essential to enable the accurate lateral translation of the distal fragment to maintain the mechanical axis. The Wiltse triangle is now complete (**Fig. 12**).

Preoperative templating of your chosen fixed-angle fixation plate is recommended.

SURGICAL TECHNIQUE & OUTCOMES

The patient is placed supine on a padded radiolucent table after which general anesthesia is used together with a regional, ultrasound-guided popliteal nerve block. Alternatively, according to host-specific preferences and/or risk factors, spinal/epidural anesthesia is used to provide intra and postoperative analgesia.

A bump is placed under the ipsilateral hip to rotate the lower limb with the patella facing anteriorly and a padded thigh tourniquet is applied to provide a bloodless field. The extremity is prepped above the level of the knee to assess limb alignment.

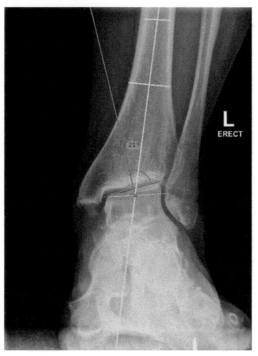

Fig. 7. Step 1 of preoperative templating: The magnitude of the valgus deformity is measured at 21°.

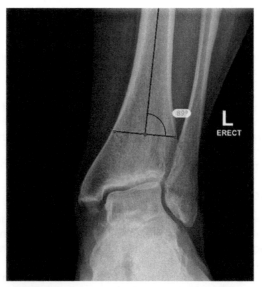

Fig. 8. Step 2 of preoperative templating: the transverse line represents the base of Wiltse's triangle and is situated immediately proximal to the syndesmosis.

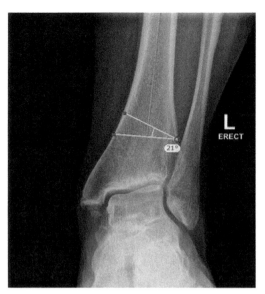

Fig. 9. Step 2 of preoperative templating: The lateral base angle (LBA) as indicated measuring 21°.

Fluoroscopy with sterile sleeves should be available from the start of the procedure to ensure correct positioning of the limb, to aid with the accurate placement of the Wiltse Triangle, performing the tibial and fibular osteotomies, evaluation of restoration of the normal mechanical axis, and correct and accurate fixation of the osteotomy (**Fig. 13**).

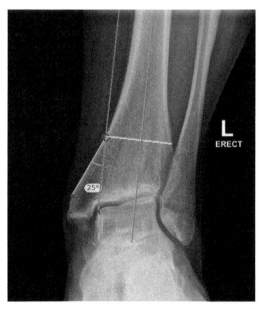

Fig. 10. Step 3 of preoperative templating: the medial flare angle (MFA) is calculated at 25°.

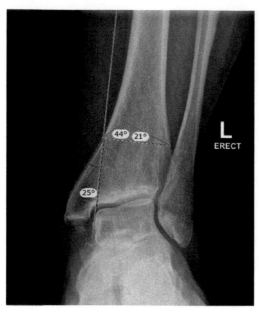

Fig. 11. Step 3 of preoperative templating: The Medial Base Angle (MBA) is calculated by subtracting the sum of the medial flare angle (MFA) and lateral base angle (LBA) from 90°: 90° − (25° + 21°) = 44°.

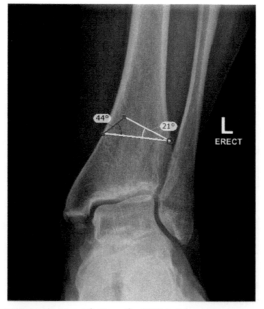

Fig. 12. Step 3 of preoperative templating: the Wiltse triangle is now completed.

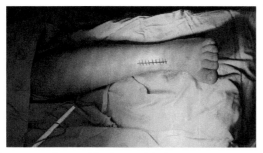

Fig. 13. Standard intraoperative positioning and incision.

A standard anterior surgical ankle approach is used to expose the distal tibia with a separate lateral fibula approach with safe skin bridges being used to expose the distal fibula. The structure most at risk during the standard anterior ankle approach is the anterior neurovascular bundle and should be protected.

The incision can be extended distally to the level of the ankle joint to enable excision of the capsule, synovium, or osteophytes around the ankle joint and/or proximally to aid with the osteotomy cuts placement or the seating of a custom cutting block.

Three options can be considered intraoperatively to accurately reproduce the preplanned Wiltse Triangle:

1. Drawing the Wiltse osteotomy on transparent paper and superimposing this over the fluoroscopy image to guide Kirchner-wire placement (**Fig. 14**).
2. Using a sterilized triangle set to guide K-wire placement (**Fig. 15**).
3. Using a 3-dimensional (3D) printed, patient-specific cutting jig: CT scan data from the patient are used to construct a 3D digital model of the anterior surface of the distal tibia. The Digital Imaging and Communication in Medicine (DICOM) data generated by medical CT scanners is converted into 3D Computer Assisted Drawing (CAD) data that can be used to manipulate the bone structure digitally and to design and print the custom cutting jig. Slots are created to act as exact cutting guides for the saw blade, thus mimicking the Wiltse triangle (**Fig. 16**).

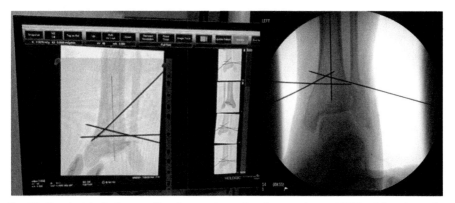

Fig. 14. Surgical technique option 1: superimposing the preplanned Wiltse triangle on the fluoroscopy screen guiding Kirchner-wire placement.

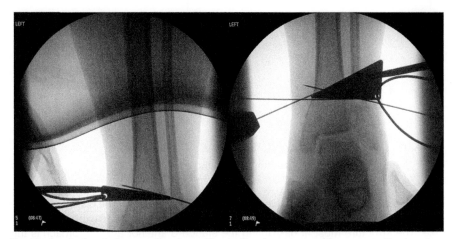

Fig. 15. Surgical technique option 1: sterilized triangle set to enable accurate K-wire placement to reproduce the Wiltse triangle.

The current preferred method in our unit is using sterilized triangles to guide the insertion of K-wires and completing the osteotomies with an oscillating saw. Under fluoroscopic guidance, the level of the base of the osteotomy is marked on the proximal border of the syndesmosis after which a 1.8-mm wire is inserted perpendicular to the anatomic long axis of the tibia at the lateral cortical border of the tibia. The LBA is replicated by placing a K-wire under fluoroscopic guidance from lateral-distal to medial-proximal crossing the 1st wire at the lateral tibial border. The MBA is replicated by placing a K-wire under fluoroscopic guidance from medial-distal to lateral-proximal. Subsequently, a triangle is formed. A K-wire can be placed in an anterior–posterior plane at the apex of the Wiltse triangle, to aid in performing an accurate osteotomy.

An oscillating saw is used to perform the cuts along each wire, taking care to disrupt the integrity of the medial and lateral cortex and to stay in the sagittal plane. An

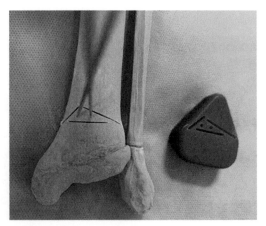

Fig. 16. Surgical technique option 3: a 3D printed, patient-specific cutting jig reproducing the Wiltse triangle.

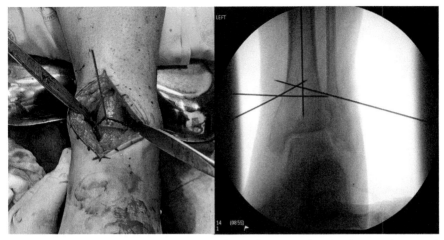

Fig. 17. Surgical technique: reproducing the Wiltse triangle via the sterile triangle technique.

oscillating saw blade with specific dimensions of 44x10 × 0.9 mm is recommended. The removed bony triangle is retained in case a supplemental bone graft is indicated (**Fig. 17**). A standard lateral fibula surgical approach is used to expose the distal fibula. A long oblique osteotomy is performed from proximal-medial to lateral-distal taking care to maintain the integrity of the syndesmosis (**Fig. 18**).

The distal tibial segment is slightly distracted, then rotated and laterally translated to enable the distal transverse tibial surface to keystone on the lateral proximal triangular surface and the medial malleolus flare to fit onto the medial proximal triangular surface. This creates a stable reduction (**Fig. 19**).

The mechanical axis, deformity correction, and translation should be evaluated. An advantage of this osteotomy is the ability to increase or decrease the translation to further restore the anatomic axis. An increase in lateral translation is obtained by lateral inferior translation of the distal tibial segment with the resultant medial gap filled with bone graft. In turn, a decrease in lateral translation is obtained by removing bone from the medial border. The resultant osteotomy will remain stable in both these adjustments (**Fig. 20**).

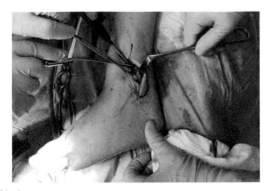

Fig. 18. Oblique fibula osteotomy.

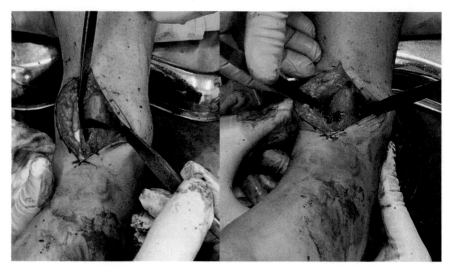

Fig. 19. Surgical technique: the Wiltse triangle is completed and removed and the oblique fibula osteotomy performed - completion of the stable Wiltse osteotomy.

The lateral distal fibula prominence may be removed if indicated and is frequently the case with large deformities and the proximal fibula can be shortened in the same plane as your oblique osteotomy if adequate bone contact needs to be facilitated (**Fig. 21**).

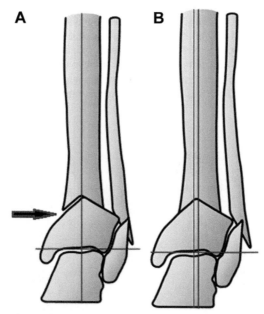

Fig. 20. Surgical technique: (*A*) Bone is removed from the medial border of the triangle, with subsequent (*B*) medial translation of the talus and anatomic axis.

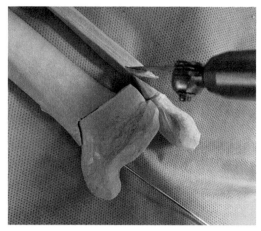

Fig. 21. Surgical technique: shortening of the fibula enables stable lateral fixation.

Routinely, the tibia is stabilized with a low-profile, fixed-angle T-plate. Fibula fixation can either be performed via intramedullary K-wire fixation or a low-profile, fixed-angle plate. External fixation can be considered due to host factors (**Fig. 22**).

POSTOPERATIVE CARE

A well-padded below-knee backslab is applied in the operating room. Strict elevation is prescribed for the immediate postoperative period. Early range of motion exercises of the hip and knee is initiated immediately postoperatively. A wound inspection is performed at 2 weeks and a walking cast is applied.

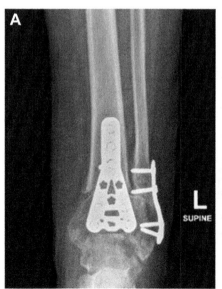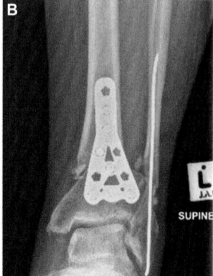

Fig. 22. Surgical technique: low-profile, fixed-angle plate for tibial fixation. Fixation options for the fibula using a (A) low-profile, fixed-angle plate, or a (B) intramedullary K-wire.

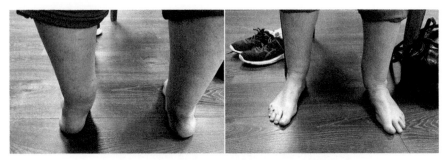

Fig. 23. Preoperative clinical photos indicating a valgus deformity of the ankle.

Subsequently, 6 weeks of toe-touch weight-bearing is prescribed with the cast being removed after this period. A moon boot is prescribed if sufficient evidence of radiographic healing is present. Partial weight-bearing for 6 weeks is then allowed, followed by full weightbearing and early resistance training. At 12 weeks osseous healing is confirmed, and resistance training is added to the exercise regime. Due to the inherent stability of the osteotomy and fixed-angle plate fixation, a more aggressive rehabilitation program can be used.

AUTHORS' EXPERIENCE
Case 1

A 55-year-old woman sustained a right ankle fracture after falling from a flight of stairs. She was treated conservatively in a below-knee cast for 6 weeks and a subsequent moonboot for 2 months. Despite extensive rehabilitation, her ankle pain and swelling persisted. She presented with anterolateral ankle pain and a progressive valgus ankle (**Fig. 23**). The range of motion was comparable to the contralateral side. Standard

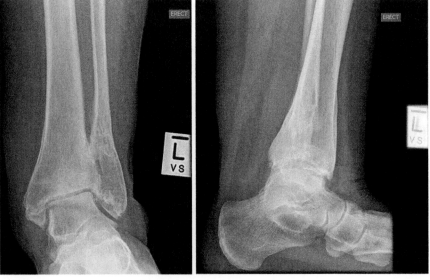

Fig. 24. Standardized preoperative x-rays reveal a 13° valgus deformity within the ankle joint.

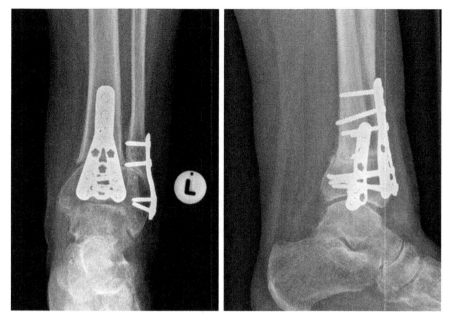

Fig. 25. Postoperative x-rays confirming the realignment of the mechanical axis.

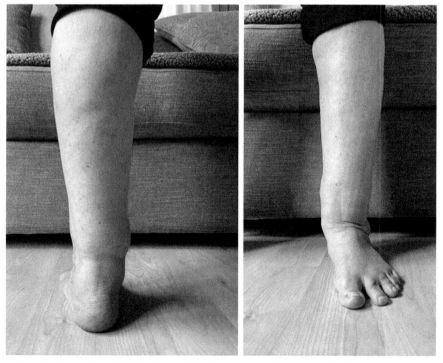

Fig. 26. Postoperative clinical photos indicating a corrected mechanical axis.

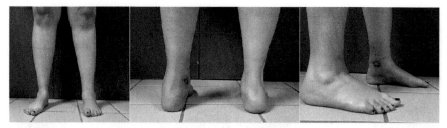

Fig. 27. Preoperative clinical photos indicating a mild valgus deformity of the ankle with a compensatory cavus deformity of the foot.

radiographs demonstrated a 13° intraarticular valgus deformity (**Fig. 24**). A Wiltse osteotomy was performed, correcting the valgus deformity and maintaining the mechanical axis (**Fig. 25**). At the 1-year follow-up, she reported no pain or discomfort in the ankle joint and active participation in her preinjury activities (**Fig. 26**).

Case 2

A 25-year-old female involved in a pedestrian-vehicle accident sustained a bimalleolar, left ankle fracture. She was treated conservatively in a below-knee cast and presented 6-months postinjury with progressive ankle deformity and significant anterolateral mechanical ankle pain. On examination, she had an acceptable range of motion with a valgus deformity of the ankle and a flexible, compensatory cavus

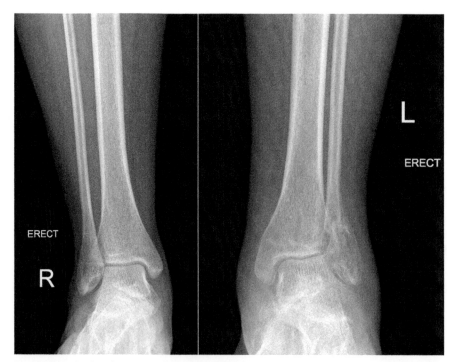

Fig. 28. Standardized preoperative x-rays reveal a 13° valgus deformity within the ankle joint (no translatory deformity was present).

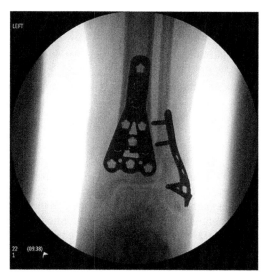

Fig. 29. Intraoperative x-ray confirm realignment of the mechanical axis.

deformity of the foot (**Fig. 27**). Preoperative x-rays revealed a 13° valgus deformity within the ankle joint with no translatory deformity (**Fig. 28**). A Wiltse osteotomy was planned and performed. Postoperative x-rays confirm realignment of the mechanical axis (**Fig. 29**).

Clinical overview

The authors performed, on average, 2 to 3 Wiltse osteotomies per year over the past 15 years. Of these patients, no nonunions were reported, all maintained their corrected intraoperative mechanical axis, and no metal hardware failure was observed. All patients had adequate pain relief. One patient experienced postoperative progression of symptomatic osteoarthritis and pain, whereafter a successful fusion was performed.

As this is an anecdotal review of the authors' experience, no functional scores were measured.

SUMMARY

The reconstituting of normal anatomy in the presence of a valgus deformity is complicated by the position of the CORA and the soft tissue limitations. The Wiltse osteotomy correctly uses osteotomy rule 2 to accurately reconstitute normal angular- and maintaining mechanical alignment. Due to the inherent stability of the Wiltse osteotomy, this procedure can be used in a wide range of patients, including the pediatric population.

CLINICS CARE POINTS

- Careful patient selection with a significant distal valgus deformity (isolated coronal plane deformity).
- Meticulous preoperative planning using adequate, standardized x-rays – "Plan the operation and operate the plan."

- Perform accurate anterior–posterior cuts with the patella facing forward, thus preventing an oblique osteotomy due to the sloping distal tibial anatomy
- Review and address the lateral fibula prominence after performing the Wiltse Osteotomy and consider additional shortening of the fibula.
- Objectively measure your corrected anatomic axis intraoperatively (templating)

ACKNOWLEDGMENTS

Our sincere gratitude to Dr Marilize Burger for her invaluable aid in the editing and formatting of the article and to Dr Ryno du Plessis and Prof Nando Ferreira for aiding with the mathematical design and planning of the "Wiltse Triangle." The authors would like to thank Mr Marius Vermeulen (CEO of Aditiv Solutions (Pty) Ltd.) and Mr Devon Hagedorn-Hansen (Technical Manager: Stellenbosch Technology Centre - Laboratory for Advanced Manufacturing) for their aid in the design and printing of the cutting jigs. TraumaCad software was used in measuring, calculating, and demonstrating the Wiltse Triangle and osteotomy. Lastly, our thanks to Dr Mark Meyerson who contribute so much in the field of foot and ankle surgery and who saw the potential of the Wiltse osteotomy.

DISCLOSURE

The authors have nothing to disclose.

REFERENCES

1. Gibson V, Prieskorn D. The Valgus Ankle. Foot Ankle Clin 2007;12(1):15–27.
2. Bluman EM, Chiodo CP. Valgus Ankle Deformity and Arthritis. Foot Ankle Clin 2008;13(3):443–70.
3. Barg A, Pagenstert GI, Horisberger M, et al. Supramalleolar osteotomies for degenerative joint disease of the ankle joint: Indication, technique and results. Int Orthop 2013;37(9):1683–95.
4. Valderrabano V, Paul J, Monika H, et al. Joint-preserving surgery of valgus ankle osteoarthritis. Foot Ankle Clin 2013;18(3):481–502.
5. Krause F, Veljkovic A, Schmid T. Supramalleolar Osteotomies for Posttraumatic Malalignment of the Distal Tibia. Foot Ankle Clin 2016;21(1):1–14.
6. Barg A, Pagenstert GI, Leumann AG, et al. Treatment of the Arthritic Valgus Ankle. Foot Ankle Clin 2012;17(4):647–63.
7. Merchant T, Dietz F. Long term follow-up after fractures of the tibial and fibular shafts. J Bone Joint Surg Am 1989;71:599–606.
8. Puno RM, Vaughan JJ, Stetten ML, et al. Long term effects of tibial angular malunion on the knee and ankle joints. J Orthop Trauma 1991;5(3):247–54.
9. Valderrabano V, Horisberger M, Russell I, et al. Etiology of ankle osteoarthritis. Clin Orthop Relat Res 2009;467(7):1800–6.
10. Pagenstert GI, Hintermann B, Barg A, et al. Realignment surgery as alternative treatment of varus and valgus ankle osteoarthritis. Clin Orthop Relat Res 2007; 462:156–68.
11. Ting AJ, Tarr RR, Sarmiento A, et al. The role of subtalar motion and ankle contact pressure changes from angular deformities of the tibia. Foot Ankle Int 1987;7(5): 290–9.

12. Knupp M, Stufkens SAS, Van Bergen CJ, et al. Effect of supramalleolar varus and valgus deformities on the tibiotalar joint: A cadaveric study. Foot Ankle Int 2011; 32(6):609–15.
13. Thordarson D, Motamed S, Hedman T, et al. The effect of fibular malreduction on contact pressures in an ankle fracture malunion model. J Bone Joint Surg Am 1997;79(12):1809–15.
14. Stamatis ED, Cooper PS, Myerson MS. Supramalleolar osteotomy for the treatment of distal tibial angular deformities and arthritis of the ankle joint. Foot Ankle Int 2003;24(10):754–64.
15. Siddiqui NA, Herzenberg JE, Lamm BM. Supramalleolar Osteotomy for Realignment of the Ankle Joint. Clin Podiatr Med Surg 2012;29(4):465–82.
16. Dabis J, Templeton-Ward O, Lacey AE, et al. The history, evolution and basic science of osteotomy techniques. Strateg Trauma Limb Reconstr 2017;12(3): 169–80.
17. Wiltse LL. Valgus deformity of the ankle: a sequel to acquired or congenital abnormalities of the fibula. J Bone Joint Surg Am 1972;54(3):595–606.
18. Paley D. Osteotomy rules. In: Herzenberg JE, editor. Principles of deformity correction. First edition. Berlin Heidelberg: Springer; 2002. p. 102–12.
19. Paley D. Principles of deformity correction. First edition. Berlin Heidelberg: Springer; 2002.

Joint Preservation Surgery for Varus and Posterior Ankle Arthritis Associated with Flatfoot Deformity

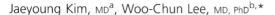

Jaeyoung Kim, MD[a], Woo-Chun Lee, MD, PhD[b],*

KEYWORDS

- Flatfoot deformity • Progressive collapsing foot deformity
- Joint preservation surgery • Realignment • posterior ankle arthritis • Ankle arthritis

KEY POINTS

- Flatfoot deformity can be associated with varus or posterior ankle arthritis as well as valgus ankle arthritis.
- Varus ankle arthritis and hindfoot valgus in flatfoot demonstrate opposing movement vectors of the talus and calcaneus at the talocalcaneal joint.
- Reduction of talocalcaneal subluxation may correct varus talar tilt.
- Posterior ankle arthritis is commonly associated with posterior translation and plantarflexion of the talus.
- Flatfoot correction may restore posterior talar translation and narrowing of the posterior ankle joint.

INTRODUCTION

A flatfoot deformity is characterized by medial longitudinal arch collapse, forefoot abduction, and hindfoot valgus, the combination of which leads to the failure of the posterior tibial tendon and medial ligaments.[1] Deltoid ligament insufficiency from long-standing flatfoot deformity can result in valgus talar tilt, and the subsequent eccentric load within the ankle joint may cause valgus ankle arthritis which is described as stage IV posterior tibial tendon dysfunction by Myerson.[2–5] In this regard, valgus ankle arthritis has been frequently described in the advanced flatfoot deformity, and deltoid ligament and/or spring ligament reconstruction with flatfoot correction has been reported as a salvage procedure.[2,4,6,7]

[a] Department of Orthopaedic Surgery, Hospital for Special Surgery, 535 East 70th Street, New York, NY 10021, USA; [b] Seoul Foot and Ankle Center, Dubalo Orthopaedic Clinic, 45, Apgujeong-ro 30 gil, Gangnam-gu, Seoul, 06022 Republic of Korea
* Corresponding author.
E-mail address: leewoochun@gmail.com

Foot Ankle Clin N Am 27 (2022) 115–127
https://doi.org/10.1016/j.fcl.2021.11.010
1083-7515/22/© 2021 Elsevier Inc. All rights reserved.

foot.theclinics.com

Varus ankle arthritis, however, is unlikely to develop with flatfoot deformity as eccentric loading would occur on the lateral aspect of the ankle joint from heel valgus in flatfoot deformity. Therefore, to date, only valgus ankle arthritis has been regarded as the result of flatfoot deformity, and the possible relationship between flatfoot deformity and varus ankle arthritis has anecdotally received no attention.[8]

Nevertheless, varus ankle arthritis is associated with a varus heel with or without cavus, and hindfoot valgus observed in the early stages of progression to arthritis was hitherto understood only as a compensatory mechanism for varus talar tilt.[9–11] However, Lee and colleagues argue that some cases of varus ankle arthritis demonstrate valgus hindfoot alignment too significant to be explained as compensation for proximal deformities, which implicates the possibility of preceding hindfoot valgus alignment before the development of varus ankle arthritis.[12] **Fig. 1** demonstrates the progression of varus ankle arthritis in a patient with a lower medial longitudinal arch and valgus heel alignment. In some cases with bilateral involvement, different directions of talar tilt may develop in the same patient, varus ankle arthritis in one ankle, and valgus ankle arthritis in the contralateral ankle (**Fig. 2**).

Varus talar tilt in flatfoot implies opposing vectors of the talus and hindfoot alignment, which can be explained by the opposite direction of deformity at the subtalar joint (**Fig. 3**). Three-dimensional (3D) instability of the talus may arise from the subtalar joint as the talus rotates on the calcaneus around an oblique axis.[12–14] The talus may varus angulate in the coronal plane, internally rotate in the axial plane, and plantarflex in the sagittal plane, while the calcaneus valgus angulates, externally rotates, and dorsiflexes at the subtalar joint.

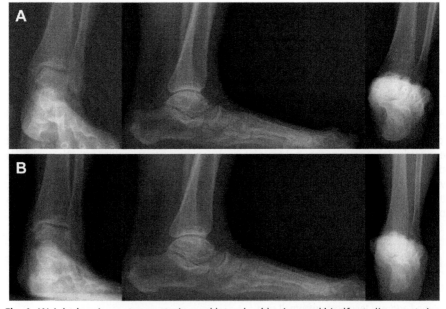

Fig. 1. Weight-bearing anteroposterior and lateral ankle view and hindfoot alignment view show progression of varus ankle arthritis over the course of 7 years in a patient with flatfoot deformity. (*A*) Initial presentation. (*B*) Progression of varus ankle arthritis 7 years after initial presentation.

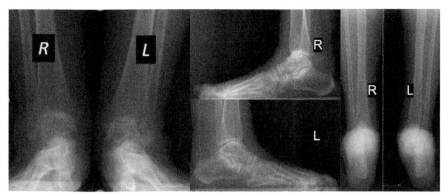

Fig. 2. Weight-bearing radiographs show varus and valgus ankle arthritis in one patient with flatfoot deformity on both sides.

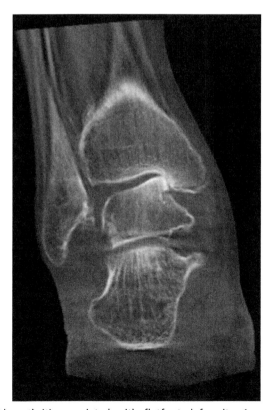

Fig. 3. Varus ankle arthritis associated with flatfoot deformity. A coronal image from weight-bearing computed tomography shows varus talar tilt at the tibiotalar joint and valgus tilt at the talocalcaneal joint.

Another novel form of ankle arthritis described in flatfoot deformity is posterior ankle arthritis. Here, arthritis is seen whereby the posterior aspect of the joint is narrow in the sagittal plane, without varus or valgus talar tilt on anteroposterior (AP) radiographs. These patterns were named posterior ankle arthritis by Kim and colleagues.[15,16] They observed that in most of their cases, ankles with eccentric posterior narrowing of the ankle joint were associated with flatfoot deformity (**Fig. 4**). Although both flatfoot deformity and ankle arthritis are known as 3D deformities with coronal, sagittal, and axial involvement, much of the radiographic emphasis has been put on evaluating and addressing the coronal plane deformity.[17] This eccentric narrowing of the posterior joint space in the sagittal plane may appear as end-stage ankle arthritis on the AP radiograph. However, there may still be utility in joint preservation surgery, as the cartilage at the anterior portion of the ankle joint remains intact. Some ankles may have a combination of varus and posterior ankle arthritis (**Fig. 5**).

While pathways in the approach of valgus ankle arthritis in flatfoot deformity are well understood and researched, this review features the mechanism and possible management pathway in the select cases of varus- and or posterior ankle arthritis associated with flatfoot. This novel approach may prove an acceptable salvage alternative to ankle joint replacement. More specifically, the correction of subtalar subluxation with or without medial longitudinal arch reconstruction may effectively preserve varus and/ or posterior ankle arthritis associated with flatfoot.

RADIOGRAPHIC FINDINGS OF VARUS ANKLE ARTHRITIS ASSOCIATED WITH FLATFOOT

Current literature has suggested that late-stage varus ankle arthritis will demonstrate varus hindfoot alignment. Valgus angulation of the hindfoot observed in the earlier stages of varus ankle arthritis has been understood as a compensation for varus talar tilt.[9,10] However, Park and colleagues recently reported advanced varus ankle arthritis associated with hindfoot valgus which was assumed to be caused by opposite directional motion at the subtalar joint.[18]

In varus ankle arthritis associated with flatfoot deformity, the degree of medial arch collapse or hindfoot valgus may not reliably reflect the preexisting degree of flatfoot deformity or hindfoot valgus before the development of varus ankle arthritis. As the

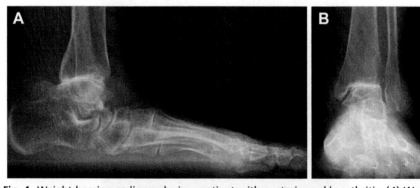

Fig. 4. Weight-bearing radiographs in a patient with posterior ankle arthritis. (*A*) Weight-bearing lateral ankle radiograph shows severe flatfoot deformity with posterior joint space narrowing. (*B*) Weight-bearing anteroposterior ankle view shows no coronal plane talar tilt, while diffuse narrowing is observed due to the visualization of the posterior aspect of the tibiotalar joint.

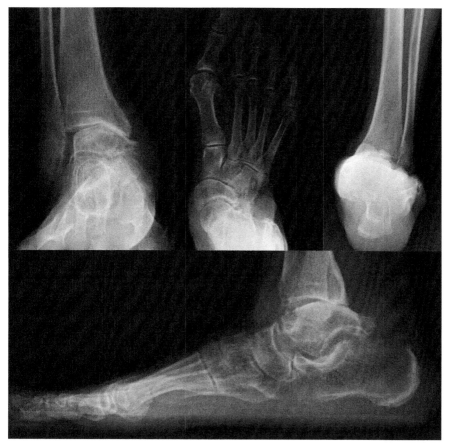

Fig. 5. End-stage ankle arthritis with flatfoot shows combined varus and posterior joint space narrowing.

varus talar tilt increases, the apparent degree of hindfoot valgus may decrease or even be tipped into a mild varus. The increased varus talar tilt also may change the profile of the longitudinal arch into slight cavus. Therefore, it is difficult to draw accurate inference for the deformity progression to varus ankle arthritis. However, we found that varus ankle arthritis associated with flatfoot showed a varus, adducted, and plantar-flexed talus, which can be assessed with varus talar tilt, degree of medial translation of the talus relative to the tibial axis, and Meary angle (**Fig. 6**).

BIOMECHANICS OF VARUS ANKLE ARTHRITIS ASSOCIATED WITH FLATFOOT

Varus ankle arthritis is caused by an eccentric load on the medial aspect of the ankle joint by varus deformities either proximal or distal to the ankle. Therefore, in early and mid-stage varus ankle arthritis, correction of proximal varus or hindfoot varus has been used to shift the weight-bearing load from the medial to the lateral aspect of the ankle joint.[19–21] However, late-stage varus ankle arthritis with a large talar tilt is challenging to manage with coronal plane correction, as this does not mean that the talus is deformed only in the coronal plane. Simultaneous internal rotation in the

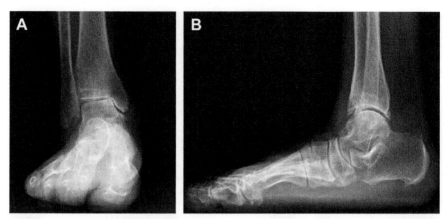

Fig. 6. Varus ankle arthritis associated with flatfoot deformity. (*A*) Weight-bearing antero-posterior ankle radiograph shows varus talar tilt and the medial translation of the talus relative to the tibial axis. (*B*) Weight-bearing lateral ankle radiograph shows plantarflexed talus with low calcaneal pitch angle.

axial plane and anterior translation in the sagittal plane may be present, which must be treated with 3D correction as demonstrated in the joint preservation of paralytic varus ankle arthritis using posterior tibial tendon transfer.[22]

In the flatfoot deformity, it has been understood that 3D talocalcaneal movement occurs mainly from the movement of the calcaneus underneath the talus, which is regarded as normally positioned in the ankle mortise. Therefore, the term peritalar subluxation was used to describe this conceptual motion.[23,24] We suggest that the mechanism of varus ankle arthritis with valgus hindfoot deformity is that the talus and the calcaneus may rotate to each other; the talus may be inverted while the calcaneus is everted (**Fig. 7**). Therefore, talocalcaneal subluxation rather than peritalar subluxation may be a better term to describe this phenomenon.

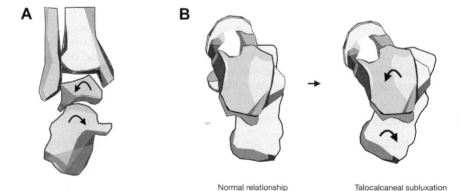

Normal relationship   Talocalcaneal subluxation

Fig. 7. Schematic drawings of talocalcaneal subluxation. (*A*) Supination of the talus and pronation of the calcaneus in the coronal plane. (*B*) Rotation of the talus and calcaneus in opposite direction in the axial plane.

JOINT PRESERVATION SURGERY IN VARUS ANKLE ARTHRITIS ASSOCIATED WITH FLATFOOT DEFORMITY

Load shifting to the lateral side of the ankle joint is the principal method of joint preservation for varus ankle arthritis.[21] However, in varus ankle associated with hindfoot valgus, lateral shifting of the weight-bearing load may aggravate the hindfoot valgus. It would not change the talocalcaneal relationship, which was suggested above as a possible etiology.

Varus talar tilt in varus ankle arthritis associated with flatfoot deformity is a rigid deformity that does not decrease with valgus angulating force, and correction at the subtalar joint would be the direct method of restoring the talocalcaneal relationship. Therefore, repositioning subtalar arthrodesis was performed by the inversion of the calcaneus. The longitudinal arch may need restoration in the presence of severe symptomatic sagging of the medial arch, which was achieved with dynamic reconstruction with flexor hallucis longus transfer to the first metatarsal base, and was named dynamic medial column stabilization.[25] In literature, repositional subtalar arthrodesis has been used as an adjunct to flatfoot reconstruction with favorable patient outcomes.[26–29] However, the loss of hindfoot motion following subtalar arthrodesis in late-stage ankle arthritis should be carefully weighed against the benefits it brings. In patients with varus ankle arthritis with heel valgus, the talocalcaneal impingement is often the chief complaint of the patient, which can be demonstrated by significant pain relief after lidocaine infiltration into the sinus tarsi. Therefore, subtalar arthrodesis would be justified to preserve the ankle joint while achieving severe pain relief from lateral talocalcaneal impingement.

Often medial opening wedge supramalleolar osteotomy was added to the subtalar arthrodesis because lateral load shifting after the flatfoot correction may benefit the joint preservation of varus ankle arthritis (**Fig. 8**). However, we believe the correction of talar tilt may have resulted mostly from subtalar arthrodesis because the decrease of varus talar tilt and lateral translation of the talus was shown on intraoperative radiographs after subtalar reduction before performing SMO (**Fig. 9**).

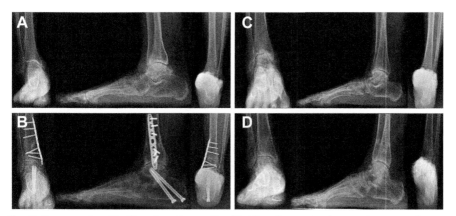

Fig. 8. Preoperative (A, C) and postoperative (B, D) radiographs show a decrease of varus talar tilt and the appearance of tibiotalar joint space after repositional subtalar arthrodesis and supramalleolar osteotomy.

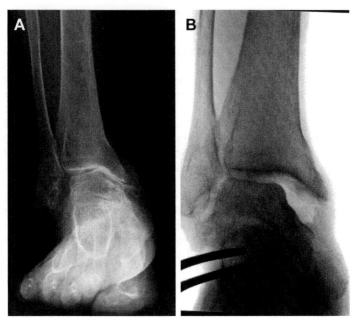

Fig. 9. The decrease of varus talar tilt and lateral translation of the talus was shown on intraoperative radiographs after temporary subtalar fixation before performing supramalleolar osteotomy. (*A*) Preoperative weight-bearing ankle anteroposterior view. (*B*) Intraoperative fluoroscopic image after spreading the subtalar joint at the sinus tarsi with a laminar spreader.

RADIOGRAPHIC FINDINGS OF POSTERIOR ANKLE ARTHRITIS

Kim and colleagues defined posterior ankle arthritis as having (1) eccentric narrowing of the joint space at the posterior aspect of the tibiotalar joint on weight-bearing ankle lateral radiograph and (2) talar tilt angle less than 4° on weight-bearing ankle AP radiographs.[15,16] This cutoff for the talar tilt angle was chosen because advanced deformity in the coronal plane accompanies the translation of the talus in the sagittal plane in a previous WBCT study.[30] In their study, radiographic characteristics in 16 ankles with posterior ankle arthritis were analyzed. Radiographic findings demonstrated that posterior ankle arthritis was associated with posterior translation and plantarflexion of the talus. As the definition of posterior ankle arthritis implicates, the talar tilt angle (TT) was nearly normal. Valgus angulation of the hindfoot and varus lower limb alignment was additional radiographic findings.[15,16]

Posterior ankle arthritis often appears as end-stage ankle arthritis on AP ankle radiographs because the narrowed posterior aspect of the tibiotalar joint is visualized, oftentimes projecting a pan articular arthritic picture. Therefore, lateral radiographs should be carefully evaluated to explore the possibility of joint preservation surgery in these ankles with asymmetric joint space narrowing in the sagittal plane.

BIOMECHANICS OF POSTERIOR ANKLE ARTHRITIS ASSOCIATED WITH FLATFOOT

As demonstrated by several cadaveric studies, sagittal plane malalignment places more kinematic impact on the ankle joint than the coronal plane malalignment.[31–33] While coronal plane malalignment can be compensated by the subtalar joint motion, sagittal plane malalignment cannot be compensated by subtalar motion.[31-33] Additionally, altered talus position relative to the tibial axis would change the moment arm of the Achilles pull, which will aggravate eccentric loading at the tibiotalar joint.[34] Therefore, we believe the restoration of the tibiotalar relationship at its earlier stage is as important and crucial for joint preservation of posterior ankle arthritis as coronal alignment correction.

It is well documented in the literature, that the ankle joint is relatively stable in the sagittal plane given its bony conformity and posterior projection of the distal tibia.[35] Besides, the talus is wider anteriorly and narrower posteriorly within the mortise. As such, the posterior translation of the talus seems unlikely to occur. The authors assume that plantarflexion of the talus places a narrower posterior portion of the talar dome within the mortise, which results in susceptibility of the talus to posterior translation and giving rise to increased peak pressures. Consequently, this concentrated weight-bearing load on the posterior aspect of the tibiotalar joint may lead to eccentric narrowing of the posterior joint space and posterior translation of the talus.

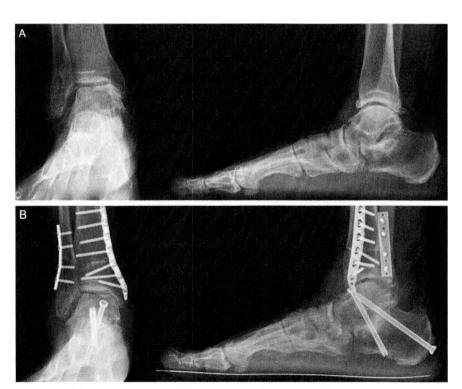

Fig. 10. Pre (*A*) and postoperative (*B*) radiographs of a patient with posterior ankle arthritis. Dorsiflexion of the talus through flatfoot reconstruction might shift the weight-bearing load from the degenerated posterior aspect of the joint to the uninvolved anterior aspect of the joint in the setting of posterior ankle arthritis. In patients demonstrating varus distal tibial plafond and medial translation of the talus, an additional supramalleolar osteotomy was performed.

JOINT PRESERVATION SURGERY FOR POSTERIOR ANKLE ARTHRITIS ASSOCIATED WITH FLATFOOT

The fundamental principle of joint preservation surgery is shifting the weight-bearing load from the degenerated area to the uninvolved area. For example, valgus angulation of the tibial plafond or hindfoot for varus ankle arthritis resulted in the unloading of the medial articular surface and increased weight-bearing load onto the lateral articular surface, and vice versa in patients with valgus arthritis.[36]

Posterior ankle arthritis was associated with the plantarflexion of the talus, lower medial longitudinal arch, and valgus hindfoot alignment, all of which suggest its association with flatfoot deformity. Dorsiflexion of the talus through flatfoot reconstruction could shift the weight-bearing load from the degenerated posterior aspect of the joint to the uninvolved central and anterior aspect of the joint in the setting of posterior ankle arthritis. We previously performed subtalar arthrodesis and dynamic reconstruction of the medial longitudinal arch with flexor hallucis longus transfer to the base of the first metatarsal for flatfoot reconstruction.[25] Intraoperative observations indicated that articular cartilage was preserved in the anterior aspect of the joint, substantiating that posterior ankle arthritis is a type of eccentric arthritis in which joint preservation can be attempted. In patients demonstrating varus distal tibial plafond and medial translation of the talus, an SMO was performed in addition to flatfoot reconstruction (**Fig. 10**). Subtalar arthrodesis was performed due to rigid hindfoot deformity and talocalcaneal

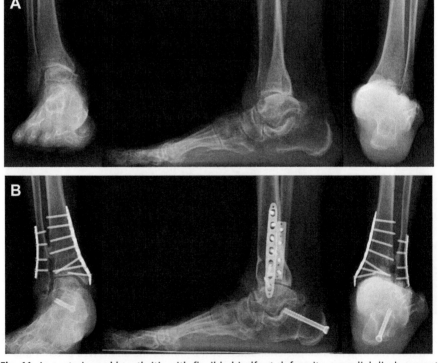

Fig. 11. In posterior ankle arthritis with flexible hindfoot deformity, a medial displacement calcaneal osteotomy and dynamic medial column stabilization were performed in addition to supramalleolar correction. (*A*) Preoperative. (*B*) Postoperative.

impingement. If the hindfoot deformity is flexible, joint preserving osteotomy of the hindfoot such as medial displacement calcaneal osteotomy may be applicable (**Fig. 11**).

Radiographic parameters indicated anterior repositioning and dorsiflexion of the talus following flatfoot reconstruction. None of the patients required conversion to joint sacrificing surgery at a minimum 2-year follow-up.

SUMMARY

Flatfoot is often associated with varus or posterior ankle arthritis as well as valgus ankle arthritis. The theoretic basis of the varus and posterior ankle arthritis associated with flatfoot was discussed based on the radiological findings. Varus ankle arthritis and hindfoot valgus in flatfoot demonstrate the opposite directional movement of the talus and the calcaneus at the subtalar joint. Reduction of this talocalcaneal subluxation may correct the varus talar tilt. Posterior ankle arthritis is mostly associated with posterior translation and plantarflexion of the talus. Correction of flatfoot may restore proper load distribution within the tibiotalar joint.

CLINICS CARE POINT

- Varus ankle arthritis or posterior ankle arthritis may be associated with flatfoot, therefore alignment on lateral radiograph or hindfoot alignment view should be carefully assessed.

DISCLOSURE

J. Kim and W-C. Lee have nothing to disclose pertaining to this topic.

REFERENCES

1. Deland JT. Adult-acquired flatfoot deformity. J Am Acad Orthop Surg 2008;16(7): 399–406.
2. Ellis SJ, Williams BR, Wagshul AD, et al. Deltoid ligament reconstruction with peroneus longus autograft in flatfoot deformity. Foot Ankle Int 2010;31(9):781–9.
3. Smith JT, Bluman EM. Update on stage IV acquired adult flatfoot disorder: when the deltoid ligament becomes dysfunctional. Foot Ankle Clin 2012;17(2):351–60.
4. Williams BR, Ellis SJ, Joseph CY, et al. Stage IV adult-acquired flatfoot deformity deltoid ligament reconstruction. Oper Tech Orthop 2010;20(3):183–9.
5. Myerson M. Adult acquired flatfoot deformity: treatment of dysfunction of the posterior tibial tendon. Instr Course Lect 1997;46:393–405.
6. Deland JT, Ellis SJ, Day J, et al. Indications for deltoid and spring ligament reconstruction in progressive collapsing foot deformity. Foot Ankle Int 2020;41(10): 1302–6.
7. Patel MS, Barbosa MP, Kadakia AR. Role of spring and deltoid ligament reconstruction for adult acquired flatfoot deformity. Tech Foot Ankle Surg 2017;16(3): 124–35.
8. Dabash S, Buksbaum JR, Fragomen A, et al. Distraction arthroplasty in osteoarthritis of the foot and ankle. World J Orthop 2020;11(3):145.
9. Hayashi K, Tanaka Y, Kumai T, et al. Correlation of compensatory alignment of the subtalar joint to the progression of primary osteoarthritis of the ankle. Foot Ankle Int 2008;29(4):400–6.

10. Wang B, Saltzman CL, Chalayon O, et al. Does the subtalar joint compensate for ankle malalignment in end-stage ankle arthritis? Clin Orthop Relat Res 2015; 473(1):318–25.

11. Krähenbühl N, Siegler L, Deforth M, et al. Subtalar joint alignment in ankle osteoarthritis. Foot Ankle Surg 2019;25(2):143–9.

12. Lee W-C, Moon J-S, Lee HS, et al. Alignment of ankle and hindfoot in early stage ankle osteoarthritis. Foot Ankle Int 2011;32(7):693–9.

13. Sangeorzan A, Sangeorzan B. Subtalar joint biomechanics: from normal to pathologic. Foot Ankle Clin 2018;23(3):341–52.

14. Sangeorzan B. Subtalar joint: morphology and functional anatomy. Inman's Joints of the Ankle. Baltimore: Williams & Wilkins; 1991. p. 31–8.

15. Kim J, Kim J-B, Lee W-C. Clinical and radiographic results of ankle joint preservation surgery in posterior ankle arthritis. Foot Ankle Int 2021. 10711007211011182. [Epub ahead of print].

16. Kim J, Kim J-B, Lee W-C. Eccentric ankle arthritis in the sagittal plane: a novel description of anterior and posterior ankle arthritis. Foot Ankle Surg 2021; S1268-7731(20):30283–6.

17. Coetzee JC. Management of varus or valgus ankle deformity with ankle replacement. Foot Ankle Clin 2008;13(3):509–20.

18. Park CH, Kim J, Kim JB, et al. Repositional subtalar arthrodesis combined with supramalleolar osteotomy for late-stage varus ankle arthritis with hindfoot valgus. Foot Ankle Int 2021. 10711007211036699. [Epub ahead of print].

19. Tanaka Y, Takakura Y, Hayashi K, et al. Low tibial osteotomy for varus-type osteoarthritis of the ankle. J bone Jt Surg Br 2006;88(7):909–13.

20. Knupp M, Stufkens SA, Bolliger L, et al. Classification and treatment of supramalleolar deformities. Foot Ankle Int 2011;32(11):1023–31.

21. Lee W-C, Moon J-S, Lee K, et al. Indications for supramalleolar osteotomy in patients with ankle osteoarthritis and varus deformity. J Bone Joint Surg Am 2011; 93(13):1243–8.

22. Lee W-C, Ahn J-Y, Cho J-H, et al. Realignment surgery for severe talar tilt secondary to paralytic cavovarus. Foot Ankle Int 2013;34(11):1552–9.

23. Toolan BC, Sangeorzan BJ, HANSEN ST. Complex reconstruction for the treatment of dorsolateral peritalar subluxation of the foot. Early results after distraction arthrodesis of the calcaneocuboid joint in conjunction with stabilization of, and transfer of the flexor digitorum longus tendon to, the midfoot to treat acquired pes planovalgus in adults. JBJS 1999;81(11):1545–60.

24. Hintermann B, Knupp M, Barg A. Peritalar instability. Foot Ankle Int 2012;33(5): 450–4.

25. Kim J, Kim J-B, Lee W-C. Dynamic medial column stabilization using flexor hallucis longus tendon transfer in the surgical reconstruction of flatfoot deformity in adults. Foot Ankle Surg 2020. S1268-7731(20)30277-30280. [Epub ahead of print].

26. Johnson JE, Cohen BE, DiGiovanni BF, et al. Subtalar arthrodesis with flexor digitorum longus transfer and spring ligament repair for treatment of posterior tibial tendon insufficiency. Foot Ankle Int 2000;21(9):722–9.

27. Murley GS, Menz HB, Landorf KB. Foot posture influences the electromyographic activity of selected lower limb muscles during gait. J Foot Ankle Res 2009;2:35.

28. Steiner CS, Gilgen A, Zwicky L, et al. Combined subtalar and naviculocuneiform fusion for treating adult acquired flatfoot deformity with medial arch collapse at the level of the naviculocuneiform joint. Foot Ankle Int 2019;40(1):42–7.

29. Stephens HM, Walling AK, Solmen JD, et al. Subtalar repositional arthrodesis for adult acquired flatfoot. Clin Orthop Relat Res 1999;(365):69–73.
30. Kim J-B, Yi Y, Kim J-Y, et al. Weight-bearing computed tomography findings in varus ankle osteoarthritis: abnormal internal rotation of the talus in the axial plane. Skeletal Radiol 2017;46(8):1071–80.
31. McKellop HA, Llinás A, Sarmiento A. Effects of tibial malalignment on the knee and ankle. Orthop Clin North Am 1994;25(3):415.
32. Paley D, Herzenberg JE, Tetsworth K, et al. Deformity planning for frontal and sagittal plane corrective osteotomies. Orthop Clin North Am 1994;25(3):425–66.
33. Ting AJ, Tarr RR, Sarmiento A, et al. The role of subtalar motion and ankle contact pressure changes from angular deformities of the tibia. Foot Ankle 1987;7(5):290–9.
34. Scheidegger P, Horn Lang T, Schweizer C, et al. A flexion osteotomy for correction of a distal tibial recurvatum deformity: a retrospective case series. bone Jt J 2019;101(6):682–90.
35. Brockett CL, Chapman GJ. Biomechanics of the ankle. Orthopaedics and trauma 2016;30(3):232–8.
36. Pagenstert GI, Hintermann B, Barg A, et al. Realignment surgery as alternative treatment of varus and valgus ankle osteoarthritis. Clin Orthop Relat Res 2007; 462:156–68.

Correction of Sagittal Plane Deformity of the Distal Tibia

Emilio Wagner, MD*, Pablo Wagner, MD

KEYWORDS

- Supramalleolar osteotomy • Distal tibia deformity • Localized ankle osteoarthritis
- Anterior ankle arthritis • Posterior ankle arthritis • Sagittal deformity

KEY POINTS

- Sagittal distal tibia deformities produce a greater change in tibiotalar joint contact areas than with valgus or varus deformities.
- Talar anterior or posterior translation occurs secondary to a distal tibia sagittal deformity and worsens the asymmetric joint overload and secondary cartilage damage.
- Distal tibial angle and talar position relative to the tibial axis should be always obtained to evaluate the deformity severity and the amount of correction needed.
- Anterior distal tibia closing or opening wedge osteotomies are the recommended treatment options for posterior or anterior ankle arthritis, respectively.
- Fibular osteotomies should be generally added to the tibia osteotomy to help with talar repositioning.

INTRODUCTION

The sagittal plane alignment of the distal tibia is not frequently analyzed, and its normal parameters are commonly forgotten. As Drs Paley and Herzenberg described years ago, seen from the lateral aspect, the middiaphyseal line of the tibia in the sagittal plane passes through the lateral process of the talus, when the plantar aspect of the foot is in 90° in relation to the tibia[1] (**Fig. 1**). Another commonly measured angle is the anterior distal tibial angle (ADTA), whose normal value is 80° (**Fig. 2**).[1]

Two different scenarios can be observed in sagittal plane deformities of the distal tibia. One scenario refers to the classic antecurvatum and recurvatum deformities, where due to a posttraumatic physeal damage or a malunited tibia fracture, a secondary anterior or posterior displacement of the talus relative to the tibial axis is seen, with no ADTA alteration. In these cases a supramalleolar apex of deformity will be found, consistent with a previous skeletal damage. Localized ankle arthrosis can coexist depending on the time elapsed since the original trauma (initially no ADTA change is seen). The second scenario, much more frequent, is observed when an asymmetric

Universidad del Desarrollo, Clinica Alemana de Santiago, Vitacura 5951, Santiago, Chile
* Corresponding author.
E-mail address: ewagner@alemana.cl

Foot Ankle Clin N Am 27 (2022) 129–144
https://doi.org/10.1016/j.fcl.2021.11.011
foot.theclinics.com

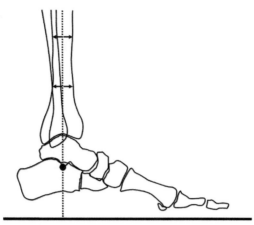

Fig. 1. The distal leg, showing a normal sagittal alignment. The axis of the tibia is represented as an intermittent dot line following the center of the diaphysis of the distal tibia, intersecting the anterolateral process of the talus, shown as a dot.

ankle joint arthritis is present compromising either the anterior or posterior aspects of the ankle joint. In these cases, a decrease in joint space is observed, with ADTA alteration and a consequent anterior or posterior displacement of the talus relative to the tibia axis. In these cases, an intraarticular apex of deformity will be found. Both scenarios share the sagittal plane deformity of the ankle consisting in a malalignment between the tibia and the talus: in one case due to a posttraumatic malunited distal tibia (antecurvatum or recurvatum deformities) and in the other case due to loss of cartilage in the anterior or posterior aspect of the ankle joint.[2]

In this article, we will use the term "anterior ankle arthritis" to refer to patients with an anterior displacement of the talus relative to the tibia, with a mechanical overload of the anterior aspect of the ankle joint, with or without changes in the anterior joint space or ADTA values. The term "posterior ankle arthritis" will refer to patients with a posterior displacement of the talus relative to the tibia, with a mechanical overload of the posterior

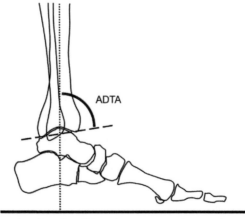

Fig. 2. The distal leg, showing the tibia axis represented as an intermittent dot line. The distal tibia articular surface is represented by a dashed line. The ADTA angle is measured anteriorly between the 2 previously mentioned lines.

aspect of the ankle joint, with or without changes in the posterior joint space or ADTA values. We will analyze the biomechanical changes happening in ankle sagittal plane malalignments, with their clinical consequences and present alternatives of treatment.

BIOMECHANICAL BACKGROUND

In cadaveric studies malunited tibia fractures show significant changes when greater than 15° of deformity is applied to the distal tibia.[3] Anterior and posterior bow deformities produce a greater change in tibiotalar joint contact areas than with valgus or varus deformities of the tibia.[4] These facts highlight the importance of identifying sagittal plane malalignments of the ankle joint.

Ankle arthrosis is usually posttraumatic in origin, explaining the frequent asymmetric presentation, as cartilage damage will manifest where most of the energy and destruction occurred.[5] Ankle joint pressure changes depending on the damaged area of the ankle, for example, the center of pressure shifts posterolaterally in ankle fractures with interosseus membrane damage.[6] Another fact to remember is that the bone resistance of the tibia and talus is not uniform on its surface, with the tibia showing greater subchondral resistance in its posteromedial aspect than in the anterolateral one.[7] Whenever there is an asymmetric damage on the ankle joint, besides the concurrent ligament damage, the talus will tend to shift to the damaged cartilage area. This will create either a coronal plane or a sagittal plane malalignment, depending on where the joint damage/deformity is located. Sagittal ankle malalignment is common in end-stage ankle arthrosis, with up to 56% of the cases presenting either anterior or posterior displacement of the talus in relation to the tibia.[8]

The most referred angle of the distal tibia in the sagittal plane corresponds to the ADTA, whose normal value is 80°.[1] The lateral process of the talus can be considered to represent the axis of rotation of the ankle on a lateral ankle radiograph, although this is not exact, as the ankle joint acts as a truncated cone, with an axis passing through both malleoli, thus having a dynamic axis of rotation. The distance between the tibial axis and the center of rotation of the ankle therefore can be measured and will represent the sagittal alignment of the ankle in relation to the tibia.[9] A comparison between 3 different ways of measuring the alignment of the talus in relation to the tibia in the sagittal plane has been published.[9] The tibial axis to talus ratio (TT), which corresponds to the ratio into which the midlongitudinal axis of the tibial shaft divides the longitudinal talar length, is the measure that tolerates the better perturbations of ankle positioning. The longitudinal talar length is defined as a line parallel to the floor, beginning at the intersection between the posterior subtalar joint and the posterosuperior cortex of the calcaneus, ending at the vertical projection of the most anterior aspect of the talus[9] (**Fig. 3**). The average normal value for the TT ratio (expressed as a percentage) has been reported to be 34 ± 2.[8] In a consequent study the TT ratio was shown to be a reliable radiographic measure to determine the position of the talus relative to the tibia, regardless of the condition of the ankle surface.[10]

CLINICAL DIAGNOSIS AND RADIOLOGICAL CHARACTERISTICS

Patients with sagittal plane deformities of the distal tibia will present clinically with arthritic symptoms, resembling any patient with localized ankle arthritis. Initially they will present with ankle pain associated with changes in physical activity, differences in footwear, changes in body weight, and so forth. The pain may begin immediately after physical activity and subside in the following hours or persist for hours or days

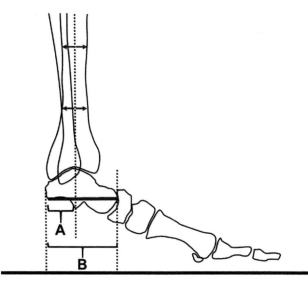

Fig. 3. The distal leg, showing the tibia axis represented as an intermittent dot line. The longitudinal talar length is represented by a horizontal continuous line beginning at the most posterior aspect of the subtalar joint and ending at the most distal aspect of the talus (its most distal aspect if projected vertically to the floor). The tibia axis divides the longitudinal talar length line into two. The TT ratio, generally expressed as a percentage, is obtained dividing distance "A" (distance along the longitudinal talar length *line* beginning at the most posterior aspect of the subtalar joint and ending at the intersection of the tibial axis and the longitudinal talar length *line*) over "B" (longitudinal talar length) and multiplied by 100.

after completing the physical activity. With worsening arthritis, pain may become continuous during the day. Recurvatum is less tolerated than procurvatum deformities because the articular surface of the talus is not well covered with the tibia, leading to pressure concentration in the anterior aspect of the ankle joint (**Fig. 4**). Procurvatum of the distal tibia should be less destructive for the ankle, as the talus is well covered by the mortise.[5] Having said this, procurvatum may be more painful for patients as a result of anterior ankle impingement. Two sagittal plane malalignment examples are provided in **Fig. 5**.

The study of patients with ankle malalignment should consider standing long leg radiographs, in addition to ankle radiographs. Patients in early stages of sagittal plane deformities may have joint angles within normal values but will have ankle pain in the area affected by previous trauma, due to a mechanical overload. In these cases, an MRI or a nuclear medicine test such as single-photon emission computed tomography will provide information supporting the idea of an ankle joint overload (**Fig. 6**). In more advanced stages of localized osteoarthritis, radiological alterations will already be seen consisting in changes in the joint space, angulation of the joint line, sclerosis or osteophytes, bone cysts, or already formally advanced osteoarthritis.

We must analyze the degree of arthrosis and radiological indices such as the ADTA, lateral distal tibial angle, talar tilt, tibiotalar angle, and any other deformity present always using the apex of deformity concept. Because we are discussing sagittal plane deformities, the ADTA angle and the TT ratio should be altered. The frontal plane should always be evaluated as well. The recommended method is using the mechanical axis deviation to obtain the lateral distal tibial angle.

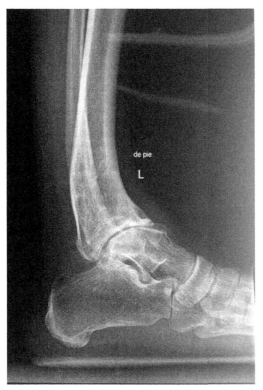

Fig. 4. Lateral ankle radiograph of a patient with a recurvatum ankle deformity. There is a clear deformity at the distal tibia due to an old distal tibia fracture. Note the uncoverage of the talus anteriorly, which leads to overload and arthritis in that area.

There are no specific classifications for ankle sagittal plane malalignments. To the best of our knowledge, the only classification for localized ankle arthritis that considers sagittal ankle position is the one published by Knupp, where on top of the analysis given to the coronal plane malalignment, a modifier is added using a letter. If there is no sagittal plane malalignment, a letter c (centered) is added to the main group. If there is any sagittal malalignment, a letter e (extruded) is added.[11]

TREATMENT

A traditional limit to use joint preserving surgery in ankle osteoarthritis is the presence of at least 50% of the talar surface still covered by cartilage. This theoretic limit is only valid for coronal plane deformities, so there is no clear limit to choose to preserve an ankle joint where there is mainly a sagittal plane deformity. Our preference is to always correct sagittal plane malalignments irrespective of the cartilage condition, considering it more important compared with coronal ankle deformities. The preferred surgery consists in a supramalleolar osteotomy of the tibia (SMOT).

ANTERIOR ANKLE ARTHRITIS

Our objective should be to correct the ankle alignment to the best we can. The coronal correction is being explained elsewhere in this issue, so we will focus on the sagittal correction. In anterior ankle arthritis, we will either find an ADTA angle less than 80°, or

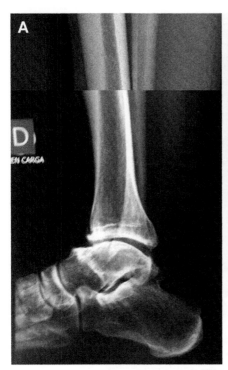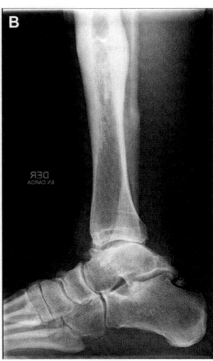

Fig. 5. Lateral radiographs of 2 clinical cases with ankle sagittal malalignment. (*A*) A case with anterior ankle arthritis, with anterior displacement of the talus relative to the tibia and anterior ankle arthrosis with a concurrent decrease of the ADTA angle. (*B*) A case with posterior ankle arthritis, with posterior displacement of the talus relative to the tibia, with an increase of the ADTA angle.

a TT ratio less than 30, or both. When planning an SMOT to correct this malalignment, we recommend using digital software to aid in the correct preoperative planning (**Figs. 7** and **8**). A correct measurement of the ADTA needs to be performed in these cases considering the removal of anterior distal tibia osteophytes to draw the joint line correctly.

If the anterior ankle arthritis case presents with an obvious extraarticular distal tibia deformity due to a malunited fracture or previous physeal damage, without any decrease in anterior joint space, the ADTA will be normal and the TT ratio will be abnormal. In these cases the apex of the deformity will be extraarticular in the distal tibia metaphysis, where the SMOT must be planned.

Most of the anterior ankle arthritis cases present with a decrease in anterior joint space, anterior distal tibia osteophytes, and abnormal ADTA and TT ratio values. In these cases, there is an intraarticular apex of deformity, and therefore, the SMOT cannot be performed at the apex of the deformity. When an SMOT is performed outside the apex, the so-called third rule of osteotomies occurs. This rule mandates that a secondary translation of the distal segment occurs when an angular correction is performed outside the deformity apex. This secondary translation occurs in the direction of correction (posterior translation in cases of operated anterior ankle arthritis), which is desirable in osteoarthritic cases. It further helps with mechanical axis correction and therefore does not need to be corrected.[12] Recovering normal angular values should not be our goal in osteoarthritic cases, as we must overcorrect the alignment, pushing the weight-bearing axis line away from the damaged cartilage. There are no

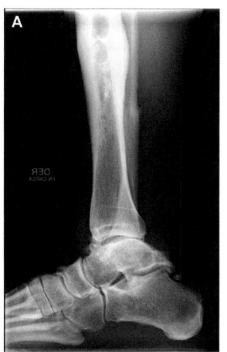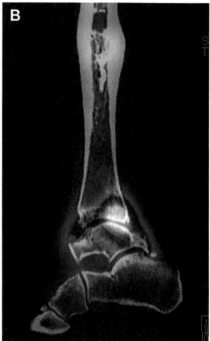

Fig. 6. Lateral ankle radiograph of a sagittal plane malalignment case. (*A*) The posterior displacement of the talus relative to the tibia, with some osteophytes present in the anterior aspect of the talus. (*B*) The same case but with an SPECT-CT image, where the posterior overload is represented by an intense yellow color.

specific recommendations relative to the amount of correction, but we recommend staying within 5° of normality to avoid creating anterior ankle impingement. For example, an anterior ankle arthritis case with an ADTA of 73° should therefore be overcorrected to 85°.

The most recommended osteotomy for anterior ankle arthritis is an anterior opening wedge osteotomy for angular corrections under 10° and a dome osteotomy for corrections greater than 10°. We recommend always adding a fibular osteotomy at the level of the syndesmosis, to aid in the correction of the TT ratio. We have seen in our experience that adding a fibular osteotomy helps the talus to relocate under the tibia, especially if there is a malunited fibula or malunited syndesmosis. A posterior distal tibia closing wedge osteotomy is also an option for deformities of 10° or less, especially if contracted soft tissues are present.

A special consideration must be given to severe recurvatum deformities, due to the posterior soft tissue contractures generally found. After performing the SMOT, the ankle will remain in plantar flexion due to posterior soft tissue contractures. Components that must be released include the posterior capsule, posterior tibial tendon, Achilles tendon, and posteromedial neurovascular sheath.

Technique

Tibial osteotomy

An anterior ankle incision is recommended, generally used also for coronal plane deformity treatment. Any anterior distal tibia osteophyte needs to be resected.

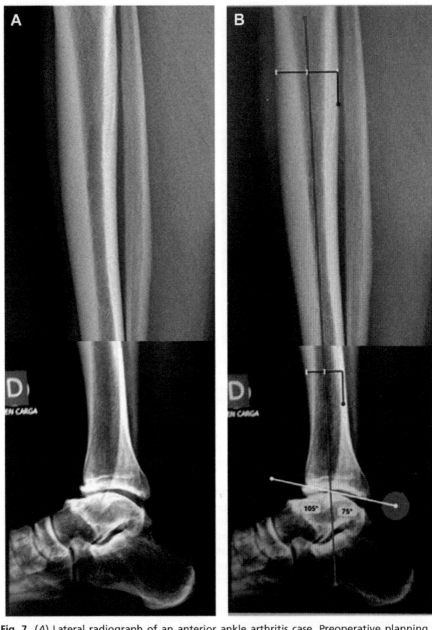

Fig. 7. (*A*) Lateral radiograph of an anterior ankle arthritis case. Preoperative planning is paramount in order to achieve the best results. (*B*) The digital measurement of the ADTA angle, in this case, 75°.

Through this approach, an anterior distal tibia opening wedge osteotomy can be performed. After protecting medial and lateral soft tissues and performing minimum periosteum dissection, an incomplete transverse distal tibia osteotomy is performed, approximately 5 cm proximal to the joint surface (**Fig. 9**). It can be performed using

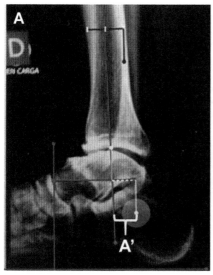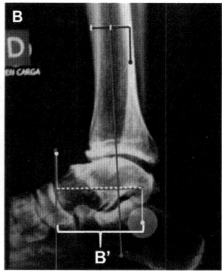

Fig. 8. Preoperative planning of the same case shown in **Fig. 6**, where the calculation of the TT ratio is exemplified. (A) The first distance to be measured, which corresponds to A′, that is, the distance measured along the longitudinal talar length line between the most posterior aspect of the subtalar joint and the intersection of the tibial axis with the longitudinal talar length line. (B) The distance B′, which corresponds to the longitudinal talar length. The TT ratio is obtained with the following formula: TT ratio: A/B*100. In this case, the TT ratio was 25.

a saw blade but in an intermittent manner and using constant cooling. The size of the opening wedge (h) is calculated with the same rule as for coronal plane correction, which considers the angle to be corrected (theta) and the width of the tibia at the osteotomy level (w) (formula: tan theta = h/w).[13] If we are correcting an anterior ankle arthritis case with an ADTA of 73°, the maximum overcorrection we could calculate would be to leave the ADTA in 85°. Using the formula, correcting 12° of the ADTA, with a tibia width of 32 mm, the wedge height size would be 6.8 mm.

An easy way to remember the SMOT wedge size needed for arthritic cases is to equal the deformity severity to the wedge size in millimeter (mm); for example, ADTA 73° is a 7° deformity (normal ADTA 80). That means a 7 mm wedge is required, and this calculation already includes the overcorrection needed. As the reader can conclude, a 6.8 mm wedge (obtained from the equation calculation previously shown) is not clinically different from a 7 mm wedge. We recommend using bone autograft if possible, obtained from the iliac crest. If this is not possible, the use of structured allografts is adequate.

When correcting anterior ankle arthritis combined with severe recurvatum deformities, we recommend performing a medial dome osteotomy (**Fig. 10**). Although technically more complex, a medial dome allows for an easier angular correction when estimating the necessary shift of the distal tibial fragment. If there is not any arthrosis or change in anterior ankle joint space, we recommend only to consider the supramalleolar apex of deformity and perform a medial dome SMOT centered on the supramalleolar apex. If there is already anterior ankle arthrosis, which is more frequent, we recommend using the intraarticular apex as the apex of deformity correction. For planning, a 4-hole third tubular plate is used. It is fixed with a pin at the medial malleolus through its first hole. Then, using it as a compass, multiple drill holes are performed

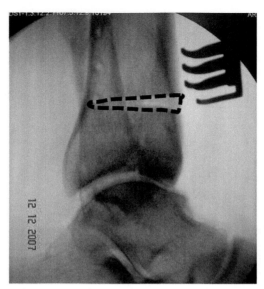

Fig. 9. Intraoperative fluoroscopy of an anterior ankle arthritic case. An incomplete transverse distal tibia opening wedge osteotomy has been performed. The size of the wedge is calculated with the same rule as for coronal plane correction, that is, 1.2° of correction for every 1 mm wedge size.

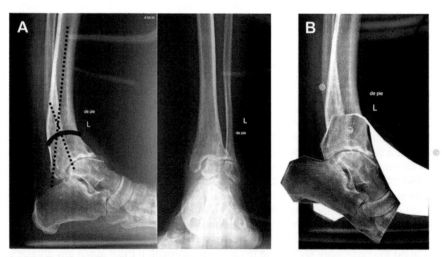

Fig. 10. Radiographic views of an anterior ankle arthritis case with a severe recurvatum deformity. (*A*) The measurement of the apex of the deformity (follow the intersection of the *dotted lines* representing the proximal and distal tibia axes) and consequent planning of a medially based dome SMOT. In the anteroposterior view, a mild varus deformity can also be seen. (*B*) The digital planning of a medial dome SMOT, where after the deformity correction, we can assume how difficult it will be to lengthen the posterior soft tissue contractures to achieve a neutral dorsiflexion.

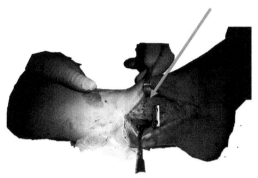

Fig. 11. Intraoperative view of the same clinical case shown in the previous images. Patient is laying supine; proximal is at the left-hand side of the picture. A medial approach was performed, and a medial dome osteotomy is being performed. Please note theone third semitubular plate at the distal tibia, which was used as a compass to "draw" with multiple perforations a medial dome SMOT on the tibia. These multiple holes were then connected with an osteotome.

using its fourth hole. After drilling, the osteotomy is completed with a conventional osteotome (**Fig. 11**). When performing the dome osteotomy (performed from a medial distal tibia approach), as there is a broad bone contact area, there is no need in using bone graft, but the correction must be tailored intraoperatively. Checking on fluoroscopy the distal fragment must be angulated until the desired correction is achieved. Fixation is performed with small fragment locked plates.

When correcting a sagittal plane deformity generally we also encounter coronal plane deformities. These deformities need a biplanar osteotomy, which are more

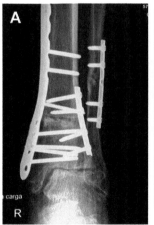
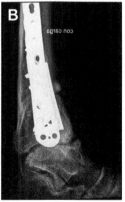
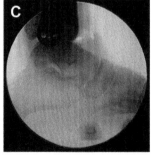

Fig. 12. Postoperative radiographs of the same patient presented in the previous figures. (*A*) The anteroposterior view of the ankle. As a correction in the sagittal and coronal plane was performed, 2 plates were used to fix the tibia. (*B*) The lateral view, where a complete correction of the recurvatum deformity was achieved. Note also the distal talar osteophytes that developed within 1 year, due to an incomplete posterior ankle soft tissue release. (*C*) The revision surgery where besides the removal of the talar osteophytes, an extensive release of posterior soft tissue was performed.

unstable than single-plane osteotomies. Our recommendation is to fix these biplanar osteotomies with 2 plates, ideally orthogonally placed (**Fig. 12**).

Fibular osteotomy

The fibula is osteotomized at the level of the syndesmosis, making sure to have enough distal fibula to be fixed later with a locking plate. The osteotomy is generally a short oblique one, resembling a Weber B fracture; this will allow an easier reorientation of the talus. A common mistake when fixing the fibula is to anatomically reduce the fragments and apply the plate. If we are correcting the TT ratio, anatomic reduction of the fibular osteotomy is not desired, as we will most probably lose all sagittal translation correction. Therefore, the fibula must remain nonreduced, and it has to be fixed with a locking plate, without interfragmentary compression. In this way we will hold the talus in the desired position.

If intraoperatively after correcting the ADTA angle and resecting the anterior tibial osteophytes, the talus seems to be too close to the anterior lip of the tibia, a talar neck plasty may be a solution to avoid future anterior ankle impingements.[5]

POSTERIOR ANKLE ARTHRITIS

In posterior ankle arthritis, we will either find an ADTA angle more than 80°, or the TT ratio higher than 38, or both (**Figs. 13** and **14**). Similar considerations must be given to

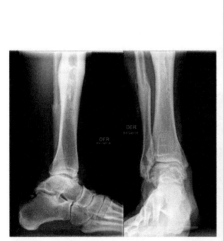
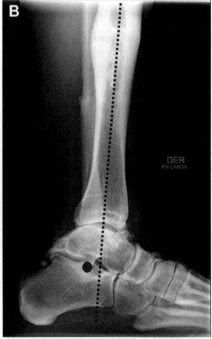

Fig. 13. Radiographic views of a posterior ankle arthritis case. (*A*) The lateral and anteroposterior view, with a clear sagittal malalignment (note the posterior position of the talus relative to the tibia). Please note that there is no significant coronal plane malalignment. (*B*) The posterior displacement of the talus relative to the tibial axis (represented by the *dotted line*). The tibia axis does not intersect the center of rotation of the ankle represented by the blue dot (located at the anterolateral talar process).

the preoperative planning, position of the apex of deformity, and desired amount of correction as already mentioned for anterior ankle arthritis.

In this case, we will indicate an SMOT using an anterior closing wedge rather than a posterior opening wedge, which is more technically challenging. The fibula must be osteotomized as already commented for anterior ankle arthritis (**Fig. 15**). In these cases, we have not seen soft tissue retractions as an additional element to be considered.

Technique

Tibial osteotomy

An anterior ankle incision is recommended, generally used also for coronal plane deformity treatment. Through this approach, an anterior tibial closing wedge can be performed, with the same calculations performed given for the anterior ankle arthritis cases. For deformities greater than 10°, a dome osteotomy is recommended using a direct distal tibia medial approach.

In posterior ankle arthritis we have seen a bigger role of a malunited fibula or syndesmosis in creating or keeping the posterior translation of the talus. The final fibular position must allow the correction of the TT ratio. Sometimes, a corrective osteotomy of the fibula should be performed forcing the distal fibula anteriorly so the talus can be anteriorized, fixing the fibula in the corrected position to hold the talus in place. The

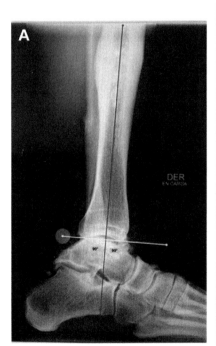
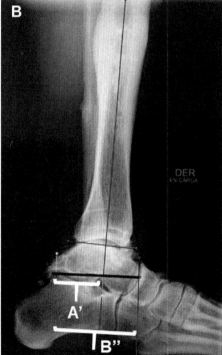

Fig. 14. Radiographic views of the same case presented in the previous figure. Preoperative planning is being performed. (A) The ADTA angle, which in this case is 90°. (B) The calculation of the TT ratio, obtained from dividing A′ over B″ and multiplying by 100. In this case, the TT ratio was 45.

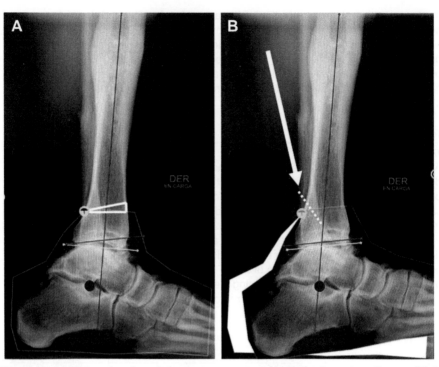

Fig. 15. Preoperative planning of the same case presented in the 2 previous figures. (*A*) A planned SMOT with an anterior closing wedge. Note the incorrect intersection of the center of rotation of the ankle (*blue dot*) and the tibia axis (*red line*). (*B*) The planned correction after removing the anterior tibial wedge. Note the correct intersection of the center of rotation of the ankle (*blue dot*) and the tibia axis (*red line*). To aid in the correction of the talar position, a fibular osteotomy must be added, allowing the talus to move forward. The fibular osteotomy is represented by a white dotted line and indicated by a white arrow.

incisura fibularis may have changed in shape, and therefore although we may see a correct reduction of the fibula in the incisura, the talar reduction may not be adequate. Therefore, we recommend using the talar reduction under the tibia and not the syndesmosis reduction to decide where to fix the fibula. It may happen in these cases that an apparent malreduction of the syndesmosis is needed to achieve a good correction of the TT ratio. A locking plate is needed to help maintain the talar position (**Fig. 16**).

RESULTS

For anterior ankle arthritis, an anterior opening wedge SMOT is the technique of choice, with good published results.[2,14] In the largest study published about anterior ankle arthritis, Scheidegger showed good results in 39 patients using either an SMOT with an opening wedge or a dome technique. The cumulative survival rate was 67% at 36 months, where 23% of the patients were converted to total ankle replacement or fusion.[15] No results have been published relative to posterior ankle arthritis.

In our experience over our last 20 cases of SMOT dealing with combined coronal and sagittal plane deformities, posterior ankle arthritis cases seem to have less

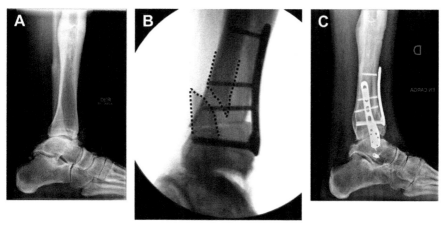

Fig. 16. Lateral radiographs of the same case presented in the previous figures. (*A*) The preoperative view with the visible sagittal ankle malalignment. (*B*) The intraoperative view after performing the SMOT with an anterior tibia closing wedge. Note the fibular contour after the fibula osteotomy, represented by the dotted lines following the proximal and distal fibular fragments. This relative "malposition" of the fibular osteotomy must be maintained and fixed with a locking plate, in order to secure the talar position. (*C*) The postoperative lateral view after the correction.

satisfactory results, due to the presence of syndesmotic damage or malunion, hindering a good result due to prolonged pain and stiffness. Our main SMOT technique for sagittal plane deformities considers adding or subtracting an anterior distal tibial wedge, which is easily combined with coronal plane corrections, using the same anterior approach. If the sagittal plane deformity prevails over the coronal deformity and presents with a magnitude of 10° or more, we prefer a medial approach to perform a medial Dome osteotomy. The medial dome SMOT is straightforward to perform, with an excellent bone-to-bone contact. In this way, we address the main deformity on its own plane, allowing an easier intraoperative correction tailoring. Smaller corrections of coronal plane deformities are possible through a medial dome, affecting some cancellous bone laterally or medially.

SUMMARY

For posterior ankle arthritis, an anterior closing wedge osteotomy is the recommended treatment option. An anterior opening wedge osteotomy is recommended for anterior ankle arthritis. If the deformity is greater than 10° in severity, a medial dome osteotomy is recommended. Special care must be taken to adequately plan the correction, in order to achieve a corrected angular position of the distal tibia and a correct centering of the talus under the tibia.

CLINICS CARE POINTS

- Anterior and posterior bow deformities produce a greater change in tibiotalar joint contact areas compared with valgus or varus deformities of the tibia.[4]
- Sagittal ankle malalignment is common in end-stage ankle arthrosis, with up to 56% of the cases presenting either anterior or posterior displacement of the talus in relation to the tibia.[8]

- Radiographically, the middiaphyseal line of the tibia in the sagittal plane passes through the lateral process of the talus when the plantar aspect of the foot is in 90° in relation to the tibia. Another commonly measured angle is the ADTA, whose normal value is 80°.[1] The TT ratio was shown to be a reliable radiographic measure to determine the position of the talus relative to the tibia, regardless of the condition of the ankle surface.[10]

- Anterior and posterior ankle arthritis have been characterized, with consequent changes in the ADTA angle and in the position of the talus relative to the tibia.[2]

- For anterior ankle arthritis, an anterior opening wedge SMOT is the technique of choice, with good, published results.[2,13]

DISCLOSURE

The authors have nothing to disclose.

REFERENCES

1. Paley, D. Chapter 18. Ankle and Foot Considerations. 571-645.
2. Kim J, Kim JB, Lee WC. Eccentric ankle arthritis in the sagittal plane: a novel description of anterior and posterior ankle arthritis. Foot Ankle Surg 2021;S1268, 7731(20)30283-6.
3. Tarr RR, Resnick CT, Wagner KS, et al. Changes in tibiotalar joint contact areas following experimentally induced tibial angular deformities. Clin Orthop Relat Res 1985;199:72–80.
4. Ting AJ, Tarr RR, Sarmiento A, et al. The role of subtalar motion and ankle contact pressure changes from angular deformities of the tibia. Foot Ankle 1987;7(5): 290–9.
5. Knupp M. The Use of Osteotomies in the Treatment of Asymmetric Ankle Joint Arthritis. Foot Ankle Int 2017;38(2):220–9.
6. Hunt KJ, Goeb Y, Behn AW, et al. Ankle Joint Contact Loads and Displacement With Progressive Syndesmotic Injury. Foot Ankle Int 2015;36(9):1095–103.
7. Jensen N, Krmer K, Hvid I. Distribution of bone strength at the distal tibia and fibula. Clin Biomech 1989;4(4):228–31.
8. Christensen JC, Schuberth JM, Powell EG. Talolisthesis in end stage ankle arthrosis. Foot Ankle Surg 2016;22(3):200–4.
9. Tochigi Y, Suh JS, Amendola A, et al. Ankle alignment on lateral radiographs. Part 1: sensitivity of measures to perturbations of ankle positioning. Foot Ankle Int 2006;27(2):82–7.
10. Tochigi Y, Suh JS, Amendola A, et al. Ankle alignment on lateral radiographs. Part 2: reliability and validity of measures. Foot Ankle Int 2006;27(2):88–92.
11. Knupp M, Stufkens SA, Bolliger L, et al. Classification and treatment of supramalleolar deformities. Foot Ankle Int 2011;32(11):1023–31.
12. Paley D, Herzenberg J, Tetsworth K, et al. Deformity planning for frontal and sagital plane corrective osteotomies. Orthop Clin North Am 1994;25(3):425–65.
13. Warnock KM, Johnson BD, Wright JB, et al. Calculation of the opening wedge for a low tibial osteotomy. Foot Ankle Int 2004;25(11):778–82.
14. Franz AC, Krähenbühl N, Ruiz R, et al. Hindfoot balancing in total ankle replacement: the role of supramalleolar osteotomies. Int Orthop 2020;44(9):1859–67.
15. Scheidegger P, Horn Lang T, Schweizer C, et al. A flexion osteotomy for correction of a distal tibial recurvatum deformity: a retrospective case series. Bone Joint J 2019;101-B:682–90.

The Role of Distraction Arthroplasty in Managing Ankle Osteoarthritis

Alirio J. deMeireles, MD, MBA[a], Ettore Vulcano, MD[b],*

KEYWORDS

- Distraction arthroplasty • Ankle distraction • Ankle osteoarthritis
- Posttraumatic arthritis

KEY POINTS

- Ankle distraction arthroplasty is a joint-preserving treatment option for moderate to severe ankle osteoarthritis.
- The ideal patient for ankle distraction arthroplasty is a young, active patient with preserved range of motion and no significant intraarticular deformity.
- There is no definitive clinical benefit to using a hinged distractor versus a fixed distractor.
- Patients should be counseled to expect maximal treatment benefit after a period of 1 year and that a significant proportion report continued, though improved, pain.

INTRODUCTION

Ankle osteoarthritis (OA), a progressive and debilitating source of chronic pain, is estimated to represent between 6% and 13% of all cases of OA.[1–3] Epidemiologic studies have found the decrease in health-related quality of life (HRQoL) from ankle OA to be comparable to that of hip or knee OA.[1,3] Importantly, when compared with OA seen in other joints, patients with ankle OA are diagnosed an average of 14 years earlier and have a more rapid progression to end-stage disease.[4] In contrast to end-stage hip or knee arthritis, however, primary OA of the ankle is rare. Valderrabano and colleagues found that posttraumatic OA (PTOA) was seen in 78% of their patients with end-stage ankle OA, while secondary OA and primary OA accounted for 13% and 9%, respectively.[5] The most common causes of ankle PTOA are lesions of the ankle ligaments, malleolar fractures, and tibial plafond fractures.[5] Historically, the main operative options for this progressive disease have been total ankle arthroplasty (TAA) or ankle arthrodesis.[6,7]

---

[a] Department of Orthopedic Surgery, Columbia University Irving Medical Center/New York-Presbyterian Hospital, 622 West 168th Street, PH 11 – 1102, New York, NY 10032-3720, USA;
[b] Department of Orthopedic Surgery, Columbia University Orthopedics at Mount Sinai Medical Center, 4302 Alton Road, Suite 220, Miami Beach, FL 33140, USA
* Corresponding author.
E-mail addresses: ettorevulcanomd@gmail.com; Ettore.Vulcano@msmc.com

Foot Ankle Clin N Am 27 (2022) 145–158
https://doi.org/10.1016/j.fcl.2021.11.006
1083-7515/22/© 2021 Elsevier Inc. All rights reserved.

TAA is an established option for the treatment of end-stage PTOA. Modern surgical implants demonstrate a 10-year survival rate of 75% to 90%.[7] Additionally, TAA allows for the arc of motion of the tibiotalar joint to be maintained as compared with ankle arthrodesis.[8] Although the 10 to 15-year outcomes studies for TAA are promising, the absence of standardized reporting tools has led to a large degree of heterogeneity within the reported data.[9] For younger, higher demand patients, the variability in long-term outcome reporting and increased reoperation rate compared with arthrodesis may limit the utility of TAA.[7] Additionally, Popelka and colleagues reported 11-year outcomes data demonstrating poorer TAA outcomes in patients with PTOA as compared with primary or secondary OA.[10]

Ankle arthrodesis is a well-established treatment of end-stage ankle OA and provides safe, reliable relief of pain.[11] Importantly, there are minimal activity restrictions after the arthrodesis. However, the loss of range of motion (ROM) seen after fusion may be unacceptable for younger, more active patients. The subsequently increased motion through the talonavicular joint seen after fusion also causes concern for the development of adjacent joint disease.[12]

In contrast to TAA and ankle arthrodesis, which irreversibly alter the native anatomy of the joint, ankle DA offers a joint-preserving technique to address end-stage ankle OA. DA uses a joint-spanning external fixator to mechanically unload the joint while concurrent complimentary procedures (ie, osteophyte removal, osteotomies, and microfracture) remove mechanical blocks to motion, provide optimal joint alignment, and encourage cartilage repair.

Given the potential limitations of TAA and ankle arthrodesis, orthopedic surgeons should be aware of ankle DA as a joint-preserving technique in the management of OA. Notably, the indications for ankle DA are expanding, with recent case reports demonstrating DA as a viable technique for the acute and definitive treatment of open ankle fractures.[13] The objective of this paper is to discuss the biomechanics, indications, surgical technique, and current outcomes data for ankle DA.

BIOMECHANICS OF DISTRACTION ARTHROPLASTY

The exact mechanism of action for cartilage repair after ankle DA is complex and has not been fully determined. The main concept is based on the hypothesis that hyaline cartilage is most likely to repair itself with the optimization of joint alignment and minimization of mechanical stress at the joint surface.[14–17] While mechanical stress at the joint is removed by the external fixator, full weight bearing by the patient allows for oscillations in the joint fluid pressure. In an in vitro study, Lafeber and colleagues demonstrated that when osteoarthritic cartilage is exposed to intermittent hydrostatic compression, proteoglycan synthesis rate is significantly increased.[18] Similarly, van Valburg performed a study examining the in vitro effect of intermittent fluid pressure gradients on articular cartilage harvested from an osteoarthritic joint versus a nonarthritic joint. The fluid pressures ranged from 0 to 13 kPa—similar to levels present with weight bearing on a distracted joint. The authors found that when the OA cartilage was subjected to intermittent fluid pressure gradients, there was a significant increase in cartilage matrix synthesis accompanied by a decrease in the production of interleukin 1 and tumor necrosis factor-alpha.

Building on this work, van Valburg and colleagues used a canine model with transected anterior cruciate ligaments to induce osteoarthritis. Their data showed that after 8 weeks of joint distraction, cartilage proteoglycan metabolism was found to closely resemble that of the nonarthritic control group.[19] Notably, on histologic examination, the tissue did not demonstrate cartilage repair. The authors hypothesized that the cartilage repair process continues after the distraction device is removed and suggest that longer follow-up would have demonstrated favorable histologic results.[19] Similarly, Wiegant evaluated the effect of joint distraction on a canine model subject to focal surgical cartilage damage. The distraction group demonstrated higher proteoglycan content, less collagen damage, and improved macroscopic and histologic damage scores compared with the control group.[20]

Other researchers have hypothesized that the biomechanical effects of joint distraction on subchondral bone resorption may contribute to cartilage healing. Intema and colleagues suggest the stress shielding exhibited by the external fixator frame results in subchondral bone resorption at the joint surface due to decreased load.[14,21] After the distractor is removed, the joint is once again subject to physiologic loads and the subchondral bone resorption normalizes (**Figs. 1** and **2**). This high degree of bone turnover may lead to increased release of factors beneficial to cartilage repair, such as transforming growth factor β, bone morphogenic protein, and insulin-like growth factors.[14] This concept would also support van Valburg's theory that cartilage repair continues to occur after the distraction device is removed.

INDICATIONS AND CONTRAINDICATIONS

Proper patient selection is critical to the success of the DA procedure. Given the highly specialized nature of ankle DA, there is currently a paucity of Level I-III evidence to guide indications.[22] Morse suggests that the ideal candidate is a young, active patient who has failed nonoperative management and who is opposed to the limitations that accompany TAA or arthrodesis.[23] Bernstein and colleagues add that an ideal candidate would also have preserved motion of greater than 20°, as ankle DA has not been shown to reliably increase ankle ROM.[24,25] Patients should be counseled on

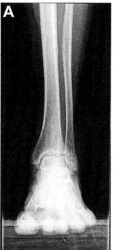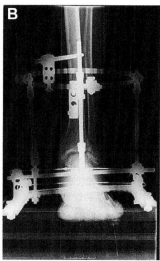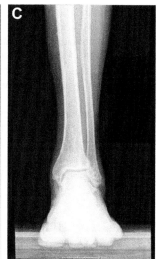

Fig. 1. AP weight-bearing (*A*) radiograph of a patient with severe posttraumatic arthritis demonstrating joint space narrowing, subchondral cyst formation, particularly in the fibula, and subchondral sclerosis. AP weight-bearing (*B*) radiograph 2 months after distraction arthroplasty with osteophyte excision. AP weight-bearing (*C*) radiograph obtained 1 year postoperatively demonstrating increased joint space, decreased subchondral sclerosis, and partial resolution of subchondral cysts.

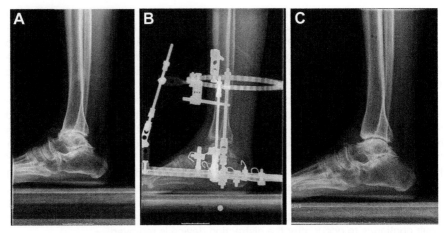

Fig. 2. Lateral weight-bearing (A) radiograph of a patient with severe posttraumatic arthritis demonstrating joint space narrowing, osteophyte formation, and marked subchondral sclerosis. Lateral weight-bearing (B) radiograph 2 months after distraction arthroplasty with osteophyte excision. Lateral weight-bearing (C) radiograph obtained 1 year postoperatively demonstrating increased joint space and decreased subchondral sclerosis.

the extended nature of the procedure and associated recovery, and understand that peak symptomatic improvement could take greater than 1 year.

While early literature viewed extraarticular deformity with resultant asymmetric wear as a relative contraindication, more recent work by Horn, Fragomen, and Rozbruch has shown ankle DA with concurrent osteotomy to be a successful option in the setting of hindfoot or distal tibia deformity.[26] Equinus contracture can be addressed concurrently and is not a contraindication.[27]

Relative contraindications include significant loss of bone stock, uncontrolled diabetes, chronic venous dermatitis, severe ankylosis of the joint with minimal remaining ROM, complete AVN of the talus, and tobacco use.[28,29] Partial avascular necrosis (AVN) of the talus is not a contraindication to surgery.[27] Absolute contraindications include arterial insufficiency, neuropathy, Charcot arthropathy, and severe intraarticular deformity.[24,28]

Notably, there are several case reports and case series demonstrating the expanding indications of ankle DA. Chan and colleagues recently published a case report demonstrating ankle DA as a viable technique for the acute and definitive treatment of open ankle fractures.[13] There is also early evidence to suggest ankle DA is safe and efficacious in the treatment of ankle joint destruction secondary to inflammatory arthritides.[30,31]

SURGICAL TECHNIQUE

There are multiple adjuvant procedures commonly performed to address complicating anatomic factors such as equinus contracture, anterior or posterior osteophyte impingement, coronal or sagittal malalignment, or intraarticular loose bodies. These include arthroscopy, arthrotomy, supramalleolar or fibular osteotomies, and soft tissue balancing procedures.

The patient is placed in the supine position on the operating table. General or spinal anesthesia may be used. Patients should receive intravenous antibiotics 30 minutes before surgery and for 24-hours postoperatively. A sterile tourniquet may be placed if performing a supramalleolar osteotomy, open arthrotomy, or arthroscopy, but should be released when attention is turned to the external fixator.[28]

The authors prefer to resect anterior osteophytes via arthroscopy performed through standard anterior portals using a 4.0 mm arthroscope.[32,33] Bulky osteophytes unable to be resected with arthroscopy should be removed with a mini-open incision through the extension of the arthroscopic portals. Saltzman and colleagues suggest the avoidance of plantarflexion during cheilectomy, as the resultant stretch of the anterior joint capsule may limit the visualization of impinging anterior osteophytes.[34] Cheilectomy is considered adequate if the anterior tibial bone spur has been resected to the anterior margin of the medial malleolus.[34] Additionally, intraoperative lateral fluoroscopic images through dorsiflexion and plantarflexion should be used to assess for residual osteophyte impingement.[28] Paley and colleagues routinely administer nonsteroidal antiinflammatory drugs (NSAIDs) for 6 weeks postoperatively to inhibit osteophyte recurrence.[27]

Arthroscopic joint lavage is performed, and all loose bodies are removed. Prior studies have suggested that compared with DA alone, adjuvant arthroscopic micro-fracture is associated with superior American Orthopedic Foot and Ankle Society (AOFAS) scores, improved pain relief, and superior radiographic improvement of arthritis.[35] However, in 2020, Gianakos and colleagues published a comparative study demonstrating no clinical benefit of concomitant microfracture with ankle DA.[36] Patients with ankle equinus contracture are treated with a gastrocnemius recession or Achilles tendon lengthening. In their 2016 review, Bernstein and colleagues reported commonly using iliac crest bone marrow autograft concentrate (BMAC) and noted that though clinical evidence is sparse, there is robust basic science literature support-ing this practice.[24,37] However, the most recent data published by Gianakos and col-leagues demonstrate no clinical benefit with the use of concentrated bone marrow aspirate with DA compared with DA alone.[36]

After adjuvant procedures, attention is turned to the application of the external fix-ator. A single circumferential tibial ring is appropriate in the absence of a supramalleo-lar osteotomy. A two-ringed tibial construct should be used if an adjuvant osteotomy is performed. Both tibial rings should be applied perpendicular to the long axis of the tibia, leaving 2 fingerbreadths of space between the skin and the inner diameter of the ring. Two 5 to 6 mm hydroxyapatite-coated half-pins are then used to secure the proximal tibial ring. Half-pins are predrilled with a 4.8 mm drill bit and should be placed bicortically. The distal tibial ring is secured with one 5 mm hydroxyapatite-coated half-pin and a 1.8 mm wire tensioned to 110 to 130lbs.

A smooth, temporary Kirschner wire (K-wire) is then used to approximate the ankle center of rotation. The K-wire approximates the Inman axis and is placed from the tip of the lateral malleolus to the tip of the medial malleolus in a posterolateral to antero-medial fashion. Positioning should be checked with fluoroscopy. Proper positioning of this wire is crucial as it provides the landmarks for placement of the medial and lateral universal hinges. The footplate is then placed in line with the foot and secured with 1.8 mm crossing wires placed across the talus, calcaneus, and metatarsals. The wires are tensioned to 70 to 90 lbs.

The external fixator can be static or allow for motion at the ankle joint (ie, hinged distraction). Saltzman and colleagues conducted a prospective randomized control trial and demonstrated superior short-term Ankle Osteoarthritis Scale (AOS) scores for patients treated with hinged distraction compared with static fixation.[34] In their follow-up study, however, they note that the positive effects seen with motion distrac-tion do not persist at the 5-year outcome mark.[38] If opting for a static construct, distraction rods without hinges are used. If hinged distraction is planned, universal hinges are applied in line with the Inman axis as described above and an unhinged posterior rod is placed. The posterior rod may be removed for motion therapy. The external fixator is typically removed at 10 to 12 weeks.[24,28]

Due to the risk of nerve injury, we avoid immediately distracting the joint to its final distance. We instead follow the protocol of Bernstein and colleagues, who recommend 3 mm of distraction while in the operating room, followed by 2 to 3 mm of distraction in the immediate postoperative period while the patient is still admitted for pain control.[24] Fluoroscopy should be used intraoperatively to ensure the appropriate distraction gap has been achieved. Any remaining distraction can be applied to the frame at the first postoperative clinic visit. Radiographs should be obtained after any adjustment to the frame.

POSTOPERATIVE MANAGEMENT

Patients are counseled on daily pin care using a 1:1 mixture of hydrogen peroxide and normal saline. They may shower after discharge from the hospital. We encourage full weight bearing through the external fixator after 3 to 5 days. If a hinged external fixator has been applied, patients are instructed to remove the posterior stabilizing bar and complete 20 repetitions of passive ROM three times per day. The frame is removed at 12 weeks.

EFFICACY OF ANKLE DISTRACTION ARTHROPLASTY

There is a growing body of evidence evaluating the efficacy of ankle DA as a treatment of osteoarthritis (**Table 1**). Current practice builds on the seminal research conducted by Judet and Judet, who demonstrated "formation of fibrous tissue" in the tibiotarsal joints of canines subject to distraction with an external fixator for 30 days.[39]

In 1995, van Valburg and colleagues published a retrospective case series detailing the outcomes of 11 patients treated with DA for severe posttraumatic arthritis. Notably, their surgical technique was different than the current standard and involved the addition of ankle hinges to a previously static frame between weeks 6 and 12.[40] At a mean follow-up of 20 months, they reported all patients had improvements in their pain, 5/11 (45%) of patients were pain free, and 6/11 (55%) patients had improved ROM. They did not report on adverse events but did note 1 patient had decreased ROM in the postoperative period.[40] The authors went on to validate these findings by conducting a prospective trial involving 17 patients with a mean age of 39.6 years (range, 17–55) who were treated with ankle DA for end-stage osteoarthritis. Evaluation at 1- and 2-year follow-up demonstrated significant improvement in patient-reported functional status, pain, and physical examination findings at the 2-year mark as compared with the 1-year results ($P < .004$).[41] Importantly, 4 of 17 patients failed treatment and went on to arthrodesis.[41]

Kanbe and colleagues published a case report detailing the use of ankle DA for the treatment of a 19-year-old woman with severe ankle arthritis.[42] At 3-year follow-up, the authors noted that the joint was pain free.[42] Importantly, the authors were able to perform an ankle arthroscopy at the time of frame removal (4 weeks after application) and directly visualized robust fibrocartilage formation.[42] Similarly, Lamm and colleagues published a case series consisting of 3 patients treated with hinged ankle DA (mean age, 41 years) who had received pre and postoperative ankle magnetic resonance imaging (MRIs) (**Fig. 3**).[43] The data showed an average of a 0.5 mm decrease in subchondral bone thickness and 0.5 mm increase in cartilage thickness.[43] These

Table 1
Summary of outcomes from studies examining ankle distraction arthroplasty

Author (Year)	Sample Size	Age[a] (yrs.)	Follow Up[a]	Level of Evidence	Study Design	Key Points	Negative Outcomes
Dabash et al,[46] 2020	1	52	9 y.	V	Case Series	Improvement in pain (no specific scale recorded); "maintenance of active lifestyle"; 15° improvement in dorsiflexion	None Reported
Greenfield et al,[29] 2019	144	48.9 ± 14.1	4.6 y (0.8–14.5 y)	IV	Retrospective Cohort	120/144 (84%) survival at 5-y - a significant improvement on prior intermediate-term data; pain scores not collected	24/144 (16.7%) patients failed treatment at 5 y; female gender and radiographic AVN of talus were predictors of failure
Xu et al,[45] 2017	16	30.3 ± 14.3	40.9 mo (17–67 mo)	IV	Retrospective Cohort	Significant improvement in average VAS score, AOFAS-AH score, and SF-36 score; joint space > 3 mm at 1 y was a predictor of treatment success; gender had no effect on prognosis	2/16 (12.5%) patients failed treatment (1 spontaneous fusion, 1 arthrodesis); 2/16 (12.5%) patients developed pin site infections
Nguyen et al,[38] 2015	29	41.5 ± 9.1	8.3 y (6.1–10.5 y)	IV	Retrospective Cohort	AOS score ≤42 at 2 y, older age at surgery, and fixed distraction were positive predictors of survival at 5 y	13/29 (44%) patients failed treatment at 5 y (8 arthrodesis, 5 TAA); 53% of patients had pin site infections
Marijnissen et al,[48] 2014	111	42.7 ± 9.8	Minimum 2 y.	IV	Combined data from prospective cohort and small RCT	At 2 years, pain scores decreased from 67% to 38% and disability scores decreased from 68% to 36%	17% of patients failed at 2 y; 44% at 5 y; female gender was predictive of failure at 2 y

(continued on next page)

Table 1
(continued)

Author (Year)	Sample Size	Age[a] (yrs.)	Follow Up[a]	Level of Evidence	Study Design	Key Points	Negative Outcomes
Saltzman et al34, 2012	29	Fixed: 42.4 (18–53) Hinged: 42.7 (27–59)	2 y.	I	Prospective RCT	At 2 years, the motion group had a mean AOS score improvement of 56.5% and the static group had a mean improvement of 22.9%	19/29 (66%) patients developed pin site infections; 2/29 (6.9%) patients developed osteomyelitis; 8/29 (28%) patients developed a nerve palsy; 1/29 (3%) developed DVT
Intema et al14, 2011	26	41 ± 9	2 y.	IV	Prospective Cohort	Significant decrease in AOS pain and disability scores; decreased subchondral bone density seen after DA is associated with clinical improvement	None reported
Lamm et al,43 2009	3	41	Minimum 1 y.	V	Case Series	Postoperatively, patients averaged a 0.5 mm decrease in subchondral bone thickness and a 0.5 mm increase in cartilage thickness	None reported
Tellisi et al,25 2009	23	43 (16–73)	30.5 mo (12–60 mo)	IV	Retrospective Cohort	21/23 (91%) patients improved their pain by an average of 19 points on AOFAS scale; improvements were greatest for patients > 60 y.	2/23 (8.7%) patients failed treatment; 100% of patients developed pin site infection
Paley et al27, 2008	23	45 (17–62)	64 mo (24–157 mo)	IV	Case Series	14/18 (78%) patients reported only mild-moderate ankle pain; 11/18 (61%) patients	2/23 (11%) patients failed treatment (1 arthrodesis, 1 TAA)

Study	N	Age[a]	Follow-up	Level of Evidence	Study Type	Results	Complications
Ploegmakers et al47, 2005	22	37 ± 11	10 y (7–15 y)	III	Retrospective Cohort	AOS scores improved from 67 to 25; disability scores improved from 20% to 73%	6/22 (27%) patients failed treatment and underwent arthrodesis
Marijnissen et al44, 2002	57	44 (18–65)	2.8 y (2.5–3.1 y)	II	Small Prospective RCT	Average improvement in pain and disability score was 35% and 69%, respectively; decrease in subchondral bone density and increase in joint space at 1 and 3 y	13/57 (23%) patients failed treatment and pursued arthrodesis; 16/57 (28%) patients had pin site infections; 8/57 (14%) patients had forefoot k-wire fracture
van Valburg et al41, 1999	17	40 (17–55)	Minimum 2 y.	II	Prospective Cohort	13/17 (76% of patients) showed significant improvement in patient-reported functional status, pain, and physical examination	4/17 (24%) went on to arthrodesis; "Occasional" pin-site infections; 4/17 (24%) had broken forefoot Kirschner wires
Kanbe et al42, 1997	1	19	3 y.	V	Case Report	Arthroscopy at time of frame removal demonstrated robust fibrocartilage formation; joint space increased 2 mm on radiographs; no pain at 3 y	None reported
van Valburg et al40, 1995	11	35 (20–70)	20 mo (10–60 mo)	III	Retrospective Case Series	6/11 (55%) patients had improved ROM; all patients noted improvement in pain; 5/11 were pain free; reported occasional use of NSAIDs	ROM decreased in 1 patient

Abbreviations: AOFAS-AH, American Orthopedic Foot and Ankle Society Ankle-Hindfoot scoring system; AOS, ankle osteoarthritis scale; AVN, avascular necrosis; DA, Distraction Arthroplasty; DVT, deep vein thrombosis; NSAIDs, nonsteroidal antiinflammatory drugs; ROM, range of motion; SF-36, short form-36; TAA, total ankle arthroplasty; VAS, visual analog scale.
[a] Mean (range)

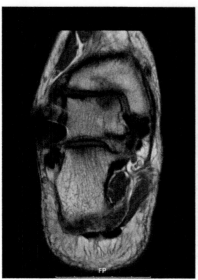 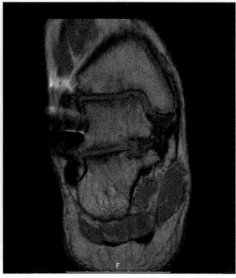

Fig. 3. Preoperative (L) and postoperative (R) MRI scans demonstrating increased joint space and improved cartilage thickness.

data further support the theory that ankle DA allows for fibrocartilage to replace areas of damaged cartilage in the tibiotalar joint.

The clinical benefit of hinged versus static distraction has been frequently discussed in the literature. In 2012, Saltzman and colleagues performed a prospective randomized controlled trial (RCT) involving 36 patients who were assigned to either hinged or static distraction. Of the 29 patients with available 2-year follow-up data, those assigned to the hinged distraction group had a mean AOS score improvement of 56.5% and the static group had a mean improvement of 22.9%. Both groups demonstrated a significant improvement from their baseline.[34] However, when the authors published a follow-up study of this data with a minimum follow-up period of 5 years, they found that the static distraction group had superior outcomes.[38] The authors were unable to identify the primary factor driving the difference in outcomes at the 2- and 5-year time points. Additionally, there have been multiple studies that have determined there is no difference in postoperative ROM for patients treated with fixed versus hinged distraction.[25,34]

It is important to consider adverse events and treatment failure rates associated with ankle DA. Pin site infections are extremely common and generally easily treated with oral antibiotics. The rate of pin site infection in the literature ranges from 0% to 100%.[25,34,38,40,44–47] Approximately 1.2% to 6.9% of patients will experience more severe infection such as osteomyelitis requiring treatment with intravenous antibiotics.[27,34,48] Additionally, pin breakage, most commonly at the midfoot, occurs at a rate of between 14% and 24%.[24,44]

The rate of treatment failure, defined as the progression to arthrodesis or TAA, varies widely. In 2019, Greenfield and colleagues published a robust retrospective cohort study reporting on 144 patients at a mean follow-up of 4.6 years who were treated with ankle DA. The authors report a 16.7% failure rate, and note that female gender and radiographic evidence of AVN of the talus were predictors of failure.[29] This data represents a staggering improvement on previously published 5-year outcomes data by Nguyen and colleagues, who reported a 44% failure rate and found that AOS score ≤42 at 2 years, older age at surgery, and fixed distraction were positive predictors of survival at 5 years.[38] This work was in alignment with Marijnissen's previously published 2014 data which also demonstrated a 44% failure rate.[48] In 2017, Xu and colleagues reported a retrospective cohort study involving 16 patients with ankle OA treated with DA. At a mean follow-up of 2.5 years, the authors found significant improvement in average VAS score, AOFAS score, and Short Form-36 (SF-36) score. They noted that joint space > 3 mm at 1 year was a predictor of treatment success and gender had no effect on prognosis.[45] The authors reported a 16.7% failure rate.[45]

One of the major benefits inherent to DA is its joint-sparing nature. Thus, the patient theoretically does not "burn any bridges" by electing to proceed with ankle DA as initial surgical treatment of ankle OA. Though sparse, the available data reporting on patients who failed DA and went on to arthrodesis or TAA show no increase in complication rate.[29] Further research on the outcomes of patients previously treated with DA is needed.

SUMMARY

Ankle DA is a safe, effective joint-preserving treatment of OA. The procedure involves removing mechanical stress at the joint surface through the application of a joint-spanning external fixator for a period of 10 to 12 weeks. There is an array of adjuvant procedures commonly performed to optimize healing potential—including microfracture, BMAC injections, osteophyte removal, supramalleolar or fibular osteotomies, and soft tissue balancing procedures. The exact mechanism driving clinical improvement has not been determined but is likely a result of the fibrocartilage proliferation seen after treatment and subchondral bone remodeling as a result of off-loading the joint. While short- and intermediate-term studies have been promising, the highly specialized nature of the procedure results in a lack of robust clinical evidence and wide variance in reported failure and complication rates. Further clinical evidence focused on longer-term outcomes studies as well as the complication rate of those who have undergone TAA or arthrodesis after DA is needed.

CLINICS CARE POINTS

Pearls:

Ankle distraction arthroplasty has a role in the treatment of moderate to severe ankle osteoarthritis.

- Advise patients that the benefits of distraction arthroplasty are perceived by patients about 1 year after removal of the frame.
- A two-ringed tibial construct should be used if an adjuvant osteotomy is performed and in patients with osteopenic bone.
- Space the foot and tibia ring about 12-15cm apart.

Pitfalls:

Due to the risk of nerve injury, avoid immediately distracting the joint to its final distance, instead opt for 3 mm of distraction while in the operating room, followed by 2 to 3 mm of distraction in the immediate postoperative period.

Relative contraindications include significant loss of bone stock, uncontrolled diabetes, chronic venous dermatitis, severe ankylosis of the joint with minimal remaining ROM, complete AVN of the talus, and tobacco use.

- Patients must be counseled on the extensive rehabilitation process associated with distraction arthroplasty, failure to do so may result poor patient reported outcomes despite appropriate clinical progress.
- Distraction arthroplasty has not been demonstrated to improve range of motion.

DISCLOSURE

E. Vulcano is a consultant for Vilex and Novastep. A.J. deMeireles has no disclosures.

REFERENCES

1. Glazebrook M, Daniels T, Younger A, et al. Comparison of health-related quality of life between patients with end-stage ankle and hip arthrosis. J Bone Joint Surg Am 2008;90(3):499–505.
2. Thomas RH, Daniels TR. Ankle arthritis. J Bone Joint Surg Am 2003;85(5):923–36.
3. Agel J, Coetzee JC, Sangeorzan BJ, et al. Functional limitations of patients with end-stage ankle arthrosis. Foot Ankle Int 2005;26(7):537–9.
4. Delco ML, Kennedy JG, Bonassar LJ, et al. Post-traumatic osteoarthritis of the ankle: a distinct clinical entity requiring new research approaches. J Orthop Res 2017;35(3):440–53.
5. Valderrabano V, Horisberger M, Russell I, et al. Etiology of ankle osteoarthritis. Clin Orthop Relat Res 2009;467(7):1800–6.
6. Rabinovich RV, Haleem AM, Rozbruch SR. Complex ankle arthrodesis: Review of the literature. World J Orthop 2015;6(8):602–13.
7. Morash J, Walton DM, Glazebrook M. Ankle arthrodesis versus total ankle arthroplasty. Foot Ankle Clin 2017;22(2):251–66.
8. Pedowitz DI, Kane JM, Smith GM, et al. Total ankle arthroplasty versus ankle arthrodesis: a comparative analysis of arc of movement and functional outcomes. Bone Joint J 2016;98-B(5):634–40.
9. Mercer J, Penner M, Wing K, et al. Inconsistency in the reporting of adverse events in total ankle arthroplasty: a systematic review of the literature. Foot Ankle Int 2016;37(2):127–36.
10. Popelka S, Sosna A, Vavřík P, et al. [Eleven-year experience with total ankle arthroplasty]. Acta Chir Orthop Traumatol Cech 2016;83(2):74–83.
11. Chalayon O, Wang B, Blankenhorn B, et al. Factors affecting the outcomes of uncomplicated primary open ankle arthrodesis. Foot Ankle Int 2015;36(10):1170–9.
12. Wang Y, Li Z, Wong DW-C, et al. Effects of ankle arthrodesis on biomechanical performance of the entire foot. PLoS One 2015;10(7):e0134340.
13. Chan JJ, Garden E, Nordio A, et al. Distraction arthroplasty as acute and definitive treatment for open ankle fracture dislocation. Orthopedics 2020;44(1): e148–50.
14. Intema F, Van Roermund PM, Marijnissen ACA, et al. Tissue structure modification in knee osteoarthritis by use of joint distraction: an open 1-year pilot study. Ann Rheum Dis 2011;70(8):1441–6.
15. van Roermund PM, Marijnissen ACA, Lafeber FPJG. Joint distraction as an alternative for the treatment of osteoarthritis. Foot Ankle Clin 2002;7(3):515–27.
16. Kanamiya T, Naito M, Hara M, et al. The influences of biomechanical factors on cartilage regeneration after high tibial osteotomy for knees with medial compartment osteoarthritis: clinical and arthroscopic observations. Arthroscopy 2002; 18(7):725–9.

17. Waller C, Hayes D, Block JE, et al. Unload it: the key to the treatment of knee osteoarthritis. Knee Surg Sports Traumatol Arthrosc 2011;19(11):1823–9.
18. Lafeber F, Veldhuijzen JP, Vanroy JL, et al. Intermittent hydrostatic compressive force stimulates exclusively the proteoglycan synthesis of osteoarthritic human cartilage. Br J Rheumatol 1992;31(7):437–42.
19. van Valburg AA, van Roermund PM, Marijnissen AC, et al. Joint distraction in treatment of osteoarthritis (II): effects on cartilage in a canine model. Osteoarthritis Cartilage 2000;8(1):1–8.
20. Wiegant K, van Roermund PM, Intema F, et al. Sustained clinical and structural benefit after joint distraction in the treatment of severe knee osteoarthritis. Osteoarthritis Cartilage 2013;21(11):1660–7.
21. Intema F, Thomas TP, Anderson DD, et al. Subchondral bone remodeling is related to clinical improvement after joint distraction in the treatment of ankle osteoarthritis. Osteoarthritis Cartilage 2011;19(6):668–75.
22. Smith NC, Beaman D, Rozbruch SR, et al. Evidence-based indications for distraction ankle arthroplasty. Foot Ankle Int 2012;33(8):632–6.
23. Morse KR, Flemister AS, Baumhauer JF, et al. Distraction arthroplasty. Foot Ankle Clin 2007;12(1):29–39.
24. Bernstein M, Reidler J, Fragomen A, et al. Ankle Distraction Arthroplasty: Indications, Technique, and Outcomes. J Am Acad Orthop Surg 2017;25(2):89–99.
25. Tellisi N, Fragomen AT, Kleinman D, et al. Joint preservation of the osteoarthritic ankle using distraction arthroplasty. Foot Ankle Int 2009;30(4):318–25.
26. Horn DM, Fragomen AT, Rozbruch SR. Supramalleolar osteotomy using circular external fixation with six-axis deformity correction of the distal tibia. Foot Ankle Int 2011;32(10):986–93.
27. Paley D, Lamm BM, Purohit RM, et al. Distraction arthroplasty of the ankle–how far can you stretch the indications? Foot Ankle Clin 2008;13(3):471–84, ix.
28. Barg A, Amendola A, Beaman DN, et al. Ankle joint distraction arthroplasty: why and how? Foot Ankle Clin 2013;18(3):459–70.
29. Greenfield S, Matta KM, McCoy TH, et al. Ankle Distraction Arthroplasty for Ankle Osteoarthritis: A Survival Analysis. Strateg Trauma Limb Reconstr 2019;14(2): 65–71.
30. Cleary G, Pain C, McCann L, et al. Short-term outcome of surgical arthrodiastasis of the ankle with Ilizarov frame in a cohort of children and young people with juvenile idiopathic arthritis. Rheumatol Adv Pract 2019;3(2):rkz031.
31. Nakasa T, Adachi N, Kato T, et al. Distraction arthroplasty with arthroscopic microfracture in a patient with rheumatoid arthritis of the ankle joint. J Foot Ankle Surg 2015;54(2):280–4.
32. Vega J, Dalmau-Pastor M, Malagelada F, et al. Ankle Arthroscopy: An Update. J Bone Joint Surg Am 2017;99(16):1395–407.
33. Golanó P, Vega J, Pérez-Carro L, et al. Ankle anatomy for the arthroscopist. Part I: The portals. Foot Ankle Clin 2006;11(2):253–73, v.
34. Saltzman CL, Hillis SL, Stolley MP, et al. Motion Versus Fixed Distraction of the Joint in the Treatment of Ankle Osteoarthritis. J Bone Joint Surg Am 2012; 94(11):961–70.
35. Zhang K, Jiang Y, Du J, et al. Comparison of distraction arthroplasty alone versus combined with arthroscopic microfracture in treatment of post-traumatic ankle arthritis. J Orthop Surg Res 2017;12(1):45.
36. Gianakos AL, Haring RS, Shimozono Y, et al. Effect of Microfracture on Functional Outcomes and Subchondral Sclerosis Following Distraction Arthroplasty of the Ankle Joint. Foot Ankle Int 2020;41(6):631–8.

37. Yanai T, Ishii T, Chang F, et al. Repair of large full-thickness articular cartilage defects in the rabbit: the effects of joint distraction and autologous bone-marrow-derived mesenchymal cell transplantation. J Bone Joint Surg Br 2005;87(5): 721–9.

38. Nguyen MP, Pedersen DR, Gao Y, et al. Intermediate-term follow-up after ankle distraction for treatment of end-stage osteoarthritis. J Bone Joint Surg Am 2015;97(7):590–6.

39. Judet R, Judet T. [The use of a hinge distraction apparatus after arthrolysis and arthroplasty (author's transl)]. Rev Chir Orthop Reparatrice Appar Mot 1978; 64(5):353–65.

40. van Valburg AA, van Roermund PM, Lammens J, et al. Can Ilizarov joint distraction delay the need for an arthrodesis of the ankle? A preliminary report. J Bone Joint Surg Br 1995;77(5):720–5.

41. van Valburg AA, van Roermund PM, Marijnissen AC, et al. Joint distraction in treatment of osteoarthritis: a two-year follow-up of the ankle. Osteoarthritis Cartilage 1999;7(5):474–9.

42. Kanbe K, Hasegawa A, Takagishi K, et al. Arthroscopic findings of the joint distraction for the patient with chondrolysis of the ankle. Diagn Ther Endosc 1997;4(2):101–5.

43. Lamm BM, Gourdine-Shaw M. MRI evaluation of ankle distraction: a preliminary report. Clin Podiatr Med Surg 2009;26(2):185–91.

44. Marijnissen ACA, Van Roermund PM, Van Melkebeek J, et al. Clinical benefit of joint distraction in the treatment of severe osteoarthritis of the ankle: proof of concept in an open prospective study and in a randomized controlled study. Arthritis Rheum 2002;46(11):2893–902.

45. Xu Y, Zhu Y, Xu X-Y. Ankle joint distraction arthroplasty for severe ankle arthritis. BMC Musculoskelet Disord 2017;18(1):96.

46. Dabash S, Buksbaum JR, Fragomen A, et al. Distraction arthroplasty in osteoarthritis of the foot and ankle. World J Orthop 2020;11(3):145–57.

47. Ploegmakers JJW, van Roermund PM, van Melkebeek J, et al. Prolonged clinical benefit from joint distraction in the treatment of ankle osteoarthritis. Osteoarthritis Cartilage 2005;13(7):582–8.

48. Marijnissen ACA, Hoekstra MCL, Pré BC du, et al. Patient characteristics as predictors of clinical outcome of distraction in treatment of severe ankle osteoarthritis. J Orthop Res 2014;32(1):96–101.

The Role of Anterior Ankle Arthroscopy in the Management of Ankle Arthritis

Literature Review, Patient Evaluation, Goals of Treatment and Technique

John E. Femino, MD*, Alan Shamrock, MD

KEYWORDS

• Ankle arthroscopy • Ankle osteoarthritis • Ankle impingement • Cam impingement

INTRODUCTION

The role of arthroscopic debridement for the treatment of pain in ankle osteoarthritis (OA) has been poorly studied. A systematic review by Glazebrook and colleagues in 2009 provided recommendations for the use of ankle arthroscopy in treating different pathologies.[1] The authors recommended *against* the use of arthroscopy in treating ankle OA with an evidence level of C based on consistent poor results in available level IV and V studies.[2–5]

Conversely, the authors gave a B recommendation for arthroscopic debridement of anterior ankle impingement (AAI) due to bone and/or soft tissue impingement, provided there are minimal OA changes.

Unfortunately, there have been no higher quality outcome studies describing the use of arthroscopic debridement in the treatment of more advanced ankle OA. Studies have not provided a systematic preoperative approach to guide patient selection for arthroscopic debridement. This adds confusion to the issue as in most studies, the primary means of patient selection are ankle radiographs in a patient complaining of ankle pain. In a study of more than 5000 patients with hip OA, plain radiographs were demonstrated to be poor diagnostic tests if used in isolation.[6] The sensitivity of radiographic hip OA for predicting hip pain localized to the groin was 36.7% and the positive predictive value was only 6.0%. With regard to knee OA, a systematic search of the literature by Bedson and colleagues demonstrated that with the setting of radiographic knee OA, the proportion of pain varied highly from 15% to 81%.[7]

This discordance between the presence of radiographic OA changes and joint pain in the hip and knee is a critical concept to consider when evaluating studies involving ankle

Department of Orthopaedics and Rehabilitation, University of Iowa, 200 Hawkins Drive, Iowa City, IA, USA
* Corresponding author.
E-mail address: john-femino@uiowa.edu

Foot Ankle Clin N Am 27 (2022) 159–174
https://doi.org/10.1016/j.fcl.2021.11.007
1083-7515/22/Published by Elsevier Inc.

foot.theclinics.com

OA. The ankle and hindfoot are an anatomically complex group of joints that have inter-twined kinematics and alignment. They are, as a functional unit, more complex than a single large joint. The complaint of "ankle pain" can be due to numerous etiologies involving the ankle and hindfoot joints; bone, articular cartilage, ligaments, tendons, and nerves all have common pathologies that can cause pain in this area. In terms of postoperative pain assessment after arthroscopic debridement for impingement, there is also a disconnect in the literature, as ongoing pain or subsequent major ankle surgery have been assumed to be due to failure of arthroscopic debridement as a technique. In the absence of a systematic selection process, including a detailed preoperative phys-ical examination to detect locations of impingement with correlative 3 dimensional im-aging, no conclusions can be drawn about the arthroscopy treatment group due to possible heterogeneity. Similarly, without a systematic postoperative physical examina-tion and radiologic assessment, one cannot make any definite conclusions regarding the outcomes or appropriateness of arthroscopic debridement for the treatment of AAI in ankle OA. Continued pain may be due to unresolved/untreated impingement.

One study to consider along this line of reasoning is the UK FASHIoN study which randomized patients with femoroacetabular impingement (FAI) to hip arthroscopy or formal Physical Therapy functional rehabilitation treatment groups. Of 121 patients who underwent hip arthroscopy 14 (8.7%) were found by a surgical review panel to have suboptimal resection of bone on the femur or acetabulum on postoperative MRI scans.[8] Unfortunately, only hip-specific outcome measures were used in this study and there was no reported postoperative physical examination to correlate ongoing pain with these radiologic findings.

Intermediate joint preserving and motion sparing operative treatments are needed for patients with ankle OA. Results of intermediate procedures are commonly judged in terms of 5-year outcomes, rather than comparing them to definitive joint sacrificing procedures such as ankle arthrodesis (AA) or total ankle arthroplasty (TAA). At the time of presentation, many patients are not ideal candidates for either AA or TAA due to young age, occupational demands, wish to preserve ankle joint mobility, or medical factors such as obesity, smoking, or suboptimally controlled diabetes. Other interme-diate treatments for ankle OA include supramalleolar osteotomy, bulk allograft replacement, and ankle distraction. These may or may not have overlap with AAI. Supramalleolar osteotomy is a well-accepted intermediate treatment of ankle OA for patients with tibial malalignment. It has been shown to have good intermediate out-comes, but it has added requirements for internal fixation, bone healing, cast immo-bilization, and nonweight bearing.[9] Bulk allograft replacement of the tibia and talus is a salvage procedure that is usually reserved for younger patients with significant osteochondral loss. The indications are narrow and there is also a requirement for bone healing to incorporate the graft and subsequent postoperative nonweight bearing and casting to facilitate the union of the graft and osteotomy if performed. In addition, there is a potential for disease transmission with fresh allografts and the host immune response may play a greater role in transplant survival than previously thought.[10,11] Another intermediate treatment is ankle distraction which involves the placement of an external fixator across the ankle for 3 to 4 months. This procedure is often combined with arthroscopic ankle debridement.[12,13] The intermediate results can be good, but complications and failures are not uncommon.[14]

BACKGROUND

Historically, most reports of arthroscopic debridement for AAI have been focused on younger athletic patients who suffer repetitive ankle dorsiflexion and/or ankle ligament injuries.[15,16] As previously stated, arthroscopic debridement is recommended for ankles with minimal OA changes.[1] Degenerative changes are commonly described using the Kellgren–Lawrence (K–L) radiographic grading scale of OA which detailed OA changes in the hand, spine, hip, knee and foot.[17] This grading system was adopted by the World Health Organization in 1961 and since gained popularity in the orthopedic literature. This is a 5-level grading scale (0–4) that differentiates between minimal (grade 2) and moderate (grade 3) based on the appearance of narrowing of the joint.[17] In their original study, Kellgren and Lawrence reported that the knee joint had the highest inter and intrarater reliability (.83 for both) with knee descriptions having been the most closely correlated with ankle ratings in the past. The K–L grading system has more recently been validated as a modified grading scale for the ankle.[18] The modified K–L grading scale dropped the grade 0 which is essentially a normal joint. It also delineates between grades 2 and 3 based on the appearance of joint space narrowing (grade 3). It uses a single weight-bearing 20-degree internal rotation mortize view. Before this publication in 2015, the use of the K–L grading was used only inconsistently in publications of arthroscopic treatment of AAI. In the future, authors should strive to use the modified K–L scale of ankle OA to facilitate the comparison of results between studies, even if further modifications are made.

One study not reviewed in the previously noted systematic review by Glazebrook and colleagues shows promise if viewed with arthroscopic debridement used as an intermediate treatment of ankle OA. Hassouna, Kumar, and Bendell reported the 5-year survival of 80 ankles after arthroscopic ankle debridement for OA, with 25 patients having moderate to severe radiographic OA changes.[19] In the OA study cohort, 72% had not progressed to major surgery (AA) at 5 years with most failures occurring within 24 months of ankle arthroscopy. In a shared decision-making discussion of operative treatment options, many patients may view 72% survivorship at 5 years as favorable if their medical conditions such as smoking and morbid obesity or life circumstances such as manual labor preclude AA or TAA at the time. Younger patients with OA and AAI who do not have midrange pain would also favor a joint sparing procedure rather than AA. The minimally invasive nature of ankle arthroscopy with a quick return to weight-bearing, motion, and activity makes it a particularly attractive option for many patients.

EMERGING CONCEPTS AND ANATOMY

Sarrafian described the anterior extension of the medial facet of the talar dome beyond the margin of the central and lateral trochlea in 91% of his series of 100 cadaveric specimens.[20] In 55% of cases, the extension was isolated to the medial facet, but in 36%, it was associated with the extension of the trochlear surface (**Figs. 1–3**). The first association of this talar morphology with the pathology of AAI was described by Amendola and colleagues in 2012.[21] Both the medial extension facet and the trochlear extension types were included in the analysis. Both morphologies were found to be more common in the AAI/OA group (51%) than in controls (2.4%) without ankle complaints. This morphology has been likened to the cam-type impingement in the hip which has become widely appreciated as a likely developmental deformity that can be a primary etiology of hip OA.[22] The treatment in the hip is to reshape the femoral head into a more rounded shape, while the treatment of AAI is to turn the dorsal talar neck/body into a concave surface (**Figs. 4** and **5**). No studies to date have described addressing the cam-shaped talus using arthroscopic debridement for AAI, but all have focused on tibial and talar osteophytes and soft tissue impingement. The anterior distal tibia is described as having a convex ridge which is the insertion of the anterior

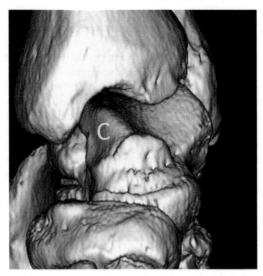

Fig. 1. 3D CT of medial talar dome extension type of Cam lesion (CC).

ankle capsule and a concavity below this that extends to the anterior articular margin. It is in this location that tibial osteophytes are typically found on lateral radiographs and easily identified by the loss of normal concavity. It is our experience that addressing the cam-shaped talus in addition to tibial osteophytes in cases of AAI can improve outcomes even in patients with higher grades of OA (3 + 4). Additionally, most ankle OA is posttraumatic and concomitant instability and alignment problems likely play a role in this common variation of morphology becoming pathologic and contributing to the symptoms of AAI.[23–25]

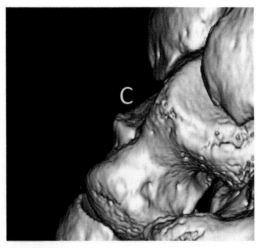

Fig. 2. Lateral view of medial talar dome extension Cam lesion (C).

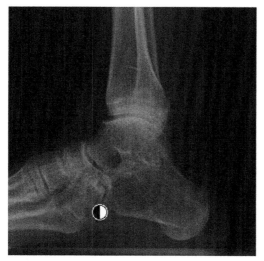

Fig. 3. Lateral radiograph of trochlear type Cam lesion.

PATIENT SELECTION
Alternatives, Shared Decision Making, Physical Examination, and Concomitant Procedures

Alternatives
The treatment of ankle OA with AA or TAA provides effective pain relief for a large number of patients. However, systematic reviews in 2007 and 2010 demonstrated that these joint sacrificing treatments also have the potential to result in significant complications, reoperation and for AA, potential long-term implications on gait and

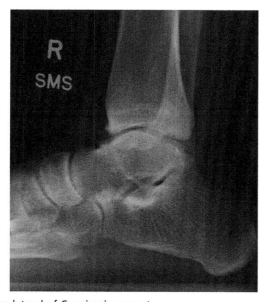

Fig. 4. Preoperative lateral of Cam impingement.

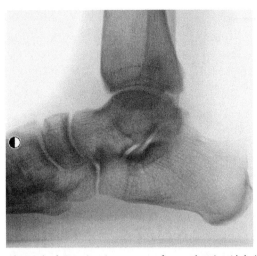

Fig. 5. Postoperative lateral of Cam impingement after reshaping/debridement.

mobility.[26,27] A 2017 study reviewing studies of third-generation TAA and AA limited to series, with a minimum of 200 and 80, respectively, demonstrated that the mean follow-up for TAA was 4.8 years (range 3.3–7.3). The mean age at the time of TAA was 61.3 years.[28] The studies reporting AA were all retrospective and the mean follow-up was 4.3 years (range 3.5–5.9). The mean patient age at the time of AA was 53.4 (range 49–56.1 years). In effect, the outcomes reported are limited to means less than 5 years and the mean ages of patients at the time of surgery of 61.3 (TAA) and 53.4 (AA), respectively. This highlights the fact that there are no definitive data to guide decision making in those patients less than 50. For this reason, the preoperative counseling should be based on shared decision making due to a paucity of data and different treatment options with different risks.[29,30] This concept has been studied in many ways but it is centered on the patient having the right to understand the limitations of the available literature and their alternatives with associated risks. The ideal patient for TAA or AA is one who would not be expected to have another major operation of their ankle in their lifetime, generally considered to be around 60 years of age. However, if a given patient for instance with a TAA experiences failure at 5 years, this assumption will have no meaning. It is for these reasons that intermediate joint and motion-preserving treatments of ankle OA are needed and are an important part of the treatment algorithm.

When evaluating a patient with ankle OA for AAI, the physical examination is crucial to determine if there is discordance between the radiographic appearance of the ankle joint and the patient's complaint of pain. The history can be confusing as many patients may have lasting pain due to impingement after they have been standing and walking for a long time. The pain likely will continue for several hours if they continued to ambulate despite increasing ankle pain. Ultimately, if the orthopedic surgeon feels that arthroscopic debridement is a good option, it should be presented as an intermediate treatment in terms of expected pain relief but balanced against the risks and limitations of TAA or AA. When deciding on an intermediate treatment of ankle OA, the patient should understand clearly that there is not an expectation that it will be the last procedure they will ever have on their arthritic ankle.

The relative intensity of the impingement compared with the midrange motion pain forms the basis of shared decision-making conversation with the patient when considering arthroscopic debridement or joint sacrificing operative treatments. Models and diagrams or printed radiographs are helpful aids for patients. The more predominant the midrange motion pain is, the less likely the patient will be to experience satisfactory relief of their pain with arthroscopic debridement. This is often a difficult discussion as are no objective measurements or strong evidence available to guide the decision. In our experience, there is a group of patients who have ankle pain with OA changes on radiographs who predominantly or solely have pain due to impingement. In that group, the recommendation for arthroscopic debridement can be made with more confidence of effective intermediate pain relief as a means of "buying time" until a definitive joint sacrificing procedure may be required to treat their ankle pain. Many patients appreciate having the option to choose this less invasive treatment, despite a lower probability of long-term satisfactory pain relief compared with TAA or AA. There is a natural attraction of joint preservation, limited time of immobilization, immediate weight bearing, and less time off from life activities.

Physical examination
The physical examination is critical for evaluating in which patients with ankle OA are good candidates for anterior arthroscopic debridement. In the literature, the selection criteria are often poorly described and sometimes not mentioned at all. Clearly, AAI is recognized as a source of pain in ankle OA, with numerous previous studies including patients with more advanced ankle OA.

In multiple studies, the diagnosis of ankle OA and the pain associated with it seems to be determined primarily by radiographic evaluation and a complaint of ankle pain. As outlined above for the hip and knee, there can often be discordance between the radiographic appearance of ankle OA and the clinical findings. It should never be assumed that the complaint of ankle pain is due to the presence of radiographic arthrosis. The concept of radiographic arthrosis with pain due to impingement has been described by Coughlin and Shurnas for the evaluation of OA in the 1st metatarsophalangeal (MTP) joint.[31] It is now well accepted that presence of midrange pain of the 1st MTP joint should be treated differently than if the midrange of motion is not painful but pain is reproduced at the limit of dorsiflexion, causing dorsal impingement. The essential question that the surgeon must answer in determining if a patient is a candidate for arthroscopic debridement is whether a patient with ankle OA has pain mainly or solely due to impingement. To first rule out the presence of midrange motion pain, the patient should be seated with the knee flexed to remove the loading effect of a tight gastrocnemius–soleus complex. The examiner then passively moves the ankle through the midrange of ankle motion without extending to the limits of motion. The examiner asks if this motion is painful or reproduces their stated pain (chief complaint). If the patient does have midrange motion pain, depending on the intensity of pain, they may not be a good candidate for anterior arthroscopic debridement. In the absence of significant midrange motion pain, the examination continues to include a 5-point impingement test across the anterior ankle. The following locations should be tested: medial gutter, anteromedial recess, anterior ankle, anterolateral recess, and lateral gutter. An impingement test is performed by providing gentle pressure over a location and asking the patient if there is tenderness and if it reproduces the patient's stated pain. Often mild or no pain will be endorsed. While holding gentle pressure, the ankle is then dorsiflexed. This maneuver places the synovium/soft tissue impingement lesion into the location of bony impingement. A positive test is elicited if sharp pain is experienced which reproduces their stated pain. In some cases, the pain is sharper or more severe than the patient's chief complaint, and they should be explicitly asked if the pain with impingement testing is similar to their stated pain in terms of character or location. If the patient indicates that it is not the pain that they are seeking help for, this should be clearly noted. Crepitus is often felt with this maneuver and may not be painful in which case this is not considered a positive impingement test as it is not symptomatic. Each location of impingement detected should be recorded and considered a distinct location of pathology. This is later helpful when interpreting radiographs and CT scans, which in turn help to guide the operative procedure. The examination should always include the examination of 2 additional locations. The adjacent sinus tarsi (anterior impingement at the subtalar joint) and the subfibular/lateral subtalar joint for associated impingement. Failure to relieve impingement in these locations can be a source of ongoing pain as well. These locations are examined in a similar fashion as the ankle except that the closing of the impingement lesions occurs with eversion. In total, 7 locations should be tested for painful impingement when evaluating a complaint of anterior ankle pain with OA.

Concomitant procedures
Another concept to consider is the optimal postoperative treatment of different procedures. Anterior arthroscopic debridement for ankle impingement in OA requires extensive bony debridement of the talus and tibia, sometimes with associated debridement of arthrofibrosis. The bleeding that occurs after debridement can lead to significant fibrosis which requires an early postop range of motion to maintain the flexibility of the peri-articular soft tissues.

Supramalleolar osteotomy is an extraarticular procedure for tibial deformity that can coexist with AAI. However, the postoperative requirement for immobilization and non-weight bearing would compromise the postoperative rehabilitation goal for ankle arthroscopic debridement of early range of motion and weight bearing, to maximize postoperative range of motion. The same conflict with postoperative rehabilitation occurs with large allograft replacements which also require prolonged nonweight bearing and immobilization, particularly when a tibial or fibular osteotomy is performed for exposure. Procedures for foot realignment such as osteotomies and arthrodesis have similar restrictions. In these cases of coexistent pathologies with conflicting postoperative needs, the procedures should be staged in most cases to optimize the outcome of each procedure.

Key Points of Physical Examination for Anterior Ankle Impingement in Osteoarthritis

- Midrange motion does not reproduce the patient's stated pain
- Mild to moderate pain with gentle pressure over the anterior joint line or gutters of the anterior ankle
- Pain is sharply increased at terminal dorsiflexion with gentle pressure held in these locations (positive impingement test)
- An impingement test is performed at the following locations
  - Medial gutter
  - Anteromedial recess
  - Anterior ankle
  - Anterolateral recess
  - Lateral gutter
- The anterior ankle has overlying soft tissues including tendons and neurovascular structures. It is possible but not common that these structures might also be tender. Frequently there is minimal or no tenderness in this location in plantarflexion. The contrast of sharp pain is evident when the ankle is dorsiflexed. More severe pain in plantarflexion should be noted and considered for other etiologies.

- Specific locations of impingement are recorded and evaluated and compared with radiologic images for preoperative planning.

Additional Physical Examination Findings and Considerations

- Sinus tarsi, and lateral subtalar/subfibular impingement (palpated dorsal to the peroneus brevis) may be present and debridement for bony and soft tissue impingement in these locations may be indicated via arthroscopic or open techniques.
- Open debridement should not compromise the goal of early range of motion and weight bearing.
- Preoperative evaluation of gastrocnemius contracture or combined gastrocnemius/soleus contracture can be limited due to bony impingement. An intraoperative examination can confirm if there is a need for concomitant gastrocnemius/soleus lengthening which aids in improved ankle joint kinematics.
- Examination for instability which is common in ankle OA can help identify another cause of ongoing or recurrent pain after arthroscopic debridement.
- In some cases, simultaneous ligament stabilization can be performed if augmented to allow early motion.
- Osteotomies in the foot and some soft tissue reconstructions require postoperative immobilization and should be avoided as simultaneous procedures. These should be planned as staged procedures.

Radiologic Imaging

Bony AAI is typically diagnosed using a lateral ankle radiograph, which can demonstrate anterior tibial and dorsal talar osteophytes. However, the use of the lateral radiograph for grading ankle arthritis has received little attention. The Kellgren–Lawrence grading scales are based on coronal plane radiographs. The aforementioned study of cam impingement of the ankle focused on the morphology of the talus in the lateral view as an etiologic factor in AAI.[21] Another study by Veljkovic and colleagues presented a method for determining the alignment of the talus under the tibia on a lateral ankle radiograph.[32] This is an important consideration when assessing sagittal plane joint congruence which can contribute to anterior impingement in a similar way to a cam-shaped talus, as the abnormal alignment prevents normal talar roll-back in dorsiflexion.

The Canadian Orthopedic Foot and Ankle Society (COFAS) grading system for ankle OA was originally developed to allow consistent reporting of preoperative ankle OA including the alignment of the ankle and foot as well as the presence of foot joint OA.[33] While it does include the use of a lateral ankle radiograph, the lateral view is not used to describe the ankle OA but is instead used for assessing foot alignment and the presence of OA in the foot joints.[33]

The ideal grading system for AAI would include lateral radiographic measurements that categorize both morphology and alignment. The contribution of foot alignment would be another level of assessment to consider in the future. The use of weight bearing CT scan imaging may represent a method to combine these assessments into one study.

The reliance on the lateral radiograph for assessing locations of impingement in ankle OA is insufficient as has been highlighted by Tol and colleagues who emphasized the use of oblique radiographs for evaluating the ankle joint gutters.[34] Ankles with OA have progressively increased size and numbers of osteophytes across the anterior ankle as well as the medial and lateral gutters. The presence of multiple osteophytes and a cam lesion of the talus increases the complexity of preoperative planning than in typical AAI cases without OA. The use of CT scan images with 3D reconstruction has been reported to provide enhanced accuracy due to the visualization of fine surface detail to expose small osteophytes.[35] The authors found that arthroscopic debridement guided by preoperative 3D CT showed improvement in the AOFAS outcome scores in a small group of patients with stage III OA changes. Although the number of patients in the stage III group was small (n = 6), the mean improvement in patients with 3D CT was from 76.3 ± 1.5 to 96.8 ± 3.7 whereas the 2 controls increased from 81 ± 4.2 to 88.5 ± 2.1. More Recently Kvarda and colleagues have also added to the argument for CT scan and 3D evaluation of the arthritic ankle when assessing for bony impingement.[36]

Enhanced detail of the medial and lateral gutters of the ankle can be identified on axial CT imaging which may demonstrate the medial and lateral osteophyte ridges on the distal talar body and the corresponding osteophytes of the medial and lateral malleoli (**Fig. 6**). Coronal CT imaging can provide additional information about the location of more inferior peri-malleolar impingement (**Fig. 7**). This is more common in cases with concomitant valgus hindfoot deformity. Weight bearing CT has been shown to be advantageous for assessing subfibular and subtalar impingement as it places the foot in a neutral-everted position.[37] We have found ultrasound examination to be a particularly helpful aid to the evaluation and diagnosis of impingement in the ankle and hindfoot. The dynamic nature of ultrasound examination and the ability to sono-palpate painful locations provides nuanced and detailed information that is sometimes difficult to gain from static radiologic images or careful physical examination. The ability to evaluate soft tissue impingement lesions as well as bony lesions has been of great benefit. The diagnostic value of focally injecting a soft tissue lesion and assessing the pain relief is an aid to locating specific sources of pain.[38–41]

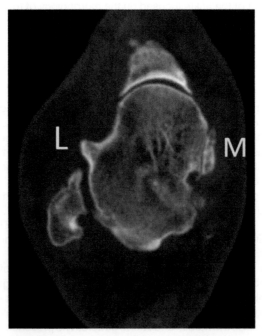

Fig. 6. Axial CT of gutter impingement: lateral (L) medial (M).

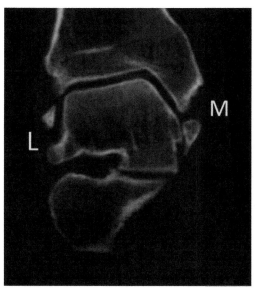

Fig. 7. Coronal CT of gutter impingement: lateral (L) medial (M).

Key Points of Radiologic, CT, 3D CT, and Ultrasound Evaluation

- A Lateral radiograph provides critical information to the diagnosis of cam impingement, alignment, and anterior osteophytes
- AP and oblique radiographs may mislead the evaluation by focusing on coronal plane sites of apparent impingement without providing axial plane detail
- True anterior impingement in the medial and lateral gutters occurs at the anterior aspect of the medial malleolus and fibula in the axial plane
- These locations correspond to osteophytes of the medial and lateral talar body–neck junction
- Oblique radiographs (internal and external rotation) can provide additional information regarding gutter impingement
- Osteophytes and bony impingement in the gutters are best evaluated with axial plane CT imaging but can be further appreciated with 3D CT
- Ultrasound can be helpful in evaluating locations of bony impingement and correlating with pain using sono-palpation. Soft tissue impingement is often a component of bony impingement pain and ultrasound-guided diagnostic injections can be helpful

Technique of Anterior Arthroscopic Debridement for Anterior Ankle Impingement in Ankle Ankle Osteoarthritis

Preoperative planning before arthroscopic debridement of AAI is vital as the talar morphology of cam impingement must be addressed. Further work is needed to fully understand how much normal articular surface and subchondral bone should be resected to appropriately address bony impingement. Our experience is that the talus should easily rollback under the anterior lip of the tibia after resection of tibial osteophytes (**Figs. 8–10**). While gastrocnemius/soleus contracture can limit the normal rollback of the talus with dorsiflexion, the understanding of when to perform gastrocnemius/soleus lengthening and what procedure to use remains a clinical

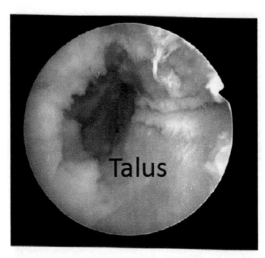

Fig. 8. Postdebridement of Cam lesion and talar osteophytes.

judgment. Specific locations of bony impingement of the tibia, talus, and fibula are addressed, and the decompression of the gutters is performed to the most inferior level necessary to relieve the axial plane impingement that creates gutter impingement pain with dorsiflexion. The use of various sized shavers and burrs is important to consider in different locations. We typically use a 3.8 mm end-shaver and a 4.0 mm bone-cutting shaver with a 4.0 mm round-cutting burr. In some cases, these are upsized to a 5.5 mm bone-cutting shaver and round-cutting burr. In tighter locations, a smaller or finer shaver like a torpedo shaver or 3.0 mm shaver might be needed to protect articular cartilage.

The 70-degree arthroscope has become indispensable in our practice as its use allows unobscured visualization directly down into the opposite gutter while using a working portal on the side of the gutter being debrided. The absence of direct visualization can lead to incomplete debridement and subsequent continued pain. We have found that a bony impingement lesion as small as 2 mm can cause ongoing pain. The procedure should be systematic, first addressing the anterior tibial osteophyte which creates more working space. Then the cam lesion is then addressed. Debridement progresses to the anteromedial and anterolateral recesses, with a focus on the inferior fascicle of the anterior tibio-fibular ligament laterally which is often previously injured and can cause abrasion to the lateral talar dome. Finally, the medial and lateral gutters are fully decompressed, and the ankle is taken to maximal dorsiflexion with visualization using the 70-degree arthroscope. If a tendon lengthening is performed to improve dorsiflexion, then the arthroscope should be used to re-evaluate the gutters after the lengthening to see if the improved motion leads to further impingement.

Key Points of Arthroscopic Debridement in Anterior Ankle Impingement

- The management of AAI in OA are often more complex with multiple sites of impingement requiring treatment
- Systematic debridement is based on a systematic evaluation (physical examination and radiologic studies)
- Preoperative planning is essential to avoid missing an impingement lesion
- Both branches of the superficial peroneal nerve (SPN) are palpated and marked

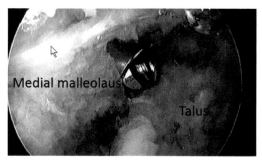

Fig. 9. 70-degree scope view from anterolateral portal looking down into medial gutter of the right ankle. Note the presence of remaining medial talar impingement lesion and medial malleolar impingement lesion with 4.0 mm burr in place.

- A 30-degree scope is used initially for the debridement of the anterior, anteromedial, and anterolateral locations
- The removal of the anterior tibial osteophyte allows more working space
- Accessory portals are frequently used to properly reshape the talar neck/body and to access the gutters (noting the branches of the SPN)
- Ankle distraction should not be used as plantarflexion decreases the anterior capsular distention and makes assessing impingement in dorsiflexion more difficult
- An end-shaver is helpful for soft tissue debridement which is typically "end-on" rather than from the side
- A bone shaver and round-cutting burr are helpful for debridement of bone
- A 70-degree scope is necessary to completely visualize and perform a thorough debridement in the medial and lateral gutters. The orientation of "looking down" into the gutter and performing an impingement test is necessary to assess the adequacy of debridement
- An arthroscopic cautery (burner) can be helpful in defining bony lesions when arthrofibrosis is covering bone
- The use of a 3D CT is critically helpful in evaluating this preoperatively
- Cam impingement is assessed after the debridement of the osteophytes and requires a preoperatively planned reshaping of the talus

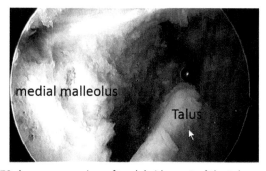

Fig. 10. The same 70-degree scope view after debridement of the talar and medial malleolar impingement lesions. Maximal ankle dorsiflexion confirmed complete debridement.

- Lateral view fluoroscopy is used to guide the creation of a more concave shape distal to the convex portion of the body and should be an iterative process
- When the cam impingement is resolved, the talar body should be easily reduced into the mortize so that the anterior margin of the talar articular surface rolls back behind the anterior tibial plafond
- It has been common early in our experience to underestimate the extent of debridement needed and leaving even 3 mm of cam impingement can have a negative impact on pain relief

Thoughts on the Performance of Concomitant Procedures

- In some cases of equinus contracture, lengthening of the gastrocnemius/soleus (Modified Strayer or Modified Vulpius) can be performed at the same time as the ankle arthroscopic debridement
- It may not always be easy to know how flexible an ankle will be after the removal of anterior impingement due to the preoperative anterior bony block to motion
- An intraoperative examination to determine the position and elasticity of the endpoint of dorsiflexion can be used to determine the potential for postoperative stretching to improve the condition
- Sinus tarsi impingement and subfibular/lateral subtalar impingement can be treated simultaneously with either arthroscopic or open techniques providing early ROM can be safely performed
- Osteotomies and soft tissue procedures that require prolonged immobilization should be avoided as concomitant procedures as the bony bleeding after thorough anterior arthroscopic debridement will create a stiffer joint if immobilized for more than a few days.

SUMMARY

The current body of literature regarding anterior ankle arthroscopic debridement for AAI cases with ankle OA has significant limitations. The reported poor outcomes lack the necessary rigor in patient selection, preoperative evaluations, and in most reports the use of a systematic operative approach. Furthermore, the lack of systematic postoperative evaluation by authors using physical examination and radiologic studies to determine the etiology of ongoing pain leaves open the possibility that treatment of impingement was incomplete. For these reasons, it would be inappropriate to conclude that anterior arthroscopic debridement has no role in the treatment of ankle OA. Critical Analysis of some studies provides encouragement that this can be a useful intermediate treatment of appropriately selected patients with AAI and ankle OA. The level of required detail in the physical examination and radiologic evaluation is much greater than for more straightforward cases of soft tissue impingement or simple osteophyte impingement in otherwise healthy joints. The success of the treatment requires a comprehensive and systematic approach to the evaluation and performance of the procedure; This could explain why results in the literature have been suboptimal in most series. Future studies should apply a rigorous approach to patient selection, procedure performance, and postoperative analysis to help clarify which patients can be best served with this procedure as part of the various intermediate treatment options for ankle OA.

DISCLOSURE

J.E. Femino received research support from Arthrex for an unrelated study. A. Shamrock has nothing to disclose.

REFERENCES

1. Glazebrook MA, Ganapathy V, Bridge MA, et al. Evidence-based indications for ankle arthroscopy. Arthroscopy 2009;25(12):1478–90.
2. Amendola A, Petrik J, Webster-Bogaert S. Ankle arthroscopy: outcome in 79 consecutive patients. Arthroscopy 1996;12(5):565–73.
3. Cerulli G, Caraffa A, Buompadre V, et al. Operative arthroscopy of the ankle. Arthroscopy 1992;8(4):537–40.
4. Martin DF, Baker CL, Curl WW, et al. Operative ankle arthroscopy. Long-term followup. Am J Sports Med 1989;17(1):16–23 [discussion: 23].
5. Ogilvie-Harris DJ, Sekyi-Otu A. Arthroscopic debridement for the osteoarthritic ankle. Arthroscopy 1995;11(4):433–6.
6. Kim C, Nevitt MC, Niu J, et al. Association of hip pain with radiographic evidence of hip osteoarthritis: diagnostic test study. BMJ 2015;351:h5983.
7. Bedson J, Croft PR. The discordance between clinical and radiographic knee osteoarthritis: a systematic search and summary of the literature. BMC Musculoskelet Disord 2008;9:116.
8. Griffin DR, Dickenson EJ, Wall PDH, et al. Hip arthroscopy versus best conservative care for the treatment of femoroacetabular impingement syndrome (UK FASHIoN): a multicentre randomised controlled trial. Lancet 2018;391(10136): 2225–35.
9. Hintermann B, Knupp M, Barg A. Supramalleolar Osteotomies for the Treatment of Ankle Arthritis. J Am Acad Orthop Surg 2016;24(7):424–32.
10. Raikin SM. Fresh osteochondral allografts for large-volume cystic osteochondral defects of the talus. J Bone Joint Surg Am 2009;91(12):2818–26.
11. Vannini F, Buda R, Pagliazzi G, et al. Osteochondral Allografts in the Ankle Joint: State of the Art. Cartilage 2013;4(3):204–13.
12. Nguyen MP, Pedersen DR, Gao Y, et al. Intermediate-term follow-up after ankle distraction for treatment of end-stage osteoarthritis. J Bone Joint Surg Am 2015;97(7):590–6.
13. Saltzman CL, Hillis SL, Stolley MP, et al. Motion versus fixed distraction of the joint in the treatment of ankle osteoarthritis: a prospective randomized controlled trial. J Bone Joint Surg Am 2012;94(11):961–70.
14. Bernstein M, Reidler J, Fragomen A, et al. Ankle Distraction Arthroplasty: Indications, Technique, and Outcomes. J Am Acad Orthop Surg 2017;25(2):89–99.
15. Ross KA, Murawski CD, Smyth NA, et al. Current concepts review: Arthroscopic treatment of anterior ankle impingement. Foot Ankle Surg 2017;23(1):1–8.
16. Tol JL, Verheyen CP, van Dijk CN. Arthroscopic treatment of anterior impingement in the ankle. J Bone Joint Surg Br 2001;83(1):9–13.
17. Kellgren JH, Lawrence JS. Radiological assessment of osteo-arthrosis. Ann Rheum Dis 1957;16(4):494–502.
18. Holzer N, Salvo D, Marijnissen AC, et al. Radiographic evaluation of posttraumatic osteoarthritis of the ankle: the Kellgren-Lawrence scale is reliable and correlates with clinical symptoms. Osteoarthritis Cartilage 2015;23(3):363–9.
19. Hassouna H, Kumar S, Bendall S. Arthroscopic ankle debridement: 5-year survival analysis. Acta Orthop Belg 2007;73(6):737–40.
20. Sarrafian S. Anatomy of the foot and ankle: descriptive, topographic, and functional. 2nd edition. Philadelphia (PA): J.B. Lippincott Company; 1993.
21. Amendola N, Drew N, Vaseenon T, et al. CAM-type impingement in the ankle. Iowa Orthop J 2012;32:1–8.

22. Ganz R, Parvizi J, Beck M, et al. Femoroacetabular impingement: a cause for osteoarthritis of the hip. Clin Orthop Relat Res 2003;417:112–20.

23. Brown TD, Johnston RC, Saltzman CL, et al. Posttraumatic osteoarthritis: a first estimate of incidence, prevalence, and burden of disease. J Orthop Trauma 2006;20(10):739–44.

24. Saltzman CL, Salamon ML, Blanchard GM, et al. Epidemiology of ankle arthritis: report of a consecutive series of 639 patients from a tertiary orthopaedic center. Iowa Orthop J 2005;25:44–6.

25. Valderrabano V, Horisberger M, Russell I, et al. Etiology of ankle osteoarthritis. Clin Orthop Relat Res 2009;467(7):1800–6.

26. Gougoulias N, Khanna A, Maffulli N. How successful are current ankle replacements?: a systematic review of the literature. Clin Orthop Relat Res 2010; 468(1):199–208.

27. Haddad SL, Coetzee JC, Estok R, et al. Intermediate and long-term outcomes of total ankle arthroplasty and ankle arthrodesis. A systematic review of the literature. J Bone Joint Surg Am 2007;89(9):1899–905.

28. Lawton CD, Butler BA, Dekker RG 2nd, et al. Total ankle arthroplasty versus ankle arthrodesis-a comparison of outcomes over the last decade. J Orthop Surg Res 2017;12(1):76.

29. Elwyn G, Frosch D, Thomson R, et al. Shared decision making: a model for clinical practice. J Gen Intern Med 2012;27(10):1361–7.

30. Shinkunas LA, Klipowicz CJ, Carlisle EM. Shared decision making in surgery: a scoping review of patient and surgeon preferences. BMC Med Inform Decis Mak 2020;20(1):190.

31. Coughlin MJ, Shurnas PS. Hallux rigidus. Grading and long-term results of operative treatment. J Bone Joint Surg Am 2003;85(11):2072–88.

32. Veljkovic A, Norton A, Salat P, et al. Lateral talar station: a clinically reproducible measure of sagittal talar position. Foot Ankle Int 2013;34(12):1669–76.

33. Krause FG, Di Silvestro M, Penner MJ, et al. Inter- and intraobserver reliability of the COFAS end-stage ankle arthritis classification system. Foot Ankle Int 2010; 31(2):103–8.

34. Tol JL, Verhagen RA, Krips R, et al. The anterior ankle impingement syndrome: diagnostic value of oblique radiographs. Foot Ankle Int 2004;25(2):63–8.

35. Takao M, Uchio Y, Naito K, et al. Arthroscopic treatment for anterior impingement exostosis of the ankle: application of three-dimensional computed tomography. Foot Ankle Int 2004;25(2):59–62.

36. Kvarda P, Heisler L, Krahenbuhl N, et al. 3D Assessment in Posttraumatic Ankle Osteoarthritis. Foot Ankle Int 2021;42(2):200–14.

37. Malicky ES, Crary JL, Houghton MJ, et al. Talocalcaneal and subfibular impingement in symptomatic flatfoot in adults. J Bone Joint Surg Am 2002;84(11):2005–9.

38. McCarthy CL, Wilson DJ, Coltman TP. Anterolateral ankle impingement: findings and diagnostic accuracy with ultrasound imaging. Skeletal Radiol 2008;37(3): 209–16.

39. Nazarian LN, Gulvartian NV, Freeland EC, et al. Ultrasound-Guided Percutaneous Needle Fenestration and Corticosteroid Injection for Anterior and Anterolateral Ankle Impingement. Foot Ankle Spec 2018;11(1):61–6.

40. Pesquer L, Guillo S, Meyer P, et al. US in ankle impingement syndrome. J Ultrasound 2014;17(2):89–97.

41. Talusan PG, Toy J, Perez JL, et al. Anterior ankle impingement: diagnosis and treatment. J Am Acad Orthop Surg 2014;22(5):333–9.

Arthroscopic Ankle Arthrodesis

Anna-Kathrin Leucht, MD[a], Andrea Veljkovic, MD, MPH(Harvard), BComm, FRCSC[b],*

KEYWORDS

- Ankle arthrodesis • Ankle fusion • Arthroscopic • Tibiotalar fusion • Ankle arthritis

KEY POINTS

- Arthroscopic ankle arthrodesis leads to shorter hospital stay, faster rehabilitation, and decreased time to union than open ankle arthrodesis.
- Arthroscopic ankle arthrodesis compared to total ankle replacement (TAR) yield similar results in end-stage ankle arthritis without deformity (COFAS type I).
- Deformity correction in both coronal and sagittal planes can reliably be achieved with arthroscopic ankle arthrodesis.
- The deformity predicts the sequence of screw positioning.
- The goal is to achieve a plantigrade foot position.

INTRODUCTION

End-stage ankle arthritis (ESAA) has a substantial impact on life due to limited function and pain. Ankle arthrodesis is a reliable treatment option for ESAA with consistently good outcomes. Arthroscopic ankle arthrodesis (AAA) has gained popularity due to low postoperative morbidity, less blood loss, shorter hospital stay, faster rehabilitation and mobilization, and decreased time to union.[1,2]

NATURE OF THE PROBLEM

In general, patients that are candidates for ankle fusion tend to be younger and active with a diagnosis of posttraumatic osteoarthritis, which is the most frequent etiology of ESAA (78%).[3] Therefore, ankle arthritis is a major source of morbidity impacting a younger working-age population than hip or knee arthritis,[4] with the mean age of presentation being 55 years of age in the ankle arthrodesis group compared with 63.2 years in patients with total ankle replacements.[5]

[a] Department of Orthopaedics and Traumatology, Cantonal Hospital of Winterthur, Brauerstrasse 15, Winterthur 8401, Switzerland; [b] Department of Orthopaedics, University of British, Footbridge Center for Integrated Foot and Ankle Care, Footbridge Clinic, Unit 221, 181 Keefer Place, Vancouver, British Columbia V6B6C1, Canada
* Corresponding author.
E-mail address: docveljkovic@yahoo.com

Foot Ankle Clin N Am 27 (2022) 175–197
https://doi.org/10.1016/j.fcl.2021.11.008
1083-7515/22/© 2021 Elsevier Inc. All rights reserved.
foot.theclinics.com

The morphologic presentation of ESAA in this patient population is seldom concentric like that seen in rheumatoid arthritis instead it is often associated with posttraumatic deformity.

Ankle arthrodesis leads to relevant alterations in gait kinematics.[6–14] Due to tibiotalar fusion, overall sagittal plane motion decreases. The increase of sagittal motion through the subtalar joint partially compensates for the absence of motion in the ankle. In general, patients with ankle arthrodesis present with lower walking velocity due to shortened stride length and lower cadence. In addition, decreased hindfoot range of motion leads to earlier heel rise, increased forefoot plantar pressure, and increased hip flexion while walking.

Altered gait mechanisms in patient with ankle arthrodesis, especially increased shear forces that are now transmitted through the subtalar and midtarsal joints, subsequently lead to the development of adjacent joint arthritis over time.[8–10,15–17] The development of adjacent joint arthritis postankle fusion is seen in multiple hindfoot and midfoot joints, but is specifically seen in the subtalar joint.[8–10,15–17] However the correlation with clinical symptoms and pain remains unclear.[15,17–20]

INDICATIONS/CONTRAINDICATIONS

Over years, open ankle arthrodesis (OAA) has been the standard surgical management of ESAA and considered the gold standard. Nowadays, the open technique is increasingly being replaced by arthroscopic ankle fusion.

In general, the indication for ankle arthrodesis is end-stage ankle arthritis nondependent on etiology, though it is often used as the surgical option for young patients with posttraumatic disease.

There are obvious advantages of less invasive arthroscopic joint preparation. These include minimal soft tissue stripping around the ankle and the potential healing benefits of less soft tissue violation and preservation of vascularity that can likely result in diminished wound complications. Therefore arthroscopic techniques are favorable in patients with concerns for healing such as those with compromised vascularity, diabetes, previous surgeries of the ankle with resultant scars, prior skin grafts or flaps, and even previous history of infection or mild avascular necrosis. Nevertheless, the presence of an active infection is considered to be an absolute contraindication.

A coronal deformity greater than 15° is considered a relative contraindication for AAA.[21,22] Newer studies have demonstrated that arthroscopic ankle fusion yields reliable fusion rates and deformity correction in ankles with larger coronal and sagittal deformity.[23–26] In a comparative series by Schmid and colleagues,[25] patients with higher tibial plafond angles (>19°) received an OAA due to the necessity of bony deformity correction. In contrast, malalignment of the ankle caused by tilting of the talus (high tibiotalar angle, incongruent deformity) is not considered a contraindication for an arthroscopic procedure as the tilting of the talus can reliably be addressed arthroscopically with strategic soft tissue releases and appropriate screw positioning.

In the authors' experience, once one becomes facile with the arthroscopic technique cases with higher tibial plafond angles (congruent deformity), whereby proper correction is more difficult to achieve, can be treated arthroscopically with good postoperative alignment and satisfaction. To achieve anatomic alignment, one must either strategically burr down the lower side or allow the higher side to the gap by strutting it out with a fully threaded screw in addition to tactically positioning structural grafts that are inserted via mini arthrotomies or extensions of portals. Gaps can also be filled with conductive scaffolds such as a demineralized bone matrix.

Severe avascular necrosis of the talus exceeding 30% is found to be one of the risk factors for failure of AAA by Zvijac and colleagues[27] Similar to this, bone defects larger than one-third of the talar dome are regarded as another relative contraindication as shown by Myerson and Quill.[1]

In the setting of adjacent joint arthritis-like subtalar or talonavicular arthritis (COFAS type 4), the indication for a total joint replacement should be considered to allow for any ankle motion which will hypothetically shield the adjacent joints.

PREOPERATIVE PLANNING

Deformity assessment is performed on weightbearing anterior to posterior, lateral, and mortise view of both ankles, additional x-ray planes and cross-sectional imaging of the foot are inevitable. The hindfoot alignment is assessed on the Saltzman view. If a diaphyseal deformity is present, a long leg view is beneficial.

On the lateral view, the ADTA (anterior distal tibial angle) and the lateral talar station are measured. On the AP view, the talar tilt angle shows the varus/valgus incongruency of the joint. The medial tibiotalar surface angle is the angle between the long axis of the tibia and the talar subchondral plane, measured on the medial side. It shows the combined deformity of talar tilting and additionally bony deformity.

The distal tibial plafond angle (or MDTA) is the angle between the tibial axis and the subchondral plane of the tibia, measured also on the medial side. This angle displays the amount of bony deformity of the distal tibia.

In general, the ankle deformity usually results from a varus or valgus tilting of the talus, especially in cases with chronic ankle instability leading to EAA and is less likely a pure bony deformity in the tibia measured with the tibia plafond angle.[28]

Additionally, CT scans can detect larger defects of the tibial or talar joint surface as well as concomitant adjacent joint arthritis. An MRI is helpful to estimate the size of a talar necrosis as it can reveal unvital bone.

Optimal Ankle Arthrodesis Position

The desired position of the ankle fusion is 5° – 10° hindfoot valgus, neutral dorsiflexion and 5° – 10° of external rotation, corresponding to the contralateral side. Especially, the subtle valgus is beneficial as it unlocks the transverse tarsal joints.[29] An equinus position of the talus needs to be prevented as it leads to knee recurvatum[7] and midfoot overload.

A posterior shift of the talus is beneficial for the foot mechanics[7] and diminishes the lever arm on the midfoot.

In addition, the foot has to be balanced under the ankle fusion to allow for a plantigrade position. Therefore, further bony and soft tissue procedures may need to be performed were necessary.

Varus Deformity

In a varus deformity, the talus is typically tilted and translated away from the lateral malleolus with lateral gaping. To correct this deformity, compression has to be performed on the lateral side with a partially threaded screw (first screw). As a second step, while keeping the optimum position of the ankle, a partially threaded screw is used on the medial side. In case of a defect, a fully threaded screw, which struts the construct is used. The third partially threaded screw is placed from the posterior malleolus, it crosses the ankle joint posteriorly and runs in axis with the talar neck (home run screw[30]). This home run screw can be placed in a typical manner from the posterolateral tibia to the neck of the talus, or from the posteromedial tibia by retracting the tibialis posterior to the anterolateral neck of the talus (modified home run screw). This can be either a long partially threaded screw or if you are concerned about micromotion, the authors advocate for a fully threaded screw. A medial soft tissue release is performed if necessary (**Figs. 1** and **2**).

Valgus Deformity

In contrast, in a valgus deformity, the talus is tilted and translated away from the medial malleolus, resulting in medial gaping. Therefore, a partially threaded

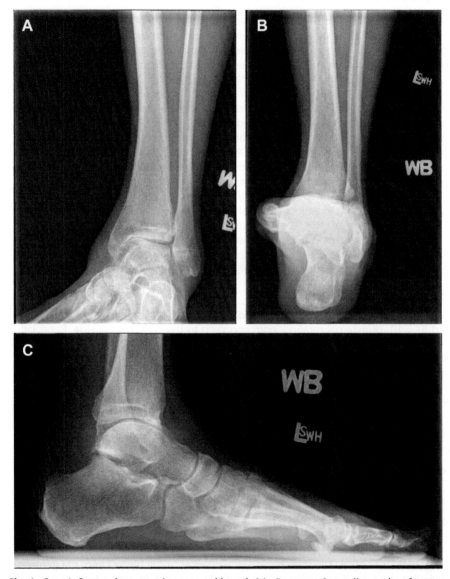

Fig. 1. Case 1: Screw placement in varus ankle arthritis. Preoperative radiographs of a varus non-concentric end-stage ankle arthritis. (*A*) Anteroposterior view; (*B*) hindfoot alignment view; (*C*) lateral view.

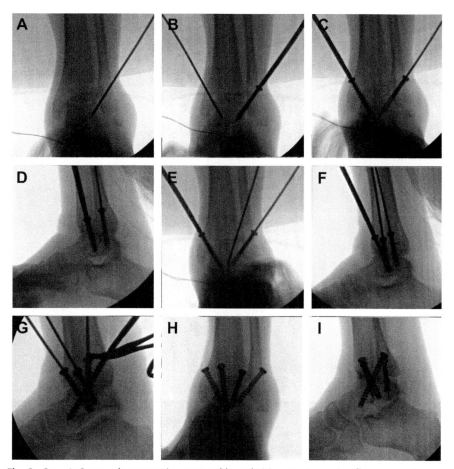

Fig. 2. Case 1: Screw placement in varus ankle arthritis. Intraoperative fluoroscopy images showing the sequence of screw positioning. (*A, B*) The first screw was inserted from lateral under compression to reduce the varus tilt. (*C, D*) The second, fully threaded screw was inserted from the medial to strut out the deformity followed by (*E, F*) an additional compression screw from lateral and finally (*G*) a home run screw. (*H*) Anteroposterior and (*I*) lateral view of final construct.

compression screw is placed on the medial side (first screw) and the ankle is strut out laterally, second screw with either a partially or in larger deformity is a fully threaded screw. Routinely the typical, or modified, home run screw is used, which runs from posterior to anterior in the talar neck axis. A lateral soft tissue release is helpful in severe deformities (**Figs. 3** and **4**).

Anterior Translated Talus

In ankle arthritis due to chronic lateral ankle instability, the talus is frequently anterior translated in the sagittal plane. This anterior translation needs to be addressed in deformity correction to reduce the length of the lever arm of the foot and thus the load of the adjacent joints of the foot during push-off. To be able to shift the talus backwards, the posterior tibial articular lip is resected. Often a gastrocnemius recession is

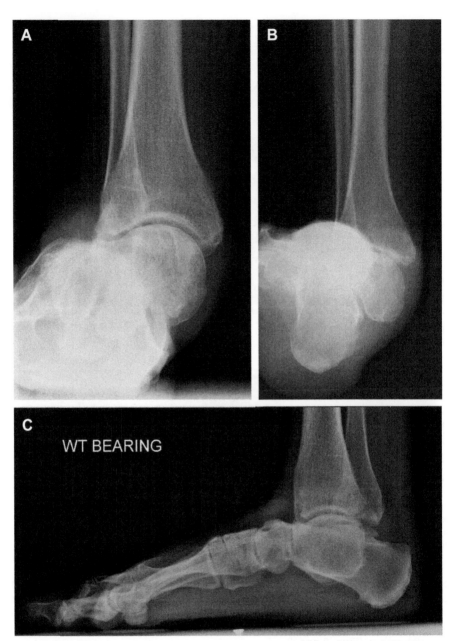

Fig. 3. Case 2: Screw placement in valgus ankle arthritis. Preoperative radiographs of a valgus concentric end-stage ankle arthritis with ball-and-socket deformity. (*A*) Anteroposterior view; (*B*) hindfoot alignment view; (*C*) lateral view.

required to detether the heel and allow for posterior translation of the talus. The home run screw is eminent for proper reduction of the talus and typically requires a short or long partially treaded screw to capture the talus and pull it back while at the same time levering the talus back with instruments from the front via arthroscopic portals and

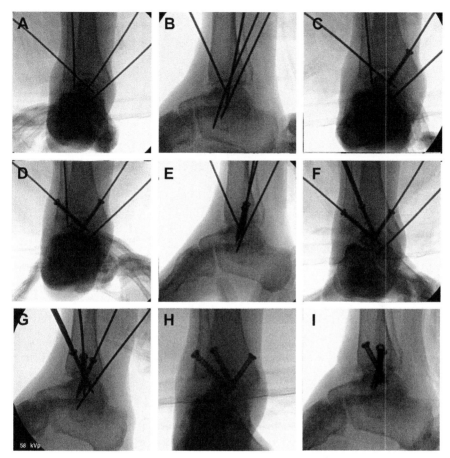

Fig. 4. Case 2: Screw placement in valgus ankle arthritis. Intraoperative fluoroscopy images showing the sequence of screw positioning. (*A, B*) The reduction of the valgus deformity was preliminary hold with k-wires. (*C*) The medial screw was inserted first under compression. (*D, E*) A fully threaded screw was used laterally to hold the position. (*F, G*) The third screw was inserted from anterolateral as a compression screw. (*H, I*) Final screw placement in anteroposterior and lateral view.

fluoroscopic guidance. It is critical to place a bump under the posterior tibia with the heel free to allow mechanical advantage when translating the talus posterior. In addition, one may need to strut out the anterior defect with a fully threaded screw from anterolateral or anteromedial tibia to posterior in the talus (**Figs. 5** and **6**).

As mentioned above, in long-standing equinus or anterior shifting of the talus an endoscopic gastrocnemius recession is critical, sometimes even a tendo-Achilles lengthening (TAL) is favorable to achieve adequate reduction.

PREPARATION AND PATIENT POSITIONING

The patient is positioned supine with the heel resting over the end of the operating table. The ipsilateral hip is slightly elevated with a beanbag, so that the corresponding leg is internally rotated and the foot is positioned straight. A thigh tourniquet is used

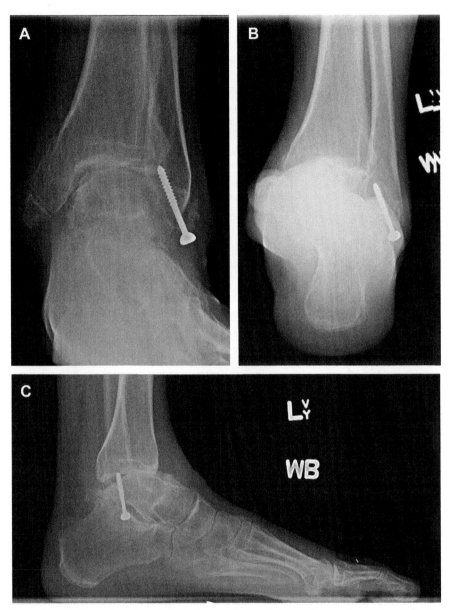

Fig. 5. Case 3: Correction of anterior talar translation. Preoperative radiographs of an anterior translated end-stage ankle arthritis. (*A*) Anteroposterior view; (*B*) hindfoot alignment view; (*C*) lateral view.

with appropriate padding. A distractor is not routinely used (authors' preference) but can be incorporated via strap traction to the foot when required in tight cases.

Antibiotic prophylaxis is given before surgery according to the hospital protocol.

The leg is prepped and draped up to the knee to enable the harvest of cancellous bone from the proximal tibia if required for certain bone defects. If anticipated by

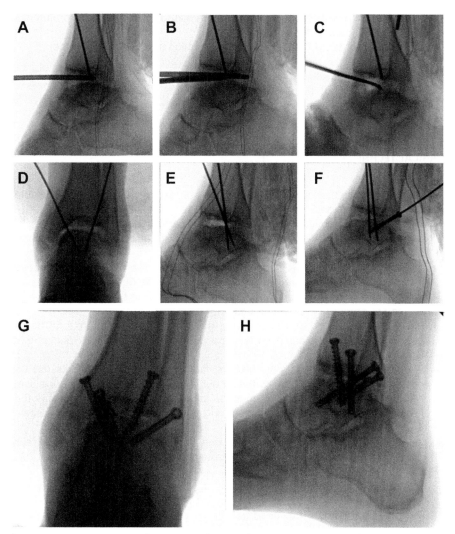

Fig. 6. Case 3: Correction of anterior talar translation. Intraoperative fluoroscopy images showing the (*A, B*) resection of the posterior tibial articular lip. Previously a gastrocnemius recession was performed to enhance posterior translation. (*C*) After levering the talus backwards the position was secured with k-wires (*D, E*). (*F*) A partially threaded home run screw is inserted to pull the talus backwards. (*G, H*) Final screw positioning in anteroposterior and lateral view. Note the neutral talar station in the lateral view.

preoperative planning that a structural auto or allograft is required to correct significant valgus or varus deformity, ipsilateral inguinal region is additionally prepped and draped for possible bulk iliac crest autograft harvest.

Instruments
- 4.0 mm arthroscope (30°) or 2.9 mm arthroscope (30°)
- Arthroscopic resector and bur, (soft tissue ablator only if inflammation is present)
- Osteotomes, curettes (straight and bent)

- An array of short and long partially and fully threaded screws (authors' preference: 6.7 mm or 6.5 cannulated screws)
- Ankle distractor strap PRN (can use body traction or a distractor device)

Extras

- Cancellous bone graft
- Iliac crest bone graft (auto- or allograft)
- Platelet-derived growth factor bone graft substitute
- Demineralized bone matrix

SURGICAL TECHNIQUE

Portals

- The intermediate branch of the superficial peroneal nerve is marked in full plantar flexion and inversion.
- Standard anteromedial and anterolateral portals are used and marked on the skin at the level of the ankle joint line. The anteromedial portal is positioned just medial to the anterior tibial tendon at the notch of Hardy.
- Through the course of the surgery additional portals like the medial and lateral gutter portals will be required. In some cases, accessory posteromedial (between tibialis posterior and FDL) and posterolateral (posterior to the peroneals) may be required to prepare the posterior talus.
- The ankle is insufflated with 20 cc normal saline via the medial approach. The anteromedial and anterolateral portals are performed using a nick and spread technique.
- If large anterior osteophytes are present, fluoroscopy might have to be used to identify the joint. Subsequent to this, a bur, curette, or osteotome can be used to debride the osteophyte. Care must be taken to elevate the soft tissues off of the spur. Failing to do this may result in damaging the anterior neurovascular structures.

  In addition removal of this anterior spur can allow for the dorsiflexion of the talus and better neutral positioning of the talus in the sagittal plane.

Preparing the joint

- In the case of arthrofibrosis or significant synovitis, an initial debridement with a resector or soft tissue ablator is performed before the joint can be assessed. The joint arthrofibrosis may need to be incised via a beaver blade under direct arthroscopic visualization.
- The remaining cartilage of the talus and tibia is removed with a soft tissue resector or bur followed by straight and curved curettes (**Figs. 7** and **8**).
- If one decides to prepare the gutters, medial and lateral gutter portals can be used to clear the medial and lateral side of the talus as well as the medial side of the distal fibula and the lateral side of the medial malleolus from cartilage (**Fig. 9**). It's the Senior Author's preference to prepare the lateral gutter as well.
- In the setting of gross syndesmotic widening, a syndesmotic fusion is recommended, specifically in valgus cases (**Figs. 10** and **11**). Thus, these articular surfaces are prepared in the same fashion as described above and portals can be made just at the top of the syndesmotic incisura to allow placement of instruments such as the shaver or bur.
- The articular surfaces are prepared with a bur to get bleeding punctuate subchondral bone.
- In addition small golf ball-like punctures are made with the high-speed bur to create areas of spot welds (**Fig. 12**).

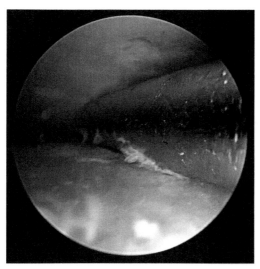

Fig. 7. Arthroscopic view of the talar dome and the tibial plateau. The articular cartilage is removed with a bur.

- A chisel can be used to create anteroposterior rails to further break the subchondral bone (**Fig. 13**).
- All debris is removed with the help of the soft tissue resector.
Addressing the deformity
- In case of a larger defect, an iliac crest bone graft is harvested. A structural iliac crest allograft can also be used.

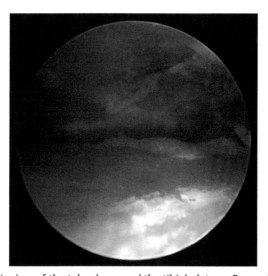

Fig. 8. Arthroscopic view of the talar dome and the tibial plateau. Bare subchondral bone is visible in front with few remaining patches of cartilage in the back of the joint, which will be removed with a curette.

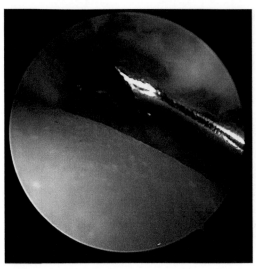

Fig. 9. Arthroscopic view of the medial talar dome and the medial gutter. A curette is used to remove the cartilage in the medial gutter.

- According to the preoperative template, a tricortical wedge is formed, with the appropriate height to correct the deformity present.
- Soft tissue release is performed, if needed.
- The tricortical wedge is then inserted either over a short anterolateral or anteromedial incision by extending the portals (**Figs. 14–16**).
- Additional cancellous bone graft can be harvested from the proximal tibia. This can be delivered via arthroscopic portals by packing the graft into a cannula and directing the graft strategically into present bone defects. In a similar fashion, bone graft substitutes can be delivered via portals under fluoroscopic guidance (**Fig. 17**).
- In the Senior Author's opinion, distances of less than 1.5 cm can be bridged with fully threaded screws to strut out the deformity and shield potential collapse. These distances can be filled with bone graft substitute or tricortical wedges inserted via mini arthrotomies as mentioned above.

Screw positioning

- The alignment of the ankle is then corrected to a subtle 5° of valgus, neutral dorsiflexion and 5° to 10° external rotation as compared with the contralateral side. This position is preliminary fixed with k-wires and confirmed with intraoperative fluoroscopy in AP and lateral planes.
- Depending on the deformity and based on preoperative planning, the typical screw placement as described above is then performed, starting with the compression screw which counteracts the deformity. In general, a minimum of 3 screws are used (Authors' preference).
- Definitive fluoroscopy films in anterioposterior, mortise, lateral of the ankle, dorsoplantar, and oblique of the foot are taken to confirm a correct reduction of the fusion and good position and length of the screws, specifically the home run screw.
- After copious irrigation, all skin incisions are closed and sterile dressing is applied.
- A well-padded trislab splint is used to immobilize the ankle.

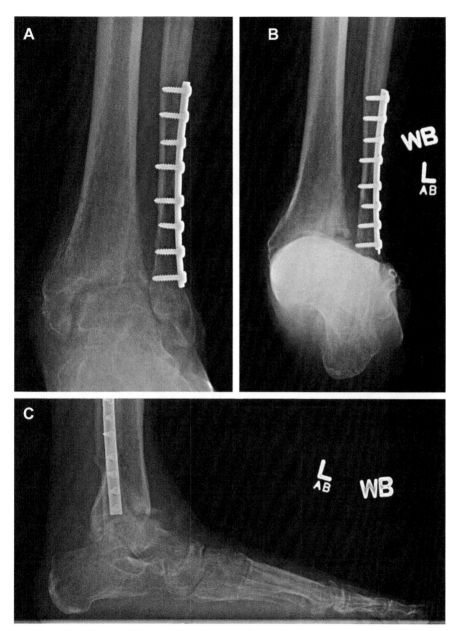

Fig. 10. Case 4: Syndesmotic fusion. Preoperative radiographs of a gross syndesmotic widening in a valgus non-concentric end-stage ankle arthritis. (*A*) Anteroposterior view; (*B*) hindfoot alignment view; (*C*) lateral view.

Adjuncts
- Endoscopic gastrocnemius recession, tendoachilles lengthening for the reduction of severe valgus, equinus, or anterior translated cases.
- Further soft tissue or bony procedures of the foot may need to be conducted to achieve a plantigrade foot position

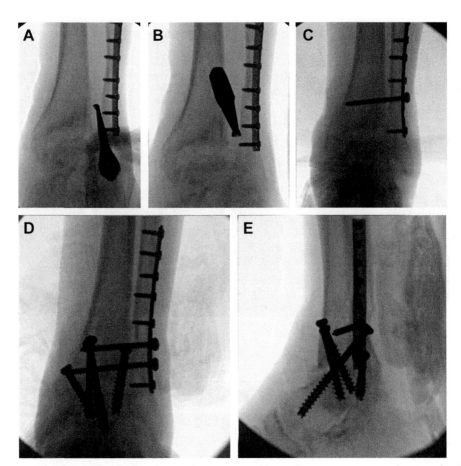

Fig. 11. Case 4: Syndesmotic fusion. (*A, B*) Intraoperative fluoroscopy images showing the preparation of the syndesmotic incisura. (*C*) The reduction was initially hold in position with one fully threaded large fragment screw. (*D, E*) Final screw positioning in anteroposterior and lateral view.

RECOVERY AND REHABILITATION

Postoperatively the ankle joint is immobilized in a well-padded trislab splint. At 2 to 3 weeks after surgery, the splint is removed for wound control and removal of stitches. A closed lower leg cast is then applied for the duration of another 4 weeks, but a boot may suffice. During these first 6 weeks, the patient is non–weight-bearing. At the Senior Author's preference, a CT scan is performed at 6-weeks postoperative consultation to confirm adequate consolidation, with greater than 50% fusion being required to start progressive weight bearing.[31] Depending on the CT result a gradual increase in weightbearing is then allowed in a walker boot. Further follow-ups are scheduled 3 months, 6 months, and 1 year after surgery.

OUTCOME
Patient Satisfaction

Functional outcomes and patient satisfaction after ankle arthrodesis remain adequate. Several studies report good outcomes in 76% to 91% of patients in mid- to long-term follow-up.[9,10,18,19,23,27,32–34]

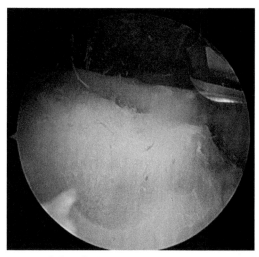

Fig. 12. Arthroscopic view of the tibial and talar joint surface. Several golf ball-like punctures can be seen.

Thomas and colleagues[9] retrospectively assessed 26 patients with ankle arthrodesis for the treatment of isolated unilateral ankle arthritis with an average follow-up of 44 months. Twenty of the 26 patients were completely satisfied or satisfied with their surgical outcome. Twenty-five patients indicated that they would undergo the surgery again. Five patients expressed the lack of noticing a gait abnormality.

With a mean follow-up of 9 years, Hendrickx and colleagues[18] demonstrated a 91% satisfaction rate with the clinical result of 60 patients with 66 ankle arthrodesis.

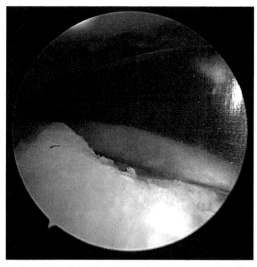

Fig. 13. Arthroscopic view of a chisel being used to create rails to break the subchondral plate.

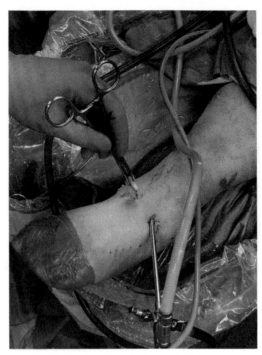

Fig. 14. Intraoperative photo of left arthroscopic ankle fusion showing the insertion of a wedged allograft to correct intraarticular deformity.

Younger and colleagues[5] evaluated the patient expectation and satisfaction as a measure for clinical outcome in patients with ESAA. A total of 654 ankles were included in the study, 204 ankles underwent ankle arthrodesis and 450 underwent TAR. The expectations met and satisfaction scores at the final follow-up were similar between both groups.

Arthroscopic Versus Open Ankle Arthrodesis

OAA has been the "gold standard" for the treatment of ankle arthritis for decades. Since the introduction of AAA by Schneider in 1983, it has been available and has gained increasing momentum over the years. Multiple recent studies have demonstrated good outcomes and even advantages compared with the open procedure.

With AAA, a high fusion rate is consistently achieved, ranging from 91% to 100% with a time to union between 8.9 weeks and 3.5 months.[23,24,26,27,35–41] In addition, several studies have shown a shorter time to union in AAA compared with OAA.[1,2,28,42] Further benefits of AAA are shorter hospital stay,[1,28,42–45] reduced blood loss[2,43] and better clinical scores.[28,43,46]

Some Level III studies exist with direct comparison of OAA and AAA, one study of Meng and colleagues[43] is only available in Chinese and therefore not included.

In 1991, Myerson and Quill[1] examined the outcome of 17 patients with AAA compared with 16 patients with OAA. A significantly faster time to union in the AAA group as well as a shorter hospital stay with an equivalent complication rate was demonstrated. However, the results of this comparison are only of limited value due to a selection bias, as the amount of deformity, the presence of prior infection, the quality of blood circulation, etc, were factors in patient selection.

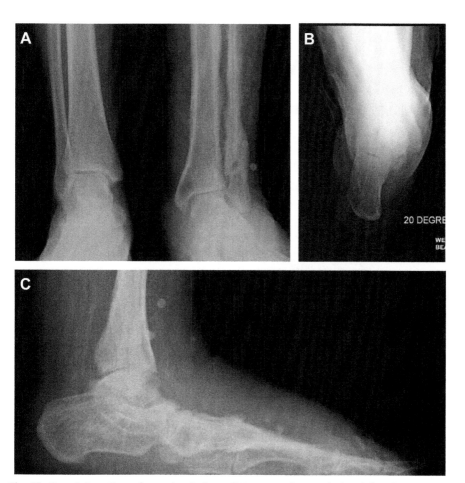

Fig. 15. Case 5: Insertion of a wedged allograft to correct intraarticular deformity. Preoperative radiographs of a valgus concentric end-stage ankle arthritis with intraarticular deformity, valgus tibial joint line. (*A*) Bilateral anteroposterior view; (*B*) hindfoot alignment view; (*C*) lateral view.

Nineteen patients with an AAA, including only limited angular deformities, and 17 patients with OAA were evaluated in a single-center retrospective review of O'Brien and colleagues.[2] AAA showed similar fusion rates to OAA, with significantly less morbidity, shorter operative times, shorter tourniquet times, less blood loss, and shorter hospital stays.

Panikkar and colleagues[46] included a total of 21 patients and found no significant difference for clinical and radiographic fusion rates or clinical scores (AOFAS) in open or arthroscopic ankle fusion.

Nielsen and colleagues[44] compared 58 arthroscopic to 49 OAA with similar inclusion criteria except that the open group had a varus/valgus malalignment exceeding 5°, resulting in the same selection bias as mentioned above (Myerson and O'Brien). The arthroscopic group had a significantly shorter hospital stay, 2.27 days less than the open group.

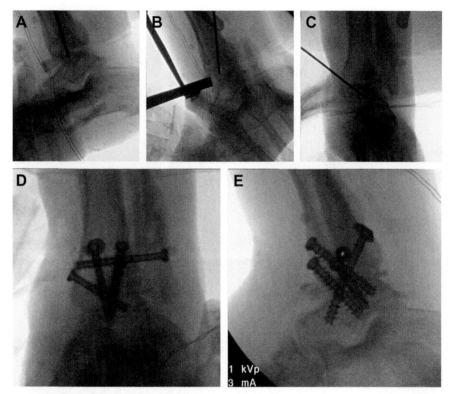

Fig. 16. Case 5: Insertion of a wedged allograft to correct intraarticular deformity. Fluoroscopy images of left arthroscopic ankle fusion showing (*A*, *B*) the insertion of a wedged allograft. (*C*) Preliminary fixation of reduction with a medial k-wire, the allograft is visible in the lateral joint space. (*D*, *E*) Final screw positioning in anteroposterior and lateral view, note that a fully threaded screw is used to strut out the deformity on the lateral side. Due to syndesmotic widening, a syndesmotic fusion was performed.

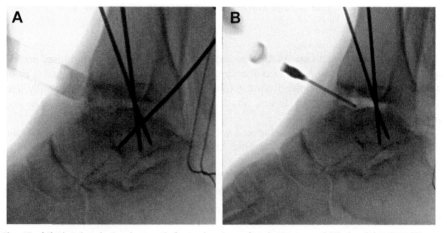

Fig. 17. (*A*) Platelet-derived growth factor bone graft substitute and (*B*) demineralized bone matrix is inserted into void via portal under fluoroscopy guidance.

The retrospective review of Quayle and colleagues[45] included 29 open and 50 AAA. It demonstrated higher complication rate and lower rate of fusion in the open group. No significant difference was found in the length of hospital stay and the ability of deformity correction.

The multicenter comparative case series of Townshend and colleagues[28] included 30 open and 30 arthroscopic arthrodesis with preoperative similar coronal and sagittal malalignment. Both techniques lead to significant improvement of pain and function, whereas the arthroscopic group showed a shorter hospital stay and better outcome at one and 2 years postoperative (ankle osteoarthritis scale (AOS) score).

Peterson and colleagues[42] evaluated the cost-effectiveness of outpatient AAA versus inpatient open technique. The outpatient AAA was significantly less expensive, with lower total site charges, but higher reimbursement for the surgeon and the hospital.

Arthroscopic Ankle Arthrodesis Versus TAR

Ankle arthrodesis is still considered a viable treatment option for ESAA regardless of the patient's age. There is no current evidence available to indicate that total ankle arthroplasty is superior to ankle arthrodesis.

Up till today, there is no Level I study available regarding this topic. The recruitment of patients for the TARVA study, a prospective randomized controlled trial comparing TAR versus AA, has been finished as well as the 1-year follow-up, the publication is pending.

The outcome of ankle arthrodesis versus TAR was examined in the following Level II and III studies.

The Level II study of Norvell and colleagues[47] including 517 patients treated either with TAR or AA, showed that both treatment options were effective at a 2-year follow-up. The improvement in several patient-reported outcomes was greater after TAR than after AA. No significant difference in the rate of revision surgery and complications was noted.

Intermediate-term clinical outcomes at a mean of 5.5 years of total ankle replacement and ankle arthrodesis were equivalent in a diverse cohort of the COFAS multicenter Level II study published by Daniels and colleagues,[48] while rates of reoperation and major complications were higher after ankle replacement.

The aim of the comparative study of SooHoo[49] was to compare the reoperation rates following ankle arthrodesis and ankle replacement based on the observational, population-based data. Including 4705 ankle fusions and 480 ankle replacements in 10 years, the study confirmed that the ankle replacement is associated with a significantly increased risk of major revision surgery but a decreased risk of requiring subtalar fusion.

The study of Saltzman and colleagues[50] compared the clinical and radiographic outcomes and the early perioperative complications of the 2 procedures. At an average follow-up of 4 years, the clinical results of both surgeries were similar. The arthroplasty group showed better pain relief but more postoperative complications requiring additional surgery.

In a multicenter prospective cohort study of Slobogean and colleagues,[51] the quality of life was assessed using health state values derived from the SF-36. A total of 107 patients treated with TAR or ankle arthrodesis expressed significantly improved health state values at 1-year follow-up, no difference between the groups was evident.

Schuh and colleagues[33] examined the participation in sports and recreational activities in patients who underwent either ankle arthrodesis (21 patients) or TAR (20 patients) at 34.5 months after surgery. No statistically significant difference was found in the activity levels, participation in sports, UCLA and AOFAS score between the arthrodesis group and the TAR group at follow-up.

In a comparative study of Krause and colleagues,[52] the impact of complications was analyzed using the AOS. A total of 114 total ankle replacements and 47 ankle arthrodesis were examined at a minimum of 2 years postoperatively and showed comparable results regarding pain relief and function. The rate of complications was significantly higher in the arthroplasty group, but the impact of complications on outcome was clinically relevant in both groups.

In a Level III study from the senior author AndreaVeljkovic,[53] AAA resulted in comparable clinical outcomes to TAR in nondeformed, COFAS Type 1 ankle arthritis. In this patient group, the short-term outcome of AAA and TAR were not significantly different, whereas TAR showed higher reoperation rates.

SUMMARY

AAA is a reliable option for the treatment of ESAA. With the arthroscopic technique a high fusion rate, reduced time to union as well as adequate deformity correction can potentially be achieved with the benefits of a shorter hospital stay and perhaps a better clinical outcome.

CLINICS CARE POINTS

- First screw corrects the deformity!
- Posterior translation of talus is eminent to reduce the lever arm of the foot and a gastrocnemius recession needs to be considered.
- Subtle valgus unlocks the transverse tarsal joint.
- Equinus position of talus needs to be prevented so as to offload stress on the midfoot and knee.
- The foot must be left plantigrade and balanced through bony and soft tissue procedures.

ACKNOWLEDGMENTS

Alastair Younger

DISCLOSURE

A-K. Leucht has nothing to disclose. A. Veljkovic has nothing to disclose pertaining this topic.

REFERENCES

1. Myerson MS, Quill G. Ankle arthrodesis. A comparison of an arthroscopic and an open method of treatment. Clin Orthop Relat Res 1991;(268):84–95.
2. O'Brien TS, Hart TS, Shereff MJ, et al. Open versus arthroscopic ankle arthrodesis: a comparative study. Foot Ankle Int 1999;20(6):368–74.
3. Valderrabano V, Horisberger M, Russell I, et al. Etiology of ankle osteoarthritis. Clin Orthop Relat Res 2009;467(7):1800–6.
4. Le V, Veljkovic A, Salat P, et al. Ankle Arthritis. Foot Ankle Orthop 2019;4(3):1–16.

5. Younger ASE, Wing KJ, Glazebrook M, et al. Patient expectation and satisfaction as measures of operative outcome in end-stage ankle arthritis. Foot Ankle Int 2015;36(2):123–34.
6. Mazur JM, Schwartz E, Simon SR. Ankle arthrodesis. Long-term follow-up with gait analysis. J Bone Joint Surg Am 1979;61(7):964–75.
7. Buck P, Morrey BF, Chao EY. The optimum position of arthrodesis of the ankle. A gait study of the knee and ankle. J Bone Joint Surg Am 1987;69(7):1052–62.
8. Beyaert C, Sirveaux F, Paysant J, et al. The effect of tibio-talar arthrodesis on foot kinematics and ground reaction force progression during walking. Gait Posture 2004;20(1):84–91.
9. Thomas R. Gait analysis and functional outcomes following ankle arthrodesis for isolated ankle arthritis. J Bone Joint Surg Am 2006;88(3):526–35.
10. Fuentes-Sanz A, Moya-Angeler J, Lopez-Oliva F, et al. Clinical outcome and gait analysis of ankle arthrodesis. Foot Ankle Int 2012;33(10):819–27.
11. King HA, Watkins TB Jr, Samuelson KM. Analysis of foot position in ankle arthrodesis and its influence on gait. Foot Ankle 1980;1(1):44–9.
12. Wu WL, Su FC, Cheng YM, et al. Gait analysis after ankle arthrodesis. Gait Posture 2000;11(1):54–61.
13. Singer S, Klejman S, Pinsker E, et al. Ankle arthroplasty and ankle arthrodesis: gait analysis compared with normal controls. J Bone Joint Surg Am 2013; 95(24):e191, 191-110.
14. Sealey RJ, Myerson MS, Molloy A, et al. Sagittal plane motion of the hindfoot following ankle arthrodesis: a prospective analysis. Foot Ankle Int 2009;30(3): 187–96.
15. Fuchs S, Sandmann C, Skwara A, et al. Quality of life 20 years after arthrodesis of the ankle. A study of adjacent joints. J Bone Joint Surg Br 2003;85(7):994–8.
16. Coester LM, Saltzman CL, Leupold J, et al. Long-term results following ankle arthrodesis for post-traumatic arthritis. J Bone Joint Surg Am 2001;83(2):219–28.
17. Ling JS, Smyth NA, Fraser EJ, et al. Investigating the relationship between ankle arthrodesis and adjacent-joint arthritis in the hindfoot. J Bone Joint Surg 2015; 97(6):513–9.
18. Hendrickx RPM, Stufkens SAS, de Bruijn EE, et al. Medium- to long-term outcome of ankle arthrodesis. Foot Ankle Int 2011;32(10):940–7.
19. Strasser NL, Turner NS. Functional outcomes after ankle arthrodesis in elderly patients. Foot Ankle Int 2012;33(9):699–703.
20. Morrey BF, Wiedeman GP Jr. Complications and long-term results of ankle arthrodeses following trauma. J Bone Joint Surg Am 1980;62(5):777–84.
21. Glick JM, Morgan CD, Myerson MS, et al. Ankle arthrodesis using an arthroscopic method: Long-term follow-up of 34 cases. Arthroscopy 1996;12(4):428–34.
22. Wasserman LR, Saltzman CL, Amendola A. Minimally invasive ankle reconstruction: current scope and indications. Orthop Clin North Am 2004;35(2):247–53.
23. Dannawi Z, Nawabi DH, Patel A, et al. Arthroscopic ankle arthrodesis: are results reproducible irrespective of pre-operative deformity? Foot Ankle Surg 2011;17(4): 294–9.
24. Winson IG, Robinson DE, Allen PE. Arthroscopic ankle arthrodesis. J Bone Joint Surg Br 2005;87(3):343–7.
25. Schmid T, Krause F, Penner MJ, et al. Effect of Preoperative Deformity on Arthroscopic and Open Ankle Fusion Outcomes. Foot Ankle Int 2017;38(12):1301–10.
26. Gougoulias NE, Agathangelidis FG, Parsons SW. Arthroscopic ankle arthrodesis. Foot Ankle Int 2007;28(6):695–706.

27. Zvijac JE, Lemak L, Schurhoff MR, et al. Analysis of arthroscopically assisted ankle arthrodesis. Arthroscopy 2002;18(1):70–5.

28. Townshend D, Di Silvestro M, Krause F, et al. Arthroscopic versus open ankle arthrodesis: a multicenter comparative case series. J Bone Joint Surg Am 2013;95(2):98–102.

29. Mann RA. Surgical implications of biomechanics of the foot and ankle. Clin Orthop Relat Res 1980;(146):111–8.

30. Holt ES, Hansen ST, Mayo KA, et al. Ankle arthrodesis using internal screw fixation. Clin Orthop Relat Res 1991;(268):21–8.

31. Glazebrook M, Beasley W, Daniels T, et al. Establishing the relationship between clinical outcome and extent of osseous bridging between computed tomography assessment in isolated hindfoot and ankle fusions. Foot Ankle Int 2013;34(12):1612–8.

32. Mehdi N, Bernasconi A, Laborde J, et al. Comparison of 25 ankle arthrodeses and 25 replacements at 67 months' follow-up. Orthop Traumatol Surg Res 2019;105(1):139–44.

33. Schuh R, Hofstaetter J, Krismer M, et al. Total ankle arthroplasty versus ankle arthrodesis. Comparison of sports, recreational activities and functional outcome. Int Orthopaedics 2011;36(6):1207–14.

34. Li Y, He J, Hu Y. Comparison of the efficiency and safety of total ankle replacement and ankle arthrodesis in the treatment of osteoarthritis: an updated systematic review and meta-analysis. Orthop Surg 2020;12(2):372–7.

35. Cameron SE, Ullrich P. Arthroscopic arthrodesis of the ankle joint. Arthroscopy 2000;16(1):21–6.

36. Saragas NP. Results of arthroscopic arthrodesis of the ankle. Foot Ankle Surg 2004;10(3):141–3.

37. Ferkel RD, Hewitt M. Long-term results of arthroscopic ankle arthrodesis. Foot Ankle Int 2005;26(4):275–80.

38. Abicht BP, Roukis TS. Incidence of nonunion after isolated arthroscopic ankle arthrodesis. Arthroscopy 2013;29(5):949–54.

39. Jones CR, Wong E, Applegate GR, et al. Arthroscopic ankle arthrodesis: a 2-15 year follow-up study. Arthroscopy 2018;34(5):1641–9.

40. Yang T-C, Tzeng Y-H, Wang C-S, et al. Arthroscopic ankle arthrodesis provides similarly satisfactory surgical outcomes in ankles with severe deformity compared with mild deformity in elderly patients. Arthroscopy 2020;36(10):2738–47.

41. Jain SK, Tiernan D, Kearns SR. Analysis of risk factors for failure of arthroscopic ankle fusion in a series of 52 ankles. Foot Ankle Surg 2016;22(2):91–6.

42. Peterson KS, Lee MS, Buddecke DE. Arthroscopic versus Open Ankle Arthrodesis: A Retrospective Cost Analysis. J Foot Ankle Surg 2010;49(3):242–7.

43. Meng Q, Yu T, Yu L, et al. [Effectiveness comparison between arthroscopic and open ankle arthrodeses]. Zhongguo Xiu Fu Chong Jian Wai Ke Za Zhi 2013;27(3):288–91.

44. Nielsen KK, Linde F, Jensen NC. The outcome of arthroscopic and open surgery ankle arthrodesis: a comparative retrospective study on 107 patients. Foot Ankle Surg 2008;14(3):153–7.

45. Quayle J, Shafafy R, Khan MA, et al. Arthroscopic versus open ankle arthrodesis. Foot Ankle Surg 2018;24(2):137–42.

46. Vivek Panikkar K, Taylor A, Kamath S, et al. A comparison of open and arthroscopic ankle fusion. Foot Ankle Surg 2003;9(3):169–72.

47. Norvell DC, Ledoux WR, Shofer JB, et al. Effectiveness and safety of ankle arthrodesis versus arthroplasty. J Bone Joint Surg 2019;101(16):1485–94.

48. Daniels TR, Younger ASE, Penner M, et al. Intermediate-Term Results of Total Ankle Replacement and Ankle Arthrodesis. J Bone Joint Surg Am 2014;96(2): 135–42.
49. SooHoo NF, Zingmond DS, Ko CY. Comparison of reoperation rates following ankle arthrodesis and total ankle arthroplasty. J Bone Joint Surg 2007;89(10): 2143–9.
50. Saltzman CL, Kadoko RG, Suh JS. Treatment of isolated ankle osteoarthritis with arthrodesis or the total ankle replacement: a comparison of early outcomes. Clin Orthop Surg 2010;2(1):1–7.
51. Slobogean GP, Younger A, Apostle KL, et al. Preference-based quality of life of end-stage ankle arthritis treated with arthroplasty or arthrodesis. Foot Ankle Int 2010;31(7):563–6.
52. Krause FG, Windolf M, Bora B, et al. Impact of complications in total ankle replacement and ankle arthrodesis analyzed with a validated outcome measurement. J Bone Joint Surg Am 2011;93(9):830–9.
53. Veljkovic AN, Daniels TR, Glazebrook MA, et al. Outcomes of total ankle replacement, arthroscopic ankle arthrodesis, and open ankle arthrodesis for isolated non-deformed end-stage ankle arthritis. J Bone Joint Surg 2019;101(17):1523–9.

Open Ankle Arthrodesis for Deformity Correction

David Vier, MD[a], Todd A. Irwin, MD[b],*

KEYWORDS

- Ankle arthritis • Ankle arthrodesis • Deformity • Technique

KEY POINTS

- Open ankle arthrodesis is a reliable way to correct deformity and achieve ankle arthrodesis
- Careful clinical and radiographic evaluation needs to be performed, keeping in mind the entire lower extremity above and below the ankle.
- Multiple approaches and fixation options are available to the surgeon, with the deformity often helping to determine which technique should be used.
- Both coronal and sagittal plane deformities are common in ankle arthritis, and achieving excellent deformity correction is paramount in achieving a plantigrade foot and successful outcome.

INTRODUCTION

Open ankle arthrodesis (OAA) is traditionally considered the most reliable way to correct deformity in ankle arthritis. This technique allows for better visualization, joint preparation access, and corrective osteotomies than other arthrodesis techniques. Open arthrodesis can be accomplished through anterior, posterior, or transfibular approaches depending on the deformity.[1–6] Other arthrodesis techniques such as arthroscopic or mini-open can be challenging to correct deformity.[7–9] Recent advancements and increased experience with total ankle replacement (TAR) implants have led some to challenge that TAR is now the gold standard for ankle arthritis even with significant deformity.[10–13] Although TAR has consistently been used with increasing frequency in the treatment of ankle arthritis over the past 15 to 20 years, OAA is still more commonly used to correct deformity and address ankle arthritis concurrently.[14–16] Surgeons should strongly consider deformity among other factors when deciding on a surgical plan to treat ankle arthritis.

a Baylor University Medical Center, 3500 Gaston Avenue, Dallas, TX 75246, USA;
b OrthoCarolina Foot and Ankle Institute, Atrium Health Musculoskeletal Institute, 2001 Vail Avenue, Charlotte, NC 28207, USA
* Corresponding author.
E-mail address: Todd.irwin@orthocarolina.com
Twitter: @ToddIrwinMD (T.A.I.)

Foot Ankle Clin N Am 27 (2022) 199–216
https://doi.org/10.1016/j.fcl.2021.11.009
1083-7515/22/© 2021 Elsevier Inc. All rights reserved.

foot.theclinics.com

CLINICAL EVALUATION/PREOPERATIVE PLANNING

- Physical examination
  - Inspection
    - Every patient should be inspected from the hip to the foot even when the chief complaint is isolated to the ankle. Deformity can occur at multiple different locations, and the clinician might also pick up on other important diagnoses such as peripheral vascular disease or a previous incision or scar which might affect surgical treatment considerations. Foot deformity should be evaluated while standing to assess for cavovarus or planovalgus deformities.
  - Palpation
    - Palpating different anatomic structures of the foot and ankle allows for the confirmation of the etiology of pain. Anterior ankle joint line tenderness helps confirm ankle arthritis, but tenderness in other areas may lead the physician to another diagnosis to consider in surgical planning such as posterior tibial or peroneal tendinitis.
  - Range of motion
    - Restricted range of motion of the ankle should be evaluated, especially when deciding between TAR and OAA. Other joints, especially the subtalar joint, should be evaluated for restricted ROM. Subtalar arthritis might influence the treating physician to consider other surgical options such as TTC or TAR.
  - Sensory
    - Evaluation for neuropathy should be conducted in every patient especially those with diabetes. This includes gross sensation to light touch as well as Semmes-Weinstein monofilament testing. Dense neuropathy might influence the surgeon to consider tibiotalocalcaneal (TTC) fusion as opposed to isolated ankle fusion or TAR.
  - Special examination
    - Silfverskiold
      - Tendoachilles lengthening or gastrocnemius recession may be important adjunct procedures in the setting of Achilles or gastrocnemius contractures to achieve appropriate tibiotalar alignment when performing OAA.
    - Ankle laxity
      - Severe ankle laxity might sway the surgeon to consider fusion over other surgical treatment options due to the additional stability it provides.
- Imaging
  - X-rays
    - Standard weight-bearing radiographs of the ankle are the recommended initial imaging assessment of ankle arthritis. This includes three views — anteroposterior (AP), mortise, and lateral views. Due to the effect of the foot alignment on the ankle and vice versa, it is strongly recommended to include AP and oblique views of the foot as well to evaluate for additional or compensatory deformity.
    - Although it is easy to be distracted by the ankle and/or foot deformity, if there is any question about another area contributing to the deformity then long leg alignment radiographs should be used. Significant deformity through the hip or knee warrants consideration of referral to an adult reconstruction colleague for correction. Many surgeons prefer to correct the deformity proximally first before correction distally. Deformity through the tibia may warrant an extraarticular osteotomy concurrently or in lieu of correction through the ankle.

- The Saltzman view, a weight-bearing hindfoot alignment view, can be useful in assessing hindfoot deformity and aid in surgical planning for the consideration of calcaneal osteotomy or subtalar fusion.[17]
- Computed tomography (CT) is an important tool in assessing deformity as well as the extent of arthritic changes. CT gives a more accurate depiction of cyst formation, sclerosis, and subchondral collapse. Weight-bearing CT provides even more information regarding dynamic deformity and can help with surgical planning, but is not as accessible as standard CT.
- Evaluation of the deformity
  - Combination of physical examination, standard foot, and ankle radiographs, long length alignment films, as well as advanced imaging should be used to evaluate deformity.
  - Varus deformity
    - Varus ankle arthritis is the most common coronal plane deformity in ankle arthritis. Isolated wear of the medial tibial plafond occurs in the setting of posttraumatic arthritis, cavovarus foot deformity, peroneal tendon tear, or ankle instability/laxity. Evaluation of the knee coronal plane alignment for deformity is important to evaluate on physical examination as well as plain radiographs. Varus ankle arthritis can develop with ipsilateral valgus knee or tibia deformity due to compensatory hindfoot/ankle alignment.[18] (**Fig. 1** A,B)
  - Valgus deformity
    - Valgus ankle arthritis is the least common coronal plane deformity. Isolated wear of the lateral plafond can occur from posttraumatic arthritis, flatfoot deformity, or an incompetent deltoid ligament. Converse to varus ankle arthritis, compensatory valgus ankle/hindfoot alignment can develop with ipsilateral varus knee deformity (**Fig. 2** A,B).

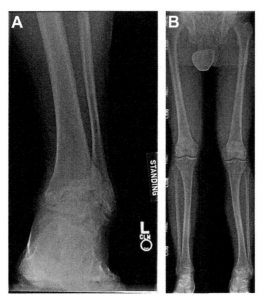

Fig. 1. (*A*) Varus ankle arthritis seen on anteroposterior (AP) ankle radiograph, with proximal deformity as potential cause seen on long-leg alignment views (*B*).

- ○ Extraarticular deformity
  - ■ Extraarticular deformity such as tibia vara/valgum would be picked up on standing clinical examination or long leg alignment films.
- ○ Concomitant foot deformity
  - ■ Evaluation of the foot deformity and its effect on the ankle cannot but understated. A standing physical examination is used to assess hindfoot valgus or varus as well as pes cavus or planus. The foot deformity can also be thoroughly assessed on weight-bearing AP and lateral foot radiographs with talar head uncoverage, talo-first metatarsal angle, and talar declination among many other parameters.

TREATMENT OPTIONS/CONSIDERATIONS

Once the decision to proceed with OAA has been made, there are several aspects of the procedure that need to be considered and carefully planned. Often the deformity will help to dictate the specific techniques that will be used. Other considerations include any prior surgery, hardware that may have to be removed, and associated skin or soft tissue concerns such as scars or flaps.

APPROACHES

- Anterior approach:
  - ○ The anterior approach has become a workhorse approach for ankle arthritis with the increased popularity of anterior plating for ankle arthrodesis and total ankle arthroplasty. Many deformities can be addressed and corrected through a standard anterior approach between the tibialis anterior (TA) tendon and extensor hallucis longus (EHL) tendon. This approach also allows for debridement of both the medial and lateral gutter which can be important to achieve intraarticular reduction in coronal plane deformity. In addition, the fibula is easily preserved with this approach to ensure future revision options.

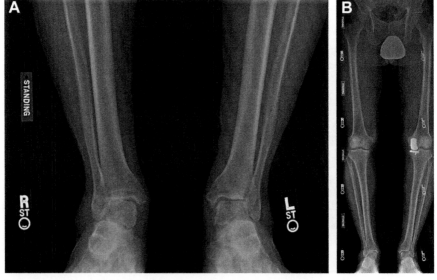

Fig. 2. (A) Valgus ankle arthritis seen on anteroposterior (AP) ankle radiograph, with varus knee deformity as potential cause seen on long-leg alignment views (B).

- Lateral approach
  - The lateral approach to the ankle offers an extensile approach with excellent access to the tibiotalar joint, as well as distal access to the subtalar joint when indicated. A fibular osteotomy is typically performed to gain access, though access can be achieved with anterior soft tissue release and posterior retraction of the fibula. Resecting the medial 1/3rd of the fibula after osteotomy, and then using the fibula as a lateral strut incorporated into the fusion can be a helpful technique. Alternatively, the fibula can be resected and used as bone graft, though this is typically only done if TTC arthrodesis is performed and conversion to total ankle arthroplasty in the future is unlikely. A separate medial incision is typically required to access the medial gutter for complete joint preparation.
- Posterior Achilles-splitting approach
  - Though less commonly needed, a posterior Achilles-splitting approach is a useful technique in particular with anterior skin or soft tissue defects that prevent other approaches. A direct posterior incision is used, followed by splitting the Achilles tendon in the coronal plane with long flaps. Access to both the tibiotalar joint and subtalar joint is achieved (**Fig. 3**).

FIXATION STRATEGIES/GRAFTING

As with many aspects of orthopedic surgery, which implants are chosen is secondary to good, sound surgical technique. This includes obtaining deformity correction before implantation and excellent joint preparation before fixation. Once this is achieved, then decisions on fixation strategies can be made.

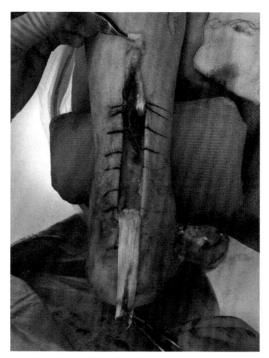

Fig. 3. Posterior approach to the ankle using a coronal split technique through the Achilles tendon.

- Screws only
  - Screw fixation alone for ankle fusion has been performed for decades and remains a viable option.[19] Considering the deformity is important when planning screw configuration, such as holding a valgus deformity corrected with a screw along the medial column of the tibiotalar joint. Currently, cannulated partially threaded screws are the most commonly used implant, though this is surgeon dependent. Other considerations include the type of metal (typically stainless steel or titanium), size of the screw, and headed or headless screws.
- Plating
  - Ankle arthrodesis plating techniques have significantly increased in popularity with the advent of ankle arthrodesis specific plating options.[19] Most current systems include anterior, lateral, and some posterior plating options, with anterior plating being the most common. Choosing which plate to use is typically dictated by the specific deformity or the preferred approach, with soft tissue considerations included in this decision-making process. Most systems have options for tibiotalar arthrodesis alone versus TTC arthrodesis. While plating can achieve a stable construct, creating excellent compression across the tibiotalar joint is paramount for a good result. Most surgeons will use lag screw fixation in addition to plating either through the plate itself, or outside of the plate, to create compression (**Figs. 4** A,B). Many systems also have the option to create compression through the plate with screws placed in a compression slot.

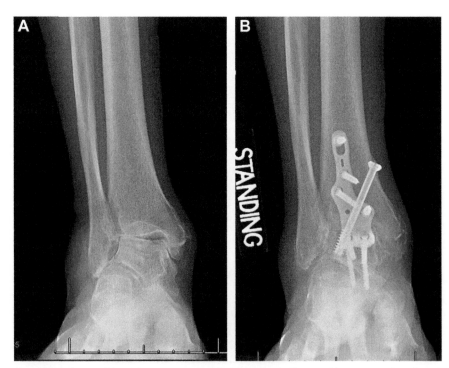

Fig. 4. (*A*) Valgus ankle arthritis treated with (*B*) anterior plate and lag screw placed medially to achieve compression and help hold the talus in a corrected position.

- Intramedullary nail
  - Some deformities or clinical conditions warrant TTC arthrodesis as opposed to isolated tibiotalar arthrodesis. In these situations, using a retrograde intramedullary nail can be an excellent option. The load sharing quality of a retrograde intramedullary nail can provide good biomechanical stability, as long as the surgeon feels sacrificing the subtalar joint is indicated or necessary Joint Preservation Surgery for Varus and Posterior Ankle Arthritis associated with Flatfoot Deformity.
- Thin-wire external fixation
  - Using a thin-wire external fixator is indicated in the setting of chronic infection, for revision when multiple other internal fixation techniques have been used, or potentially for deformity correction at the same time as ankle arthrodesis (**Fig. 5**).[20]
- Grafting options
  - To achieve solid arthrodesis, most surgeons include bone graft into the fusion construct. Options for bone graft include autograft, allograft, or a combination of both. The most common autograft options are cancellous bone taken from the calcaneus, proximal tibia, or the iliac crest. Over the past several years, a plethora of bone graft substitutes have been developed by industry and a full analysis of these options is beyond the scope of this review. When the deformity

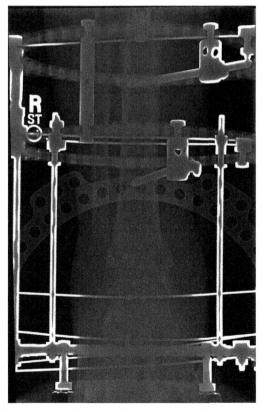

Fig. 5. AP ankle radiograph 3 weeks after thin-wire external fixator placement used for revision ankle arthrodesis.

results in bone loss, the structural bone graft may be required to help with deformity correction and stability of the construct (see Specific Techniques section).

DEFORMITY CORRECTION

Regardless of the approach or fixation options used, achieving deformity correction is paramount to achieving a good result. Ideal hindfoot position after ankle fusion is neutral in the sagittal plane, 0 to 5° of hindfoot valgus, and 0 to 5° of external rotation.[21] Intraarticular deformity is most common, though evaluating for tibia deformity proximally should also be done. Similarly, there is often compensatory foot deformity that occurs after longstanding ankle or tibia deformity. After the proximal deformity is corrected, the surgeon must be ready to correct any foot deformity or instability present to achieve a plantigrade foot underneath the ankle arthrodesis.

- Intraarticular deformity
  - Coronal plane deformity
    - Intraarticular varus and valgus deformity are the most common ankle deformity seen in ankle DJD. Most of the time this deformity can easily be corrected through the joint with good reduction and stable fixation constructs.
    - Varus deformity is very common. Once the deformity is reduced and the tibiotalar joint is in a neutral position, a lag screw can be placed along the lateral column of the joint to hold it in position as part of the construct. Alternatively, if anterior plating is being utilized the plate itself can hold the joint reduced (**Figs. 6** A–D). If a lateral approach is preferred, the fibula can be used as a strut or a lateral plate can be used similar to tension side fixation in fracture management.
    - Valgus deformity is also seen with some regularity, often secondary to deltoid ligament insufficiency from prior injury or longstanding flatfoot deformity. Similar to varus, a medial column-based tibiotalar lag screw can hold the valgus deformity reduced as part of the fixation construct (see **Fig. 4** A,B).
    - Technique tips:
      - Plafond defects: In longstanding deformity, the tibial plafond can erode asymmetrically. To achieve good deformity correction, this defect needs to be addressed. Options include removing bone from the opposite side to even out the plafond to achieve the neutral position, or placing the structural graft in the defect to accommodate for the deformity and hold the talus in neutral (**Fig. 7 A**-G). The authors' preference is to use a prefabricated Evans or Cotton allograft soaked in bone marrow aspirate concentrate as a wedge graft on the side of the defect (**Fig. 8**A,B)
      - Gutter spurs: Evaluating the CT scan closely for medial or lateral gutter osteophytes is important to achieve good deformity correction (**Fig. 9**). Aggressive gutter debridement may be required to allow the talus to correct into a neutral position.
  - Sagittal plane deformity
    - Careful evaluation of the talus position in the sagittal plane is very important and can be difficult intraoperatively due to the motion at the talonavicular joint. Large anterior osteophytes can prevent dorsiflexion and cause a subsequent equinus contracture of the ankle. If the neutral ankle position cannot be achieved after anterior debridement, a tendo-Achilles lengthening with or without a posterior capsular release may need to be performed.

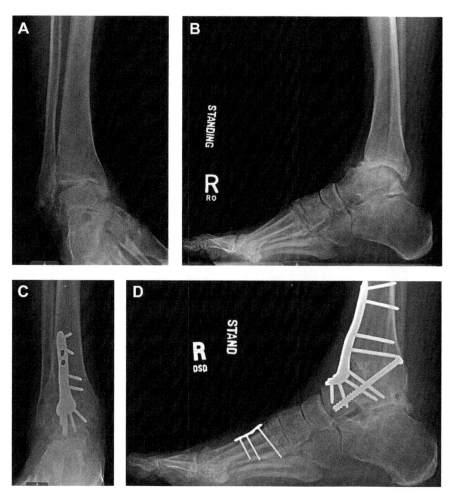

Fig. 6. (*A, B*) Preoperative radiographs showing varus ankle arthritis with associated anterior translation of the talus. (*C, D*) 6-months postoperative radiographs showing anterior plate and lag screw construct correcting both deformities.

Fusing the tibiotalar joint in equinus can result in a poor long-term outcome due to adjacent joint stress and hyperextension at the knee.

- Translation of the talus in the sagittal plane is common. Anterior translation is more common than posterior translation, likely secondary to longstanding ankle instability as the cause of arthritis (see **Figs. 6B and 7**B). However, posterior translation may be seen in posttraumatic settings secondary to posterior malleolus fracture displacement (**Fig. 10** A,B). Recognizing this translation and correcting it before fixation is important to achieve a functional position of the fusion.

- Extraarticular deformity
  - Tibia deformity
    - Deformities in the tibia can be present along the entire length of the tibia. As noted in the Evaluation section, the lower extremities should be inspected from above the knee, and long leg alignment films should be used if there

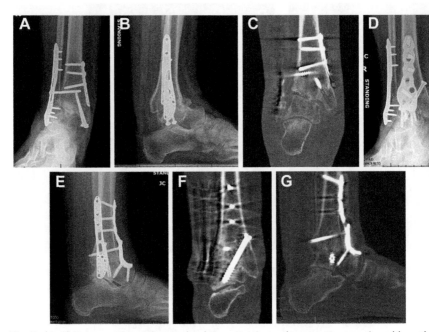

Fig. 7. (A, B) Preoperative radiographs demonstrating valgus posttraumatic ankle arthritis with anterior translation of the talus. (C) Coronal CT scan showing a collapse of the lateral tibial plafond. (D, E) 6-months postoperative radiographs demonstrating deformity correction in both planes with the use of a plate and screw construct. Structural allograft was used in the lateral tibiotalar joint to help correct the deformity. (F, G) Coronal and sagittal CT scans showing incorporation of the graft and solid arthrodesis.

is suspicion of tibial deformity or to evaluate the overall mechanical axis from hip to ankle.

- Tibial shaft deformities can be present in any plane and may be multiplanar (**Fig. 11** A, B). If the shaft deformity will ultimately affect the foot position after ankle arthrodesis, a concomitant tibial osteotomy may be required.
- Tibial plafond and supramalleolar deformities may be seen after severe distal tibia and pilon fractures. Careful preoperative evaluation needs to

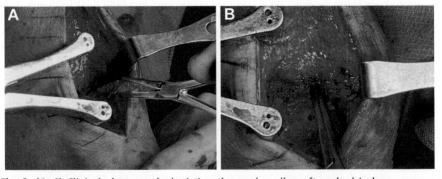

Fig. 8. (A, B) Clinical photograph depicting the wedge allograft soaked in bone marrow aspirate concentrate placed in the lateral side of the joint to hold the tibiotalar joint in the neutral position.

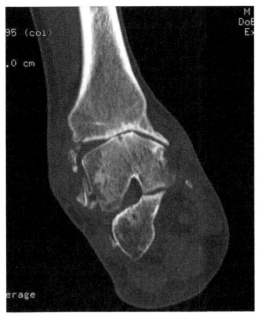

Fig. 9. Coronal CT scan showing both lateral and medial gutter osteophytes on the talus that will need to be removed to achieve the neutral position of the talus within the ankle mortise.

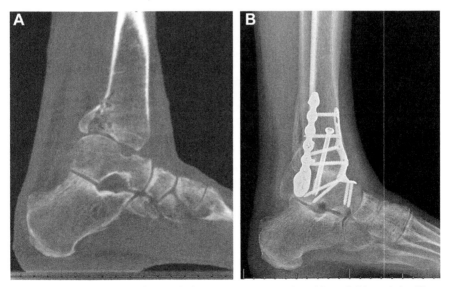

Fig. 10. (A) Lateral ankle radiograph showing posttraumatic ankle arthritis and significant posterior translation of the talus secondary to untreated posterior malleolus fracture (B).

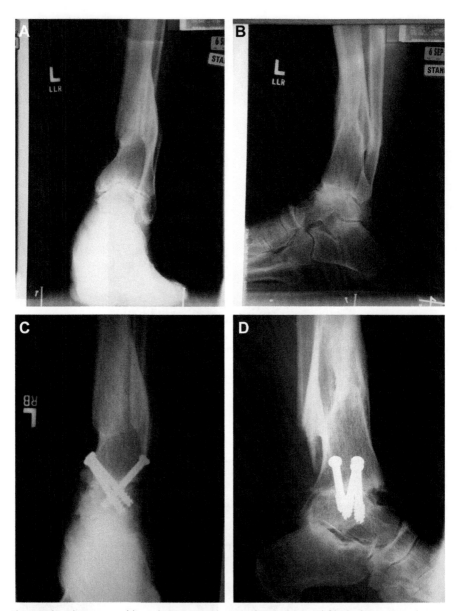

Fig. 11. (*A, B*) Severe ankle arthritis secondary to distal tibia and fibula fracture malunion. (*C, D*) Deformity correction and ankle arthrodesis achieved through flat cuts in the tibia and talus with screw fixation.

    be performed before arthrodesis to understand the deformity and plan for its correction.

- ■ Technique tip:
  - In the setting of severe plafond or supramalleolar deformity, performing flat cuts through the tibia and/or talus can be an effective technique to correct the deformity and remove unhealthy or nonviable bone (see **Fig. 11** C,D).

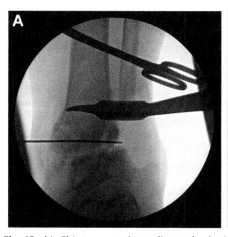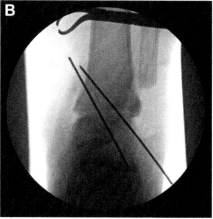

Fig. 12. (*A*, *B*) Intraoperative radiographs depicting the use of a kirschner wire to determine the appropriate orientation of the flat cut orthogonal to the longitudinal axis of the tibia.

- This technique will inevitably shorten the limb so care must be taken to minimize how much shortening is performed.
- Using a k-wire as a guide, and confirming in both the A-P and lateral fluoroscopic views before bone resection is a helpful technique to avoid pitfalls (**Fig. 12** A,B).
  ○ Foot deformity
    ■ Compensatory foot deformity is common after longstanding ankle deformity. Anticipating the foot position after ankle joint correction is important for preoperative planning.
    ■ Varus ankle deformity may result in or exacerbate a cavus or cavovarus foot position. In most cases, the hindfoot will be corrected through the ankle joint fusion once that deformity is addressed. After the ankle joint is corrected, it is important to evaluate the position and flexibility of the first ray in relation to the other metatarsal heads. When the first metatarsal is plantarflexed, a dorsiflexion first metatarsal osteotomy should be performed (see **Fig. 6**D).
    ■ Valgus ankle deformity can result in similar foot deformities seen in a progressive collapsing foot deformity, or adult-acquired flatfoot. The subtalar joint needs to be closely evaluated in this situation. If there is concomitant subtalar instability or DJD seen radiographically, then converting to a TTC arthrodesis may be required. Sometimes performing the ankle arthrodesis alone will be enough to correct the flatfoot deformity, assuming good deformity correction is achieved. If there is residual forefoot supination or first ray instability, then performing medial column stabilization may be required to achieve a plantigrade foot. The most common procedures performed in this setting are a Cotton opening wedge osteotomy through the medial cuneiform or a 1st tarsometatarsal joint arthrodesis.

RECOVERY – POSTOPERATIVE PROTOCOL

Patients are placed into a short-leg well-padded splint at neutral for the first 2 weeks postoperatively and kept non–weight-bearing. The authors prefer transitioning to a short-leg cast at the first postoperative visit, though some surgeons prefer a prefabricated tall boot at this stage. Patients are kept non–weight-bearing or toe-touch weight-bearing only for the first 6 weeks postoperatively. At 6 weeks, patients are placed into a prefabricated tall boot and allowed to transition to full weight-bearing as tolerated. Wean out of boot into regular shoewear after 12 weeks. Ankle radiographs are typically checked at 2 weeks, 6 weeks, 12 weeks, and 6 months postoperatively. Standing CT scan is ordered between 4 and 6 months postoperatively if there is a concern for delayed or nonunion clinically. Formal physical therapy is not typically required. Rocker bottom shoewear is recommended to accommodate for the loss of tibiotalar motion.

OUTCOMES

- Fusion rates
  - Ankle arthrodesis is such a successful, reliable surgery in large part due to its high union rates, ranging from 91% to 100% in many studies.[2,3,5,6,19,22,23] Similar union rates have been reported specifically in OAA, although many studies have reported higher union rates in AAA when directly compared with OAA.[9,23–28] Fixation method has not been shown to change union rates in OAA.[19] A systematic review of ankle fusion for failed TAR by Gross and colleagues demonstrated the ankle fusion rate after failed TAR was 89.4% in 193 patients overall, with the most common failure due to rheumatoid arthritis.[29–31]
- Patient-reported outcomes
  - Significant pain improvement and functional outcomes have been consistently shown after OAA, especially in patients who achieve successful bony union.[2,3,5,6,28,32–35]
- Complications
  - Overall revision rates in the literature range from 7% to 20%.[3,5,22,34,36–38] Soohoo and colleagues reported a major revision surgery rate in OAA of 5% at 1 year and 11% at 5 years, including a subtalar fusion rate of 2.8% at 5 years. Patients undergoing OAA had a higher nonunion rate with previous subtalar fusion or preoperative varus deformity.[22] The rate of subtalar arthrosis significantly progresses after ankle arthrodesis, ranging from 32.5% of patients 7 years after OAA and 91% 22 years after OAA.[32,39] Even addressing subsequent subtalar arthritis after ankle arthrodesis has increased complications. Zanolli and colleagues showed a significantly decreased subtalar fusion rate after ipsilateral ankle fusion than a native ankle, and Gross and colleagues showed a significantly decreased subtalar fusion rate after ankle arthrodesis than after TAR.[40,41]
- TAR versus fusion
  - The debate continues on which treatment is superior for end-stage ankle arthritis. More recent studies have shown improved clinical outcomes with TAR than fusion even in large deformities, but other studies have shown no difference between the 2 treatment options. In reality, patient selection is crucial for both methods. Ankle arthrodesis has a significantly higher progression to subtalar fusion and subsequent subtalar fusion nonunion rate as noted above.
  - Studies comparing OAA to TAR with intermediate and long-term results collectively have failed to show a significant difference between the 2 regarding complication rate and patient-reported outcomes; however, many report a higher reoperation rate but higher satisfaction rate with TAR.[34,37,38,42–47] Schuh and colleagues report no difference in activity level with sports or recreational activity between the 2 groups.[48] Gait in OAA with significant preoperatively deformity was similar to that in TAR without preoperative deformity but

neither were as good as controls.[49] Piriou and colleagues showed a reduction in limp but slower gait with TAR versus ankle fusion.[50] Patients with TAR preserve more anatomic and overall sagittal ROM than ankle arthrodesis. Some sagittal ROM of the foot is maintained although limited after OAA through the talonavicular joint. This supports the theory of increased stress and thus progression of arthritis of adjacent joints after fusion.[51,52]

- Open versus arthroscopic
  - Although many studies report shorter tourniquet time, less estimated blood loss, shorter hospital length of stay, increased fusion rates, and decreased time to fusion with AAA when compared with OAA, most do not compare preoperative deformity.[8,9,23–28,33,35,53,54] However, other studies are inconclusive on treatment superiority and note that OAA is much more likely to be performed in the setting of deformity than AAA.[9,35]
- Gait
  - Ankle fusion improves parameters in gait including temporal-spatial, kinematic, and kinetic measures.[55] As mentioned above, gait function was similar in patients treated with arthrodesis for deformity when compared with arthroplasty in nondeformed ankles, but neither returned to normal compared with unaffected ankles[49]

SUMMARY

OAA remains a very reliable solution for ankle arthritis, in particular in the setting of deformity. Careful preoperative evaluation needs to be performed, both clinically and radiographically. The specific deformity present helps determine the approach used as well as the fixation choices. Deformity is most commonly seen intraarticularly, though deformity can also be present anywhere along the lower extremity, including compensatory deformity in the foot. Multiple different techniques can be used to address both the deformity and achieve a successful ankle arthrodesis. Patient outcomes reported in the literature are generally good, with high union rates and improved functional outcomes, though subtalar arthritis is a common long-term complication.

CLINICS CARE POINTS

- Evaluate all aspects of the extremity for deformity including the tibia, supramalleolar, ankle joint, and any concomitant foot deformity.
- Use lag screw fixation across the medial or lateral column of the ankle joint to correct valgus or varus intraarticular deformity, respectively.
- Structural graft can be used to fill in intraarticular defects prior to definitive fixation.
- Remove medial and lateral gutter osteophytes to allow the talus to achieve neutral fixation prior to fixation.
- Avoid equinus positioning of the tibiotalar joint at the time of fixation.
- Address any compensatory foot deformity after the ankle joint fixation is performed in order to ensure a plantigrade foot.

DISCLOSURE

T.A. Irwin: Paragon 28, Consultant/Royalties; Medline, Consultant/Royalties; GLW, Consultant, AOFAS committee chair. D. Vier: Nothing to disclose.

REFERENCES

1. Abidi NA, Gruen GS, Conti SF. Ankle arthrodesis: indications and techniques. J Am Acad Orthop Surg 2000;8(3):200–9.
2. Dekker RG, Kadakia AR. Anterior Approach for Ankle Arthrodesis. JBJS Essent Surg Tech 2017;7(2):e10.
3. Gordon D, Zicker R, Cullen N, et al. Open ankle arthrodeses via an anterior approach. Foot Ankle Int 2013;34(3):386–91.
4. Nickisch F, Avilucea FR, Beals T, et al. Open Posterior Approach for Tibiotalar Arthrodesis. Foot Ankle Clin 2011;16(1):103–14.
5. Rogero RG, Fuchs DJ, Corr D, et al. Ankle Arthrodesis Through a Fibular-Sparing Anterior Approach. Foot Ankle Int 2020;41(12):1480–6.
6. Smith JT, Chiodo CP, Singh SK, et al. Open ankle arthrodesis with a fibular-sparing technique. Foot Ankle Int 2013;34(4):557–62.
7. Paremain GD, Miller SD, Myerson MS. Ankle arthrodesis: Results after the miniarthrotomy technique. Foot Ankle Int 1996;17(5):247–52.
8. Raikin SM. Arthrodesis of the ankle: Arthroscopic, mini-open, and open techniques. Foot Ankle Clin 2003;8(2):347–59.
9. Schmid T, Krause F, Penner MJ, et al. Effect of Preoperative Deformity on Arthroscopic and Open Ankle Fusion Outcomes. Foot Ankle Int 2017;38(12):1301–10.
10. Mann RA, Mann JA, Reddy SC, et al. Correction of moderate to severe coronal plane deformity with the STAR™ ankle prosthesis. Foot Ankle Int 2011;32(7):659–64.
11. Queen RM, Adams SB, Viens NA, et al. Differences in outcomes following total ankle replacement in patients with neutral alignment compared with tibiotalar joint malalignment. J Bone Jt Surg - Ser A 2013;95(21):1927–34.
12. Lee GW, Lee KB. Outcomes of Total Ankle Arthroplasty in Ankles with >20° of Coronal Plane Deformity. J Bone Jt Surg - Am 2019;101(24):2203–11.
13. Cody E, Demetracopoulos C, Adams S, et al. Outcomes of Total Ankle Arthroplasty in Moderate and Severe Valgus Deformity. Foot Ankle Orthop 2018;3(3). 2473011418S0003.
14. Pugely AJ, Lu X, Amendola A, et al. Trends in the use of total ankle replacement and ankle arthrodesis in the United States medicare population. Foot Ankle Int 2014;35(3):207–15.
15. Terrell RD, Montgomery SR, Pannell WC, et al. Comparison of practice patterns in total ankle replacement and ankle fusion in the United States. Foot Ankle Int 2013;34(11):1486–92.
16. Raikin SM, Rasouli MR, Espandar R, et al. Trends in treatment of advanced ankle arthropathy by total ankle replacement or ankle fusion. Foot Ankle Int 2014;35(3):216–24.
17. Saltzman CL, El-Khoury GY. The hindfoot alignment view. Foot Ankle Int 1995;16(9):572–6.
18. Norton AA, Callaghan JJ, Amendola A, et al. Correlation of Knee and Hindfoot Deformities in Advanced Knee OA: Compensatory Hindfoot Alignment and Where It Occurs. Clin Orthop Relat Res 2015;473(1):166–74.
19. van den Heuvel SBM, Doorgakant A, Birnie MFN, et al. Open Ankle Arthrodesis: a Systematic Review of Approaches and Fixation Methods. Foot Ankle Surg 2021. https://doi.org/10.1016/j.fas.2020.12.011.
20. Easley ME, Montijo HE, Wilson JB, et al. Revision tibiotalar arthrodesis. J Bone Jt Surg - Ser A 2008;90(6):1212–23.

21. Buck P, Morrey BF, Chao EYS. The optimum position of arthrodesis of the ankle. A gait study of the knee and ankle. J Bone Jt Surg - Ser A 1987;69(7):1052–62.

22. Chalayon O, Wang B, Blankenhorn B, et al. Factors affecting the outcomes of uncomplicated primary open ankle arthrodesis. Foot Ankle Int 2015;36(10):1170–9.

23. Ferkel RD, Hewitt M. Long-term results of arthroscopic ankle arthrodesis. Foot Ankle Int 2005;26(4):275–80.

24. Abicht BP, Roukis TS. Incidence of nonunion after isolated arthroscopic ankle arthrodesis. Arthrosc - J Arthrosc Relat Surg 2013;29(5):949–54.

25. Elmlund AO, Winson IG. Arthroscopic Ankle Arthrodesis. Foot Ankle Clin 2015; 20(1):71–80.

26. Mok TN, He Q, Panneerselavam S, et al. Open versus arthroscopic ankle arthrodesis: a systematic review and meta-analysis. J Orthop Surg Res 2020;15(1). https://doi.org/10.1186/s13018-020-01708-4.

27. O'Brien TS, Hart TS, Shereff MJ, et al. Open versus arthroscopic ankle arthrodesis: A comparative study. Foot Ankle Int 1999;20(6):368–74.

28. Veljkovic AN, Daniels TR, Glazebrook MA, et al. Outcomes of Total Ankle Replacement, Arthroscopic Ankle Arthrodesis, and Open Ankle Arthrodesis for Isolated Non-Deformed End-Stage Ankle Arthritis. J Bone Jt Surg - Am 2019; 101(17):1523–9.

29. Gross C, Erickson BJ, Adams SB, et al. Ankle Arthrodesis After Failed Total Ankle Replacement: A Systematic Review of the Literature. Foot Ankle Spec 2015;8(2): 143–51.

30. Culpan P, Le Strat V, Piriou P, et al. Arthrodesis after failed total ankle replacement. J Bone Jt Surg - Ser B 2007;89(9):1178–83.

31. Hopgood P, Kumar R, Wood PLR. Ankle arthrodesis for failed total ankle replacement. J Bone Jt Surg - Ser B 2006;88(8):1032–8.

32. Takakura Y, Tanaka Y, Sugimoto K, et al. Long term results of arthrodesis for osteoarthritis of the ankle. Clin Orthop Relat Res 1999;361:178–85.

33. Woo BJ, Lai MC, Ng S, et al. Clinical outcomes comparing arthroscopic vs open ankle arthrodesis. Foot Ankle Surg 2020;26(5):530–4.

34. Glazebrook M, Burgesson BN, Younger AS, et al. Clinical outcome results of total ankle replacement and ankle arthrodesis: a pilot randomised controlled trial. Foot Ankle Surg 2020. https://doi.org/10.1016/j.fas.2020.10.005.

35. Honnenahalli Chandrappa M, Hajibandeh S, Hajibandeh S. Ankle arthrodesis— Open versus arthroscopic: A systematic review and meta-analysis. J Clin Orthop Trauma 2017;8(Suppl 2):S71–7.

36. Lee GW, Wang SH, Lee KB. Comparison of intermediate to long-term outcomes of total ankle arthroplasty in ankles with preoperative varus, valgus, and neutral alignment. J Bone Jt Surg - Am 2018;100(10):835–42.

37. Haddad SL, Coetzee JC, Estok R, et al. Intermediate and long-term outcomes of total ankle arthroplasty and ankle arthrodesis: A systematic review of the literature. J Bone Jt Surg - Ser A 2007;89(9):1899–905.

38. Daniels TR, Younger ASE, Penner M, et al. Intermediate-Term Results of Total Ankle Replacement and Ankle Arthrodesis. J Bone Jt Surg 2014;96(2):135–42.

39. Coester LM, Saltzman CL, Leupold J, et al. Long-term results following ankle arthrodesis for post-traumatic arthritis. J Bone Joint Surg Am 2001;83-A(2): 219–28.

40. Zanolli DH, Nunley JA, Easley ME. Subtalar Fusion Rate in Patients with Previous Ipsilateral Ankle Arthrodesis. Foot Ankle Int 2015;36(9):1025–8.

41. Gross CE, Lewis JS, Adams SB, et al. Secondary Arthrodesis after Total Ankle Arthroplasty. Foot Ankle Int 2016;37(7):709–14.

42. Morash J, Walton DM, Glazebrook M. Ankle Arthrodesis Versus Total Ankle Arthroplasty. Foot Ankle Clin 2017;22(2):251–66.
43. SooHoo NF, Zingmond DS, Ko CY. Comparison of reoperation rates following ankle arthrodesis and total ankle arthroplasty. J Bone Jt Surg - Ser A 2007; 89(10):2143–9.
44. Jiang JJ, Schipper ON, Whyte N, et al. Comparison of perioperative complications and hospitalization outcomes after ankle arthrodesis versus total ankle arthroplasty from 2002 to 2011. Foot Ankle Int 2015;36(4):360–8.
45. Saltzman CL, Mann RA, Ahrens JE, et al. Prospective Controlled Trial of STAR Total Ankle Replacement versus Ankle Fusion: Initial Results. Foot Ankle Int 2009; 30(7):579–96.
46. Younger ASE, Wing KJ, Glazebrook M, et al. Patient expectation and satisfaction as measures of operative outcome in end-stage ankle arthritis: A prospective cohort study of total ankle replacement versus ankle fusion. Foot Ankle Int 2015;36(2):123–34.
47. Reb CW, Watson BC, Fidler CM, et al. Anterior Ankle Incision Wound Complications Between Total Ankle Replacement and Ankle Arthrodesis: A Matched Cohort Study. J Foot Ankle Surg 2021;60(1):47–50.
48. Schuh R, Hofstaetter J, Krismer M, et al. Total ankle arthroplasty versus ankle arthrodesis. Comparison of sports, recreational activities and functional outcome. Int Orthop 2012;36(6):1207–14.
49. Flavin R, Coleman SC, Tenenbaum S, et al. Comparison of Gait After Total Ankle Arthroplasty and Ankle Arthrodesis. Foot Ankle Int 2013;34(10):1340–8.
50. Piriou P, Culpan P, Mullins M, et al. Ankle replacement versus arthrodesis: A comparative gait analysis study. Foot Ankle Int 2008;29(1):3–9.
51. Pedowitz DI, Kane JM, Smith GM, et al. Total ankle arthroplasty versus ankle arthrodesis: A comparative analysis of arc of movement and functional outcomes. Bone Jt J 2016;98(5):634–40.
52. Sturnick DR, Demetracopoulos CA, Ellis SJ, et al. Adjacent Joint Kinematics After Ankle Arthrodesis During Cadaveric Gait Simulation. Foot Ankle Int 2017;38(11): 1249–59.
53. Stone JW. Arthroscopic Ankle Arthrodesis. Foot Ankle Clin 2006;11(2):361–8.
54. Townshend D, Di Silvestro M, Krause F, et al. Arthroscopic versus open ankle arthrodesis: A multicenter comparative case series. J Bone Jt Surg - Ser A 2013;95(2):98–102.
55. Brodsky JW, Kane JM, Coleman S, et al. Abnormalities of gait caused by ankle arthritis are improved by ankle arthrodesis. Bone Joint J 2016;98-B(10):1369–75.

Deciding Between Ankle and Tibiotalocalcaneal Arthrodesis for Isolated Ankle Arthritis

Manuel Monteagudo, MD*, Pilar Martínez-de-Albornoz, MD

KEYWORDS

- Ankle • Arthritis • Treatment • Arthrodesis • Tibiotalar • Tibiotalocalcaneal

KEY POINTS

- Osteotomies around the ankle (supramalleolar and calcaneal) and total ankle replacement are challenging arthrodesis as the "gold standard" treatment of end-stage ankle arthritis.
- Recent meta-analyses reveal that replacements and arthrodesis may achieve similar clinical outcomes, although the incidence of reoperation and major surgical complications is still higher with replacements.
- After an isolated ankle (tibiotalar) arthrodesis, the triceps will progressively shift the subtalar into varus thus blocking compensatory motion from the midtarsal joints. Subtalar varus with arthritis is the main complication after tibiotalar arthrodesis. In a tibiotalocalcaneal arthrodesis, the subtalar joint may be fixed in the correct valgus position.
- The comparison between ankle and tibiotalocalcaneal arthrodesis does not clearly favor one over another in terms of pain relief, patient satisfaction, and gait analysis. Compensatory sagittal plane motion through the midtarsal joints when the subtalar is fixed in valgus may be responsible for these matched results.
- In the last few years, our threshold for indicating tibiotalocalcaneal over isolated tibiotalar arthrodesis has been lower and lower to finally become our procedure of choice regardless of the radiographic state of the subtalar joint.

 Video content accompanies this article at http://foot.theclinics.com.

INTRODUCTION

End-stage ankle arthritis has significant effects on daily activities, with similar pain and morbidity as hip arthritis.[1] Ankle arthritis is a major source of disability affecting younger population than hip and knee arthritis. It is suffered by adults in the best

Orthopaedic Foot and Ankle Unit, Orthopaedic and Trauma Department, Hospital Universitario Quirónsalud Madrid, Faculty Medicine UEM Madrid, Calle Diego de Velazquez 1, Pozuelo de Alarcon, 28223 Madrid, Spain
* Corresponding author.
E-mail address: mmontyr@yahoo.com

Foot Ankle Clin N Am 27 (2022) 217–231
https://doi.org/10.1016/j.fcl.2021.11.012

productive years with still around 10 to 15 years away from their retirement age, some of them at the top of their careers.[2] Mean age for knee arthroplasty is 65, 66 for total hip arthroplasty, 63 for total ankle replacement (TAR), and 55 for ankle arthrodesis (AA).[3]

More than 70% of cases (unlike the hip and knee) are posttraumatic (rotational ankle fractures), with 30% being inflammatory or primary arthritis.[2] Most cases of symptomatic ankle arthritis are asymmetrical with varus or valgus malalignment. In the last decade, the focus of debate on the surgical treatment of end-stage ankle arthritis has been on joint preserving procedures that allow for the redistribution of the joint loading force with the goal of stopping or at least delaying the progression of degenerative cartilage changes.[3] Although increasingly popular, joint-preservation realignment osteotomies are not indicated in cases of symmetric arthritis and surgery for the end-stage cases is predominantly AA or TAR. Arthroscopic AA and open AA are comparable in clinical outcomes to TAR in patients with nondeformed, end-stage ankle arthritis.[4] The rate of component revision in patients with TAR is similar to the rate of revision for patients who underwent arthroscopic AA or open AA; however, patients with TAR underwent a greater number of additional procedures.[4] There is a trend toward increasing the indications for TAR, but arthrodesis is still performed more frequently.[5] New TAR designs and techniques are recently challenging arthrodesis as the "gold standard" procedure.

Treatment of the end-stage osteoarthritic ankle is often complicated by associated problems such as scarring of the thin soft-tissue envelope, stiffness, malalignment, and degenerative changes in the subtalar and talonavicular joints that may result in instability, deformity, and changes in the biomechanics of the joint(s).[6] Arthrodesis is the procedure of choice for ankle arthritis when a TAR is not indicated. The conventional rationale for TAR instead of AA (ie preventing neighboring joints from future arthritis and preserving better motion) has been recently questioned by several studies demonstrating that secondary arthritic changes around an arthrodesis are not always symptomatic and also gait analysis studies demonstrate marginal differences in the quality of gait between the 2 procedures.[7–10] In this context, arthrodesis is still the most popular surgery for end-stage-ankle-arthritis and relieves pain by eliminating motion and providing stability.[5] A recent meta-analysis revealed that TAR and AA could achieve similar clinical outcomes, although the incidence of reoperation and major surgical complications was significantly higher in the TAR group.[11] Many other studies also confirm this scenario.[12–18] Further studies of higher methodological quality with long-term follow-up are required to confirm the current data.

In cases with an established indication of arthrodesis, an isolated ankle (tibiotalar) fusion is the rule unless the subtalar joint (STJ) shows signs of arthritis. In the case of a combined tibiotalar and subtalar degeneration, a tibiotalocalcaneal (TTC) arthrodesis is the procedure of choice. Understanding the new role of a "healthy" subtalar after an isolated ankle fusion is paramount to question if the preservation of that joint adds any future benefits in terms of pain and gait improvement when planning for an AA. The analysis of biomechanical studies shows that the STJ should ideally work at around 5° of valgus to allow for the midtarsal joints to maximize their sagittal plane motion.[19,20] However, the authors have observed that when skipping STJ in an ankle fusion, action of the triceps frequently shifts the subtalar into varus thus blocking compensatory motion from the midtarsal joints.[19] Besides, the most common complication needing additional surgery after an AA is secondary degeneration of the STJ.[17,21] TTC arthrodesis allows for the control of the valgus position thus allowing potential maximized motion around the midtarsal joints. The comparison between ankle and TTC arthrodesis does not clearly favor one over another.[22] So, when deciding to fuse an arthritic ankle should we indicate an isolated ankle (tibiotalar) or rather a TTC arthrodesis?

The aim of the present article is bringing the reader up to the rationale after presenting TTC arthrodesis as a potential better indication than isolated tibiotalar fusion for end-stage ankle arthritis based on the analysis of complications after tibiotalar arthrodesis, the pathomechanics after an isolated tibiotalar arthrodesis, gait, and satisfaction of patients after these two procedures.

PATHOMECHANICS AFTER TOTAL ANKLE REPLACEMENT, ANKLE ARTHRODESIS, AND TIBIOTALOCALCANEAL ARTHRODESIS

Any surgical technique aimed to treat end-stage ankle arthritis should achieve a painless ankle and foot while preserving motion and gait parameters as close to a healthy limb as possible. The rationale under TAR is the preservation of motion and protection of adjacent joints. Regained ankle motion plus preservation of neighboring joint motion should translate into better pain relief and better parameters of gait. However, clinical results are not that different when compared with AA. A recent prospective cohort study by Daniels and colleagues showed both TAR and AA to be independently effective treatments for end-stage ankle arthritis.[23] Another recent multicenter randomized controlled trial (level II study) demonstrated a statistically significant benefit with both TAA and AA.[24] The AA cohort saw a greater improvement in average AOFAS total score when compared with the TAR cohort. However, the difference was not statistically significant.

Gait analysis after TAR versus AA is not vastly different either. In a prospective level II study, Flavin and colleagues showed that compared with AA, patients with TAR had higher walking velocity attributable to both increases in stride length and cadence as well as more normalized first and second rockers of the gait cycle.[25] Kinematic analysis showed that patients with an ankle arthroplasty had better sagittal dorsiflexion, whereas those with an arthrodesis had better coronal plane eversion. It was also apparent that total ankle arthroplasty produced a more symmetric vertical ground reaction force curve, (which was closer to that of the controls) than the curve of the AA group. The authors concluded that patients in both the arthrodesis and arthroplasty groups had significant improvements in various parameters of gait when compared with their own preoperative function.[25] Neither group functioned as well as the normal control subjects. The data suggested that the major parameters of gait after AA in deformed ankle arthritis are comparable to those after TAR in nondeformed ankle arthritis. In their rationale, the authors stated that regardless of the articulations across which sagittal plane motion occurs postoperatively, some patients experience the persistence of mobility rather than the expected (dramatic) increase in stiffness.

Other studies favor TAR over AA in terms of gait analysis. Singer and colleagues suggest that patients who had undergone arthroplasty, when compared with patients with an arthrodesis, demonstrated greater postoperative total sagittal plane motion.[26] The gait patterns of patients following three-component, mobile-bearing total ankle arthroplasty more closely resembled normal gait when compared with the gait patterns of patients following arthrodesis. Apparently, dorsal motion in the sagittal plane was primarily responsible for the differences.

The different findings previously presented focused toward the STJ and the midtarsal joints as the main factors contributing to the different results between TAR and AA. After an isolated tibiotalar arthrodesis, the triceps would no longer act on the tibiotalar but on the subtalar during the gait cycle. Invertors are almost invariably more powerful than evertors during foot contact along the gait cycle. Continuous inversion of the STJ would change overtime the normal valgus (pronation) disposition toward a varus (eversion) disposition, with the rare exception of patients with a talocalcaneal coalition or advanced subtalar arthritis (**Fig. 1**, Video 1). The varus disposition will change the shock-absorbing valgus properties of the STJ into a rigid/stiff mode.[19] STJ varus effectively blocks sagittal motion of the midtarsal joints.[27] STJ valgus maximizes sagittal motion of the midtarsal joints.[28] This scenario would explain that short follow-up studies of isolated AA in which some subtalar motion is still preserved show a compensatory increase in sagittal motion of the subtalar and medial column joints by around 6°.[29] When the STJ is fixed in slight valgus, the midtarsal joints would only take a few months to adapt by increasing their sagittal motion and compensating the loss of sagittal motion in the ankle-subtalar complex. This could also explain why patients after TTC arthrodesis show an even greater increase in midfoot load: the STJ, which has a compensatory hypermobility after AA, is fused and therefore the midfoot is loaded even more and must compensate alone for the motion in the sagittal plane.[29]

To our knowledge, there is no direct evidence to strongly support progressive STJ tilting into varus. But there is no evidence at all on the fate of the subtalar after AA, except confusing data that ranges from hypermobility to absence of motion.[6,29,30] Compensatory motion at the subtalar after tibiotalar fusion is assumed to protect tarsal joints from arthritic degeneration but this has not been proven with sound methodology (triceps function under closed chain mechanics/gait). Some authors prove that very little or no subtalar movement is registered after ankle fusion.[30,31] In the latter study,[31] the contact pressure and the transferred force at the STJ were decreased in the arthrodesis foot at the 3 gait phases. This provides a basis to speculate that

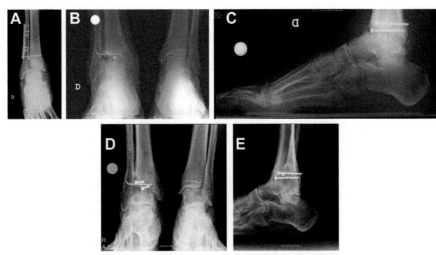

Fig. 1. Suboptimal fixation of an ankle fracture in a 40-year-old-patient. (*A*) Suboptimal fixation of the fracture almost invariably leads to ankle arthritis. (*B*) One year postoperatively after some hardware removal. Anteroposterior view of weight-bearing x-rays showing arthritis developing in the tibiotalar joint. (*C*) Lateral view x-rays of the arthritic ankle. (*D*) Two years from trauma the anteroposterior weight-bearing x-rays show ankle ankylosis in an apparent correct position. (*E*) Ankylosis is more evident in the lateral view of the weight-bearing ankle that also shows signs of subtalar varus (open sinus tarsi, posterior subtalar parallel to the floor). Video 1 clearly demonstrates hindfoot varus on visual gait analysis. Progressive varus tilting of the subtalar may be observed after tibiotalar fusion/ankylosis as invertors are more powerful than evertors.

subtalar arthritis may not be a consequence of AA, but rather a progression of preexisting degenerative changes at this joint, which are demonstrated universally in patients requiring arthrodesis.[32] A study of the relationship between hind- and midfoot arthritis and AA found that 68 of 70 patients showed preexisting arthritis, mostly in the STJs.[32] Even if we assumed a compensatory increased motion at the subtalar, the subtalar is not designed to properly compensate the loss of motion from the tibiotalar and it would do so at the expense of developing arthritis.[29]

In a TTC arthrodesis, we may effectively fix the subtalar in slight valgus thus influencing over the adaptation of the midtarsal joints compensation whereas pathomechanics of an isolated AA would induce the varus shifting of the STJ with a decreased or null compensation from the midtarsal joints. On the assumption that AA is not that far in terms of clinical and mechanical parameters to TAR, and with the existing knowledge of how the ankle, STJ, and midtarsal joints behave after different ankle joint procedures, might we consider a TTC arthrodesis as an option instead of an isolated tibiotalar arthrodesis in end-stage ankle arthritis even with a radiographically "healthy" STJ? To fully decide the answer, we should ideally know how good an isolated AA is and how good a TTC arthrodesis is, and most importantly, if a TTC arthrodesis compares favorably to an isolated AA in terms of pain relief, gait parameters, and patient satisfaction.

HOW GOOD IS ANKLE (ISOLATED TIBIOTALAR) ARTHRODESIS?

AA results in significant improvements in pain and function and has been considered the gold standard for the surgical treatment of end-stage ankle arthritis.[33] The first description of AA is attributed to Albert in 1879, who reported on the fusion of both knees and ankles in a 14-year-old boy suffering from severe palsy of the lower extremity due to poliomyelitis.[5] The use of AA as a treatment of posttraumatic osteoarthritis began in the 1930s. The ideal position for fusion is plantigrade with the hindfoot 0°-5° of valgus, 5° to 10° of external rotation and the talus posteriorly translated under the tibia. Coronal alignment should allow about 5° of hindfoot valgus, which occurs naturally through the STJ in healthy individuals. The tibiotalar surfaces should be well-apposed and parallel to the talar dome in the coronal plane. Postoperatively the ankle has been traditionally immobilized in a cast for 3 months, the first 6 weeks being non–weight-bearing, but up to 12 weeks in patients with higher-risk comorbidities such as diabetes mellitus. However, in both arthroscopic and open AA early weight-bearing at 2 weeks, provided fixation is stable, has been shown not to reduce union rates.[34]

Several AA techniques are available, and the choice depends on the surgeon's preference and experience, alignment of the ankle, quality of bone stock, soft tissue conditions, risk factors for nonunion or other complications. In the last few years, arthroscopic AA has gained popularity, reporting shorter hospital stays, shorter time to solid fusion, and equivalent union rates when compared with open arthrodesis.[34–36] Arthroscopic procedures have been shown to achieve fusion rates between 89% and 100%.[34,36] Complications specific to arthroscopic techniques include nerve injury at the portals and sinus tract formation. However, using an anterior open approach and screws, Zwipp and colleagues reported minor complications, with 5% of wound dehiscence or wound edge necrosis and 3% of postoperative hematomas with fusion rates as high as 99%.[37] In the presence of significant talar bone loss, often associated with poor bone quality as, for example, in the setting of salvage of a failed TAR or correction of severe deformity, screw fixation is unlikely to provide sufficient primary stability to achieve adequate bony fusion.[38] In that particular setting, Plaass and colleagues achieved bony fusion using anterior double-plating fixation in all of 29 patients, including 16 ankles with osteoarthritis and poor bone quality, 4 patients with nonunion of an AA, and 9 failed ankle arthroplasties.[39] In cases of severe misalignment, poor bone stock, and critical soft tissue conditions and/or poor perfusion, external fixation may be contemplated. Reports on the outcomes of the Ilizarov ring or comparable external fixation techniques for ankle fusion are rare, with the ones available accounting for fusion rates between 80% and 100%.[40,41.] Although historical series reported high rates of nonunion, infection, and amputation after AA, recent studies presented have reported good functional outcomes with low complication rates.[37–39] In general, major complications of AA are nonunion, malunions, limb shortening, and adjacent joint arthritis. Newer implants specifically built for AA have made the procedure easier for the surgeon and surely better for the patient.[39]

Function of the fused ankle is clearly important to patients. Ankle range-of-motion will be decreased in patients postoperatively, but the remaining joints in the foot, the midfoot and STJs, will maintain some degree of plantarflexion and dorsiflexion and might even be increased compared with the preoperative values.[42] Although the fused ankle will exhibit an increase in walking speed and distance compared with the osteoarthritic ankle, gait asymmetry will persist, with reduced hindfoot motion and an alteration in kinematics through the stance phase, hyperextension of the knee, and early heel lift.[43] As a result of the previous, forces through the midfoot region will be increased in late stance. Long-term outcomes of AA have also included the problem of progression of arthritis in other joints of the foot, especially the STJ.[44] However, this might not be clinically significant. Sheridan and colleagues recently reported in a retrospective review that patients that underwent AA generally had preexisting mid- and hind-foot osteoarthritic changes and suggested that prospective studies could be required to examine this phenomenon further.[32]

One of the straight-cut indications for TAR used to be bilateral end-stage ankle arthritis. It was believed that bilateral AA was an invalidating procedure for those rare cases of bilateral disease. But Vaughan and colleagues studied a group of 8 patients with bilateral AA and showed good functional results and high patient satisfaction into the medium term.[45] That review highlights that after bilateral AA the mean AOFAS score is comparable to that for bilateral TAR.[46] However, patients with bilateral AA are noted to have increased difficulty with stairs, inclines and uneven terrain when compared patients with unilateral AA.

HOW GOOD IS TIBIOTALOCALCANEAL ARTHRODESIS?

Whenever an isolated ankle (tibiotalar) arthrodesis is indicated care should be taken to address the state of the STJ. In the presence of simultaneous tibiotalar and subtalar arthritis, the combination of a TAR and a subtalar arthrodesis may work in selected cases. But when a TAR is not indicated, and there exists a combination of tibiotalar and subtalar arthritis, a TTC fusion is usually the procedure of choice to simultaneously address combined arthritis.[47,48] TTC is also indicated when poor bone stock is present in the talus because of avascular necrosis or a failed TAR and in cases of deformity, and poor soft tissue conditions. Arthrodesis following a failed TAR is almost invariably a TTC as the STJ is usually arthritic and/or there is significant bone loss from the talus. Indirectly, several studies have confirmed that salvage arthrodesis after a failed TAR perform inferior to primary AA.[49,50] Rahm and colleagues directly compared 23 patients who underwent salvage AA after failed TAR with 23 matched patients who received primary AA.[51] They concluded that salvage arthrodesis led to impaired life quality and reduced function combined with significantly higher pain when compared with primary AA. These findings can be used to counsel our patients preoperatively.

The patient should know preoperatively that failure of TAR will lead to worse pain control and function if a revision to fusion is needed.

The ideal position for TTC arthrodesis is plantigrade with the hindfoot 0°-5° of valgus, 5° to 10° of external rotation and the talus posteriorly translated under the tibia. Coronal alignment should allow about 5° of hindfoot valgus, which may be achieved directly when fixing the STJ thus avoiding secondary varus displacement frequently observed after AA (**Fig. 2**). The tibiotalar and subtalar surfaces should be well-apposed and moderate compression is achieved with the use of screws, nail, or lateral plate and screws. Postoperatively the ankle has been traditionally kept non–weight-bearing for around 6 weeks, but with a stable nail fixation early (or almost immediate) weight-bearing may be allowed. Controlled axial compression through a stable nail may help to promote union. Weight-bearing is initiated as tolerated in a protective walker boot which is usually some weeks before patients are allowed to weight bear after AA.

TTC arthrodesis with internal fixation may also be a suitable method of salvage for the treatment of a failed tibiotalar arthrodesis in selected patients.[50] In this scenario, fixation of an isolated tibiotalar AA is compromised and TTC allows for the addition of grafts and better primary stability. It is common to encounter a large bony void that needs to be filled with a bulk femoral head allograft. Achieving fusion with these structural allografts can be challenging because of the graft's inherent poor healing capacity, with fusion rates reported as low as 50% when a femoral head allograft was used with an intramedullary nail.[52–56] Compression has been shown to be important not only in stabilizing the arthrodesis sites but also in promoting bone healing and allowing for load sharing between implanted devices and native osseous tissue to prevent fatigue fracture of hardware.[57] Most modern intramedullary nails are designed to generate arthrodesis site compression at the time of surgery. An additional study reported that patients treated with second-generation nails incorporating an internal compression mechanism experienced faster times to fusion and higher fusion rates than patients treated with first-generation nails lacking an internal compression feature (**Fig. 3**).[58] The operative management of failed TARs via conversion to TTC arthrodesis is a challenging procedure with multiple reports of low patient satisfaction and function when compared with primary TTC fusion (**Fig. 4**).[49–51]

Complication rates of TTC are reported to be as high as 40%, with potential nonunion rates up to 15.8%, but there is a bias with the selection of patients as

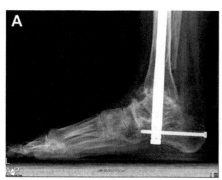
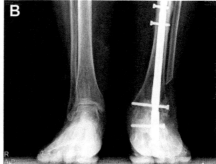

Fig. 2. Subtalar valgus positioning is crucial when performing TTC arthrodesis. (*A*) Lateral weight-bearing view of an ankle with a correct subtalar position. (*B*) Anteroposterior view of the same patient showing the right hindfoot valgus built into the arthrodesis.

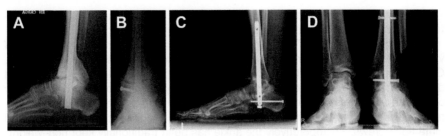

Fig. 3. First-generation nails for TTC arthrodesis lacked stable multiplanar fixation. Nonunion was relatively common. (*A*) Lateral weight-bearing view x-ray showing nonunion in a TTC fixed with a first-generation nail. (*B*) Anteroposterior view of the same case. (*C*) Lateral view of second-generation nail with posterior-to-anterior fixation. (*D*) Anteroposterior view of second-generation nail showing built-in valgus.

many of the indications are made in high-risk patients.[52] Patients in TTC studies have more comorbidities and risk factors for failure than those in AA studies.[53] Diabetes, diabetic neuropathy, high (>2) American Society of Anesthesiologists (ASA) classification, and Charcot neuroarthropathy—popular among TTC studies—all were predictive of developing a nonunion in the subtalar or tibiotalar joints.[52] Prior peripheral neuropathic conditions have strong evidence for failure to achieve union.[55] Different studies in which osteoarthritis was the main indication for patients with TTC reported more favorable outcomes with union rates close to 100%.[48,53,56] Arthroscopic TTC arthrodesis drastically reduced infections with the same union rates as conventional open TTC.[59] Carranza-Bencano et al reported on a big series of 40 patients that underwent minimally invasive (nonarthroscopic) TTC achieving bony union in 86% of cases.[60]

TTC arthrodesis with intramedullary nailing is traditionally performed with formal preparation of both the subtalar and ankle joints. Some authors believe that STJ preparation is not necessary to achieve satisfactory outcomes demonstrating a similar decline in pain, with a high rate of union, and a decrease in operative time when the preparation of the STJ was not performed.[61] However, other authors have reported on the benefits of preparing the STJ in achieving a higher union rate.[62] When a retrograde nail is used for TTC, some surgeons note a decreased STJ fusion rate compared with ankle union. Dujela and colleagues studied the STJ fusion rate of TTC with a retrograde nail. 66 retrograde TTC fusions (in 63 patients) resulted in radiographic fusion of

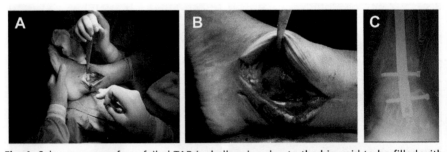

Fig. 4. Salvage surgery for a failed TAR is challenging due to the big void to be filled with grafting and higher risk of nonunion. (*A*) Lateral approach to remove failed implant. (*B*) Allograft may be fixed with the talar screw of the nail. (*C*) Second-generation nails allow for controlled compression of tibiotalar, and subtalar joints as shown in this postoperative x-ray of this case.

the ankle and STJ in 68.2% of the patients.[63] There were 11 cases of AA with STJ nonunion, 6 cases of STJ fusion but ankle nonunion, and 4 cases of nonunion of both joints. In all, a 22.8% radiographic nonunion rate of the STJ was observed. Suboptimal TTC fusion rates may result from inadequate compression of joint surfaces increasing motion (**Fig. 5**). A cadaver study comparing fixation with 3 partially threaded cannulated screws, hindfoot nail, and lateral plate showed lateral TTC plates provided increased compressive forces at the ankle and STJs (**Fig. 6**).[64]

DECIDING BETWEEN ISOLATED TIBIOTALAR VERSUS TIBIOTALOCALCANEAL ARTHRODESIS

The rationale for isolated AA versus TTC is (as with TAR) to preserve neighboring joints, especially the subtalar, from developing secondary arthritis. But there is no proven correlation between radiographic degenerative changes and pain and disability or with the need for additional fusion procedures around the ankle. The analysis of short-term complications after an isolated (AA) has shown that the most common secondary surgery was subtalar fusion.[17,21] It is not long after AA that symptomatic subtalar arthritis may develop. In a study comparing function and patient satisfaction after bilateral AA, two of the patients subsequently developed significant subtalar symptoms that required an STJ arthrodesis, one at 34 months and the other at 89 months post-AA.[45]

Pathomechanics after isolated AA includes the potential progressive varization of the STJ (invertors being more powerful than evertors) which prevents midtarsal joint compensation in the sagittal plane, resulting in a stiff foot and ankle.[19,27,28] This complication may be avoided by securing the subtalar into the correct valgus position while performing a TTC arthrodesis. A slight valgus in the TTC complex will allow the midtarsal joint to maximize its sagittal plane motion and effectively compensate for the loss of motion in the fused segment (Videos 2 and 3). That might explain the high satisfaction rate encountered in TTC series by some authors.[48,56]

Significant gait asymmetry is expected after tibiotalar and/or TTC arthrodesis. TTC arthrodesis is not as well documented as AA in terms of postoperative gait and patient satisfaction. With the current knowledge regarding ankle fusion, gait alteration should be more limited following isolated tibiotalar and greater after TTC. Chopra and Crevoisier studied gait comparing 12 isolated tibiotalar arthrodesis, 12 TTCs, and 12 controls to find that both operations led to significant gait alteration and bilateral symmetry.[65] However, the incorporation of the STJ in TTC arthrodesis did not worsen

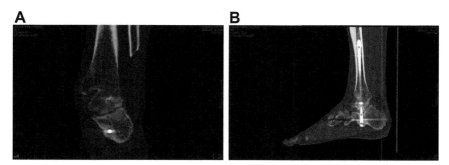

Fig. 5. Subtalar joint nonunion is more common than tibiotalar nonunion in TTC arthrodesis. (*A*) CT showing frontal view of a tibiotalar union but subtalar nonunion in a TTC arthrodesis. (*B*) Sagittal view of the same case.

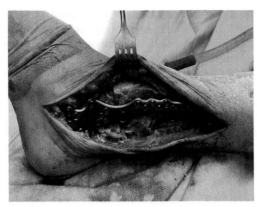

Fig. 6. Intraoperative view of a TTC arthrodesis using a specific TTC plate and screws. Plates and nails are more stable than screws when fixing tibiotalar and subtalar joints.

gait outcomes. The AA group showed a significantly higher alteration compared with controls in maximum contact force and pressure distribution and reported greater asymmetry in 29 of the 48 parameters studied. An explanation for this paradoxic result might be the preservation and maximization of sagittal plane motion in the midtarsal joints when the subtalar is fixed in valgus in a TTC arthrodesis (uncontrollable in isolated AA arthrodesis).[19] A previous study demonstrated a small loss of sagittal plane motion in the affected limb after TTC arthrodesis.[47] There were objective improvements in ambulatory function which may suggest that pain is more important than stiffness as a cause of the asymmetric gait. In a study directly comparing AA versus TTC surprising results were obtained.[66] Functional outcomes and patient satisfaction were studied after the two procedures to find that both were associated with good functional outcomes and satisfaction. No differences were found in terms of pain, satisfaction, and return to work. However, fewer patients with AA met their desired level, possibly because their index situation was not as bad as patients in the TTC group, and their expectations were higher. A recent study by Waly and colleagues found that patients with the worst scores at baseline (AOS, AAS, SF-36) made the greatest gains in function and pain postoperatively.[3] These results might be biased but surely minimize the role attributed to STJ in the global success after ankle fusion. The subtalar is not designed to properly compensate the loss of motion from the tibiotalar and apparently impingement is registered in the posterior part of the posterior facet of the subtalar which may account for the increased incidence of subtalar arthritis after AA.[29] But Chopart joints are designed to compensate the loss of motion in the hindfoot as triceps complex would act maximizing sagittal plane motion through these joints (as long as there is no subtalar varus which would block that sagittal motion).[19,27,28] The only potential explanation for all data in the previous studies should reside in the STJ and the midtarsal joints. STJ secondary varus tilting would justify the abnormal lateral shift in the peak pressure during the loading phase reported for the operated side in ankle (tibiotalar) arthrodesis but not in the TTC arthrodesis.[65] The increased loading of the lateral border of the foot on the operated side of AA has repeatedly been reported.[43,44,65] Extensive stiffness in the ankle, hindfoot and midfoot would force other segments to necessarily compensate but at the expense of gait disturbance and pain. On the contrary, controlled valgus fixation of the STJ in a TTC arthrodesis would over time maximize sagittal plane motion in the midfoot thus improving several gait parameters such as maximum contact force and pressure distribution.

All these data together with other facts such as an easier surgical technique, less wound complications, earlier weight-bearing, and less reinterventions, make TTC arthrodesis a reliable alternative to AA in patients with isolated ankle arthritis and a radiographically (but not functionally "healthy" subtalar). More data to argue in favor of TTC over isolated AA are preexisting arthritis in the STJ at the time of ankle fusion. If prevalence is higher than considered (up to 32.5% of the patients in a study by Takakura[67]) that would be another factor to decide for TTC. Our threshold for indicating TTC over isolated tibiotalar arthrodesis has been lower and lower in the last few years to finally become our procedure of choice regardless of the radiographic state of the STJ.

SUMMARY

The relative benefits of osteotomies, arthrodeses, and arthroplasties in the treatment of ankle arthritis remain uncertain. To address the void in high-quality evidence comparing arthrodesis and arthroplasty, there are currently 2 large prospective trials in progress. In the United States, a trial sponsored by the Seattle Institute for Biomedical and Clinical Research is aiming to provide 2-year follow-up data.[68] This was originally designed as a randomized controlled trial, but because of lack of patient recruitment, the trial was converted to a prospective cohort study. In the United Kingdom, the randomized control trial TARVA (total ankle replacement vs arthrodesis) is in progress.[69] Initial results are due in 2022/23.

The decision to offer the patient either AA or replacement is made on an individual patient basis according to the surgeon's indications. The older, less demanding patient is more likely to undergo TAR and the younger more active patient arthrodesis. Patients with complex ankle deformities are also more likely to be offered arthrodesis. These influences have the potential to unfavorably affect complication rates as well as survivorship in the raw data from outcome studies. An objective in the treatment of end-stage arthritis is the normalization of gait. However, gait analyses studies are not conclusive on the superiority of TAR over AA, nor of AA over TTC. Arthrodesis remains the gold standard in the treatment of end-stage ankle arthritis providing predictable results with patients with TAR having to undergo more revision surgeries. Nevertheless, there is obviously a definite place for TAR in a selected group of patients. In the next few years, in the light of the modern studies prospectively comparing TAR versus AA, we will conceivably better define the group of individuals who will benefit most from each procedure.

An isolated AA may address the severe pain at the ankle while preserving adjacent joints from the development of arthritis. However, altered biomechanics (pathomechanics) after isolated tibiotalar arthrodesis progressively force the STJ to tilt into varus, unless there is a concomitant talocalcaneal coalition or subtalar arthritis. A "radiolographycally-healthy" varus subtalar causes the locking of midtarsal joints compensation in the sagittal plane thus resulting in a stiff and nonfunctional foot. We may avoid this complication by simultaneously fixing the subtalar into the desired 5° of valgus with a TTC. The question is not to "move more" but to "move better". And TTC allows for a better sagittal plane compensatory motion in the midtarsal joint than an AA with a varus STJ. Not surprisingly, when comparing both procedures, patients are happier and present with better function with TTC arthrodesis.[60] None of the studies presented in this article is conclusive on its own about the superiority of TTC over AA, but together they present a persuasive pattern toward considering TTC as a better option than AA in the treatment of end-stage ankle arthritis regardless the radiographic state of the STJ.

CLINICS CARE POINTS

- After an isolated ankle (tibiotalar) arthrodesis, the triceps will progressively shift the subtalar joint into varus thus blocking compensatory motion from the midtarsal joints.
- In a tibiotalocalcaneal arthrodesis the subtalar may be fixed with the correct valgus.
- Comparison between ankle and tibiotalocalcaneal arthrodesis does not clearly favor one over another for pain relief, satisfaction, and gait analysis.
- Compensatory sagittal plane motion through the midtarsal joints when the subtalar is fixed in valgus may be responsible for these results.
- Tibiotalocalcaneal arthrodesis has become our procedure of choice over isolated tibiotalar arthrodesis for end-stage ankle arthritis regardless of the radiographic state of the subtalar joint.

SUPPLEMENTARY DATA

Supplementary data related to this article can be found online at https://doi.org/10.1016/j.fcl.2021.11.012.

REFERENCES

1. Bloch B, Srinivasan S, Mangwani J. Current concepts in the management of ankle osteoarthritis: a systematic review. J Foot Ankle Surg 2015;54(5):932–9.
2. Ewalefo SO, Dombrowski M, Hirase T, et al. Management of posttraumatic ankle arthritis: literature review. Curr Rev Musculoskelet Med 2018;11(4):546–57.
3. Waly FJ, Yeo EMN, Wing KJ, et al. Relationship of preoperative patient-reported outcome measures (PROMs) to postoperative success in end-stage ankle arthritis. Foot Ankle Int 2020;41(3):253–8.
4. Chan JJ, Chan JC, Poeran J, et al. Surgeon type and outcomes after inpatient ankle arthrodesis and total ankle arthroplasty: a retrospective cohort study using the nationwide premier healthcare claims database. J Bone Joint Surg Am 2019;101(2):127–35.
5. Milstrey A, Domnick C, Garcia P, et al. Trends in arthrodeses and total joint replacements in Foot and Ankle surgery in Germany during the past decade-Back to the fusion? Foot Ankle Surg 2021;27(3):301–4.
6. Coester LM, Saltzman CL, Leupold J, et al. Long-term results following ankle arthrodesis for post-traumatic arthritis. J Bone Joint Surg Am 2001;83:219–28.
7. Eerdekens M, Deschamps K, Wuite S, et al. The biomechanical behavior of distal foot joints in patients with isolated, end-stage tibiotalar osteoarthritis is not altered following tibiotalar fusion. J Clin Med 2020;9(8):2594.
8. Fuchs S, Sandmann C, Skwara A, et al. Quality of life 20 years after arthrodesis of the ankle a study of adjacent joints. J Bone Joint Surg Br 2003;85:994–8.
9. Ling JS, Smyth NA, Fraser EJ, et al. Investigating the relationship between ankle arthrodesis and adjacent-joint arthritis in the hindfoot: a systematic review. J Bone Joint Surg Am 2015;97:513–20.
10. Chopra S, Rouhani H, Assal M, et al. Outcome of unilateral ankle arthrodesis and total ankle replacement in terms of bilateral gait mechanics. J Orthop Res 2014;32(3):377–84.
11. Kim HJ, Suh DH, Yang JH, et al. Total ankle arthroplasty versus ankle arthrodesis for the treatment of end-stage ankle arthritis: a meta-analysis of comparative studies. Int Orthop 2017;41(1):101–9.

12. Anastasio AT, Patel PS, Farley KX, et al. Total ankle arthroplasty and ankle arthrodesis in rheumatic disease patients: An analysis of outcomes and complications using the National Inpatient Sample (NIS) database. Foot Ankle Surg 2021;27(3):321–5.
13. Espinosa N, Klammer G. Treatment of ankle osteoarthritis: arthrodesis versus total ankle replacement. Eur J Trauma Emerg Surg 2010;36(6):525–35.
14. Heckmann N, Bradley A, Sivasundaram L, et al. Effect of insurance on rates of total ankle arthroplasty versus arthrodesis for tibiotalar osteoarthritis. Foot Ankle Int 2017;38(2):133–9.
15. Merrill RK, Ferrandino RM, Hoffman R, et al. Comparing 30-day all-cause readmission rates between tibiotalar fusion and total ankle replacement. Foot Ankle Surg 2019;25(3):327–31.
16. Morash J, Walton DM, Glazebrook M. Ankle arthrodesis versus total ankle arthroplasty. Foot Ankle Clin 2017;22(2):251–66.
17. SooHoo NF, Zingmond DS, Ko CY. Comparison of reoperation rates following ankle arthrodesis and total ankle arthroplasty. J Bone Joint Surg Am 2007; 89(10):2143–9.
18. Younger AS, Wing KJ, Glazebrook M, et al. Patient expectation and satisfaction as measures of operative outcome in end-stage ankle arthritis: a prospective cohort study of total ankle replacement versus ankle fusion. Foot Ankle Int 2015;36(2):123–34.
19. Maceira E, Monteagudo M. Subtalar anatomy and mechanics. Foot Ankle Clin 2015;20(2):195–221.
20. Brockett CL, Chapman GJ. Biomechanics of the ankle. Orthop Trauma 2016; 30(3):232–8.
21. Stavrakis AI, SooHoo NF. Trends in complication rates following ankle arthrodesis and total ankle replacement. J Bone Joint Surg Am 2016;98(17):1453–8.
22. Cooper PS. Complications of ankle and tibiotalocalcaneal arthrodesis. Clin Orthop Relat Res 2001;(391):33–44.
23. Daniels TR, Younger AS, Penner M, et al. Intermediate-term results of total ankle replacement and ankle arthrodesis: a COFAS multicenter study. J Bone Joint Surg Am 2014;96(2):135–42.
24. Glazebrook M, Burgesson BN, Younger AS, et al. Clinical outcome results of total ankle replacement and ankle arthrodesis: a pilot randomised controlled trial. Foot Ankle Surg 2021;27(3):326–31.
25. Flavin R, Coleman SC, Tenenbaum S, et al. Comparison of gait after total ankle arthroplasty and ankle arthrodesis. Foot Ankle Int 2013;34(10):1340–8.
26. Singer S, Klejman S, Pinsker E, et al. Ankle arthroplasty and ankle arthrodesis: gait analysis compared with normal controls. J Bone Joint Surg Am 2013; 95(24):e191 (1–10).
27. Kirby KA. Methods for determination of positional variations in the subtalar joint axis. J Am Podiatr Med Assoc 1987;77(5):228–34.
28. Viladot Perice A, Dalmau A. Tratamiento de las secuelas postraumáticas del miembro inferior. Fundación Mapfre. Temas Medicina 1988;30:535–43.
29. Sealey RJ, Myerson MS, Molloy A, et al. Sagittal plane motion of the hindfoot following ankle arthrodesis: a prospective analysis. Foot Ankle Int 2009;30(3): 187–96.
30. Morrey BF, Wiedeman GP Jr. Complications and long-term results of ankle arthrodeses following trauma. J Bone Joint Surg Am 1980;62(5):777–84.
31. Wang Y, Li Z, Wong DW, et al. Effects of ankle arthrodesis on biomechanical performance of the entire foot. PLoS One 2015;10(7):e0134340.

32. Sheridan BD, Robinson DE, Hubble MJ, et al. Ankle arthrodesis and its relationship to ipsilateral arthritis of the hind- and mid-foot. J Bone Joint Surg Br 2006; 88(2):206–7.

33. Harrasser N, Gebhardt C, Südkamp NP, et al. Physical performance and quality of life after ankle fusion. Z Orthop Unfall 2020;158(6):611–7.

34. Glick JM, Morgan CD, Myerson MS, et al. Ankle arthrodesis using an arthroscopic method: long-term follow-up of 34 cases. Arthroscopy 1996;12(4):428–34.

35. Veljkovic AN, Daniels TR, Glazebrook MA, et al. Outcomes of total ankle replacement, arthroscopic ankle arthrodesis, and open ankle arthrodesis for isolated non-deformed end-stage ankle arthritis. J Bone Joint Surg Am 2019;101(17): 1523–9.

36. Winson IG, Robinson DE, Allen PE. Arthroscopic ankle arthrodesis. J Bone Joint Surg Br 2005;87(3):343–7.

37. Zwipp H, Rammelt S, Endres T, et al. High union rates and function scores at midterm follow up with ankle arthrodesis using a four-screw technique. Clin Orthop Relat Res 2010;468(4):958–68.

38. Endres T, Grass R, Rammelt S, et al. Ankle arthrodesis with four cancellous lag screws. Oper Orthop Traumatol 2005;17(4–5):345–60.

39. Plaass C, Knupp M, Barg A, et al. Anterior double plating for rigid fixation of isolated tibiotalar arthrodesis. Foot Ankle Int 2009;30(7):631–9.

40. Eylon S, Porat S, Bor N, et al. Outcome of Ilizarov ankle arthrodesis. Foot Ankle Int 2007;28(8):873–9.

41. Salem KH, Kinzl L, Schmelz A. Ankle arthrodesis using Ilizarov ring fixators: a review of 22 cases. Foot Ankle Int 2006;27(10):764–70.

42. Arno F, Roman F. The influence of footwear on functional outcome after total ankle replacement, ankle arthrodesis, and tibiotalocalcaneal arthrodesis. Clin Biomech (Bristol, Avon) 2016;32:34–9.

43. Rouhani H, Crevoisier X, Favre J, et al. Outcome evaluation of ankle osteoarthritis treatments: plantar pressure analysis during relatively long-distance walking. Clin Biomech (Bristol, Avon) 2011;26(4):397–404.

44. Schuh R, Hofstaetter JG, Hofstaetter SG, et al. Plantar pressure distribution after tibiotalar arthrodesis. Clin Biomech (Bristol, Avon) 2011;26(6):620–5.

45. Vaughan P, Gordon D, Goldberg A, et al. Patient satisfaction and function after bilateral ankle arthrodeses. Foot Ankle Surg 2015;21(3):160–3.

46. Karantana A, Martin GJ, Shandil M, et al. Simultaneous bilateral total ankle replacement using the S.T.A.R: a case series. Foot Ankle Int 2010;31(1):86–9.

47. Tenenbaum S, Coleman SC, Brodsky JW. Improvement in gait following combined ankle and subtalar arthrodesis. J Bone Joint Surg Am 2014;96(22):1863–9.

48. Perez-Aznar A, Gonzalez-Navarro B, Bello-Tejeda LL, et al. Tibiotalocalcaneal arthrodesis with a retrograde intramedullary nail: a prospective cohort study at a minimum five year follow-up. Int Orthop 2021;45(9):2299–305.

49. Hopgood P, Kumar R, Wood PL. Ankle arthrodesis for failed total ankle replacement. J Bone Joint Surg Br 2006;88(8):1032–8.

50. Easley ME, Montijo HE, Wilson JB, et al. Revision tibiotalar arthrodesis. J Bone Joint Surg Am 2008;90(6):1212–23.

51. Rahm S, Klammer G, Benninger E, et al. Inferior results of salvage arthrodesis after failed ankle replacement compared to primary arthrodesis. Foot Ankle Int 2015;36(4):349–59.

52. Kowalski C, Stauch C, Callahan R, et al. Prognostic risk factors for complications associated with tibiotalocalcaneal arthrodesis with a nail. Foot Ankle Surg 2020; 26(6):708–11.

53. Lee BH, Fang C, Kunnasegaran R, et al. Tibiotalocalcaneal arthrodesis with the hindfoot arthrodesis nail: a prospective consecutive series from a single institution. J Foot Ankle Surg 2018;57(1):23–30.
54. Levinson J, Reissig J, Schaheen E, et al. Complications and radiographic outcomes after tibiotalocalcaneal fusion with a retrograde intramedullary nail. Foot Ankle Spec 2021;14(6):521–7.
55. Patel S, Baker L, Perez J, et al. Risk factors for nonunion following tibiotalocalcaneal arthrodesis: A systematic review and meta-analysis. Foot Ankle Surg 2021. S1268-7731(21)00036-00039.
56. Pitts C, Alexander B, Washington J, et al. Factors affecting the outcomes of tibiotalocalcaneal fusion. Bone Joint J 2020;102-B(3):345–51.
57. Baumbach SF, Massen FK, Hörterer S, et al. Comparison of arthroscopic to open tibiotalocalcaneal arthrodesis in high-risk patients. Foot Ankle Surg 2019;25(6): 804–11.
58. Taylor J, Lucas DE, Riley A, et al. Tibiotalocalcaneal arthrodesis nails: a comparison of nails with and without internal compression. Foot Ankle Int 2016;37(3): 294–9.
59. Berson L, McGarvey WC, Clanton TO. Evaluation of compression in intramedullary hindfoot arthrodesis. Foot Ankle Int 2002;23(11):992–5.
60. Carranza-Bencano A, Tejero S, Del Castillo-Blanco G, et al. Minimal incision surgery for tibiotalocalcaneal arthrodesis. Foot Ankle Int 2014;35(3):272–84.
61. Mulhern JL, Protzman NM, Levene MJ, et al. Is subtalar joint cartilage resection necessary for tibiotalocalcaneal arthrodesis via intramedullary nail? a multicenter evaluation. J Foot Ankle Surg 2016;55(3):572–7.
62. Yoshimoto K, Fukushi JI, Tsushima H, et al. Does preparation of the subtalar joint for primary union affect clinical outcome in patients undergoing intramedullary nail for rheumatoid arthritis of the hindfoot and ankle? J Foot Ankle Surg 2020; 59(5):984–7.
63. Dujela M, Hyer CF, Berlet GC. Rate of Subtalar Joint Arthrodesis After Retrograde Tibiotalocalcaneal Arthrodesis with Intramedullary Nail Fixation: Evaluation of the RAIN Database. Foot Ankle Spec 2018;11(5):410–5.
64. Hamid KS, Glisson RR, Morash JG, et al. Simultaneous intraoperative measurement of cadaver ankle and subtalar joint compression during arthrodesis with intramedullary nail, screws, and tibiotalocalcaneal plate. Foot Ankle Int 2018;39(9): 1128–32.
65. Chopra S, Crevoisier X. Bilateral gait asymmetry associated with tibiotalocalcaneal arthrodesis versus ankle arthrodesis. Foot Ankle Surg 2021;27(3):332–8.
66. Ajis A, Tan KJ, Myerson MS. Ankle arthrodesis vs TTC arthrodesis: patient outcomes, satisfaction, and return to activity. Foot Ankle Int 2013;34(5):657–65.
67. Takakura Y, Tanaka Y, Sugimoto K, et al. Long-term results of arthrodesis for osteoarthritis of the ankle. Clin Orthop Relat Res 1999;(361):178–85.
68. Muller P, Skene SS, Chowdhury K, et al, TARVA Study Group. A randomised, multi-centre trial of total ankle replacement versus ankle arthrodesis in the treatment of patients with end stage ankle osteoarthritis (TARVA): statistical analysis plan. Trials 2020;21(1):197.
69. Norvell DC, Ledoux WR, Shofer JB, et al. Effectiveness and safety of ankle arthrodesis versus arthroplasty: a prospective multicenter study. J Bone Joint Surg Am 2019;101(16):1485–94.

Moving?

Make sure your subscription moves with you!

To notify us of your new address, find your **Clinics Account Number** (located on your mailing label above your name), and contact customer service at:

Email: journalscustomerservice-usa@elsevier.com

800-654-2452 (subscribers in the U.S. & Canada)
314-447-8871 (subscribers outside of the U.S. & Canada)

Fax number: 314-447-8029

Elsevier Health Sciences Division
Subscription Customer Service
3251 Riverport Lane
Maryland Heights, MO 63043

*To ensure uninterrupted delivery of your subscription, please notify us at least 4 weeks in advance of move.

Printed and bound by CPI Group (UK) Ltd, Croydon, CR0 4YY

08/05/2025

01864700-0003